Culture, Mind, and Society

Series Editor

Peter G. Stromberg
Anthropology Department
University of Tulsa
Tulsa, Oklahoma, USA

Editors
Vigdis Broch-Due
Norwegian Academy
of Science and Letters
Centre for Advanced Study
Oslo, Norway

Bjørn Enge Bertelsen
University of Bergen
Bergen, Norway

Culture, Mind, and Society
ISBN 978-3-319-39048-2 ISBN 978-3-319-39049-9 (eBook)
DOI 10.1007/978-3-319-39049-9

Library of Congress Control Number: 2016949259

Printed on acid-free paper

This Palgrave Macmillan imprint is published by Springer Nature
The registered company is Springer International Publishing AG
The registered company address is: Gewerbestrasse 11, 6330 Cham, Switzerland

Series Editor Preface

Psychological Anthropologists study a wide spectrum of human activity: child development, illness and healing, ritual and religion, selfhood and personality, political and economic systems, just to name a few. In fact, as a discipline that seeks to draw the lines connecting persons and culture, it would be difficult to come up with examples of human behavior that fall outside the purview of psychological anthropology. Yet beneath this substantive diversity lies a common commitment. The practitioners of psychological anthropology seek to answer broad questions about how peoples' inner worlds are interwoven with their outer ones. And while psychological anthropologists may focus on emotions or human biology, on language or art or dreams, they rarely stray far from the attempt to understand the mental and physical possibilities and limitations that ground human experience.

Early in the twentieth century, psychologist Robert Woodworth, a student of anthropological pioneer Franz Boas, dismantled studies purporting to show racial differences in pain tolerance by pointing out that even so basic an experience as pain varies cross-culturally based upon the context of belief in which the pain occurs. The authors whose work is collected in *Violent Reverberations: Global Modalities of Trauma* extend a similar argument into the realm of trauma, an experience that is at once universal and powerfully inflected by local understandings. These arguments have profound implications on both theoretical and practical levels. We need to better grasp the relationships between culture and emotional distress, not only to build our understanding of our species, but also to inform interventions in the tragic situations that are, sadly, a part of the human condition.

Preface

The chapters of this anthology come from a larger collection of papers presented at a workshop held in Bergen in June 2013, as part of Broch-Due's long-term research project *The Effects of Violence and Impoverishment on Psychosocial Health among Pastoralist Communities in Northern Kenya*, financed by the Research Council of Norway. Findings from these East African explorations had made it abundantly clear that the dominant theorising on trauma needed some fresh ethnographical perspectives and analytical revisions. To examine these issues, the convenors, Professor Vigdis Broch-Due, Associate Professor Bjørn Enge Bertelsen and Postdoctoral Fellow Margit Ystanes, all located at Department of Social Anthropology, University of Bergen, invited anthropologists whose work spans distinct contexts in Africa, Asia, Europe and the Americas.

The motivation for the workshop, and this volume, has been the ways in which the term trauma has dramatically changed meaning and location over time in western history. In antiquity, trauma meant a physical wound—an exterior sign of the infliction of pain. In its contemporary form, trauma has come predominantly to signify a wounded soul not only of the victims but also the witnesses of violence whether they are on the scene or watch on the screen. This journey of trauma from the exterior to the interior—from skin to soul—should alert us to the fact that experiences of pain and embodiment cannot be taken to be the same for all human beings across time and space, but rather needs fine-grained ethnographical and historical frames of analysis. The precise ways in which trauma straddles the permeable boundaries between 'interiority' and 'exteriority' depend on how the physical body itself—its intimacies, energies, agencies, matters—is lived and perceived in each place. Embodiment is of course always embedded in relations of intersubjectivity and sociality. We need thus to explore within the same analytical framework the physical, psychological and social effects of trauma across cultures and continents. This inquiry requires a new set of questions such as:

What does the notion of trauma mean in a truly global human context—in dire situations calibrated by highly different socio-cultural frameworks, changing and varied institutional set ups, or multiple forms of violence? How are we to make sense of the significant gap between the term's genealogy and disciplinary history within medicine and psychology, on the one hand, and its current multiple usages by development studies, critical theorists or even macroeconomists, on the other? And how well does the term capture the lingering and lasting dimensions of violence that endures and recurs, that ossifies and transmogrifies?

In addressing these fundamental questions, the contributions to this volume map the surprisingly multifarious circumstances in which trauma is invoked—as an analytical tool, a therapeutic term or as a discursive trope. Trauma embraces a series of social phenomena of different content, complexity and scale, thus posing analytical challenges on both epistemological and existential levels. Most significantly, the expansion of trauma into all walks of life, and its new psychological mooring in the mind, would be impossible without a western modernity, not only intellectually but also technologically and politically. Trauma-writ-large complements the industrialization of violence, and they are both characterized by a speedy and spectacular visibility. These blown-up versions, however, sidetrack the slower modes of atrocities and suffering seeping through marginalized spaces, which typically remain out of sight of global attention. This empirical diversity in the forms of violence and trauma powerfully reveals the limits of universalizing axiomatic language and interpretative frames. Our volume foregrounds sociality in its multiple forms as the canvas of trauma theorizing and thus offers a groundbreaking critique against the epistemological individualism that dominates western scripts. Whilst these modern renditions of trauma and memory are ahistorical, abstracting and atomizing devices, they also remove agency from those afflicted along with the specificity of their suffering. Our case studies across the world highlight instead the many creative ways people faced with personal and social crisis struggle to transform their situation into something more comprehensible and manageable. Through these glimpses into specific scenarios we see how the experiential effects of trauma differ not solely in the imprints on bodies and minds, but also with the workings of time, memory, narration and re-enactment. The volume takes the reader on a journey across widely differing terrains: from Norwegian institutions for psychiatric patients to the post-war emergence of speech genres on violence in Mozambique, from Greek and Cameroonian ritual and carnivalesque treatments of historical trauma to national discourses of political assassinations in Argentina, the volume provides an empirically founded antidote against claiming a universal 'empire of trauma' (Fassin and Rechtman 2007) or seeing the trauma as successfully defined by the *Diagnostic and Statistical Manual of Mental Disorders (DSM)*.

This volume demonstrates how classical anthropological theories such as rites de passage, liminality and the carnivalesque can be highly productive in order to make more penetrating and performative analysis of trauma, violence and pain cross-culturally. As will become evident reading this volume, 'trauma' always speaks its historical moment and cultural modulation, invoking different temporalities and modalities. The reader will thus be exposed to a variety of violent reverberations through landscapes, bodies and communities and their dramatic effects.

The chapters presented here have been developed further since the original workshop. We are grateful to all authors who have been so willing to rewrite and reorganize their papers along the lines suggested by the editors. We also thank Margit Ytsanes for all the work she put into the preparation for the workshop and this volume. Finally, we extend our gratitude to the Research Council of Norway's Mental Health Programme, which funded the workshop as well as the activities of the abovementioned research project.

Vigdis Broch-Due
Oslo, Norway

Bjørn Enge Bertelsen
Bergen, Norway

Contents

Notes on Contributors

Nicolas Argenti is a social anthropologist at Brunel University London. He has conducted research in Cameroon and Greece on questions of political violence and trans-generational memory. His monograph on Cameroon, *The Intestines of the State*, came out in 2007, and a monograph on the island of Chios is currently in progress.

Rania Astrinaki is an assistant professor at the Department of Social Anthropology, Panteion University Athens, Greece. She has been conducting a long-term field and archival research on the relationship between violence, power, history and identity in the mountain communities of Western Crete. Her recent research concerns political issues of the Greek crisis. Her research interests and publications focus on violence, state processes, politics, gender, identity formation and historical transformations. She has also translated anthropological works into Greek.

Bjørn Enge Bertelsen, an associate professor at the Department of Social Anthropology, University of Bergen, has researched issues such as state formation, violence, poverty and rural-urban connections in Mozambique since 1998 in addition to having had a long-standing interest in theory development within the discipline of anthropology. Bertelsen's articles have appeared in *Ethnos, Journal of Southern African Studies, Social Analysis, Anthropology Today, Urban Studies and Anthropological Quarterly*. He has authored the monograph *Violent Becomings: State Formation, Sociality, and Power in Mozambique (2016)*, as well as co-edited the three anthologies *Crisis of the State: War and Social Upheaval* (with Bruce Kapferer, [2009] 2012), *Navigating Colonial Orders: Norwegian Entrepreneurship in Africa and Oceania, ca. 1850 to 1950* (with Kirsten Alsaker Kjerland, 2015) and *Critical Anthropological Engagements in Human Alterity and Difference* (with Synnøve Bendixsen, Palgrave Macmillan, 2016).

Vigdis Broch-Due is Professor of Social Anthropology and Global Poverty Studies, University of Bergen. She is currently employed as Scientific Director at Centre for Advanced Study (CAS), Oslo. Broch-Due's academic career has taken her from teaching positions in Anthropology at the Universities of Oslo and Washington (Seattle), to the Directorship of a Poverty and Prosperity Research programme at the Nordic Africa Institute, Uppsala, to senior research positions at the Universities of Cambridge, SOAS and Rutgers. Her books include *Carved Flesh/Cast Selves: Gendered Symbols and Social Practices*; *The Poor Are Not Us: Poverty and Pastoralism in Eastern Africa*; *Producing Poverty and Nature in Africa*; *Violence and Belonging: The quest for Identity in postcolonial Africa* and *Trusting and its Tribulation: Interdisciplinary Engagements with Intimacy, Sociality and Trust*. She has published articles on gender and embodiment, cosmology, cultural models of the relations between animals, people and nature, pastoral development, colonialism and changing property relations.

Carol A. Kidron is an associate professor in the Department of Anthropology at the University of Haifa, Israel. Kidron has undertaken comparative ethnographic work with Holocaust descendants in Israel and children of Cambodian genocide survivors in Cambodia and Canada. Beyond her interest in personal and collective Holocaust and Genocide commemoration, Kidron's more recent research examines the glocalization of discourses on justice and reconciliation, victimhood, and memory in post-conflict societies. Her present field work in Cambodia explores processes of localization and friction in local–global encounters and the multi-layered responses to hegemonically imposed memorialization, organic forms of genocide commemoration and atrocity tourism. Kidron's publications include 'Toward an Ethnography of Silence: The Lived Presence of the Past in the Everyday Life of Holocaust Trauma Survivors and Their Descendants in Israel' (*Current Anthropology* 2009) and 'Alterity and the Particular Limits of Universalism: Comparing Jewish-Israeli Holocaust and Canadian-Cambodian Genocide Legacies' (*Current Anthropology*, 2012).

Antonius C.G.M. Robben is Professor of Anthropology at Utrecht University, the Netherlands, and past president of the *Netherlands Society of Anthropology*. He holds a PhD (1986) from the University of California, Berkeley, and has been a research fellow at the Michigan Society of Fellows, Ann Arbor, the Harry Frank Guggenheim Foundation, New York, and the David Rockefeller Center, Harvard University. His most recent books include *Political Violence and Trauma in Argentina* (2005), which won the Textor Prize for Excellence in Anthropology from the *American Anthropological Association* in 2006, and the edited volumes *Iraq at a Distance: What Anthropologists Can Teach Us About the War* (2010), *Ethnographic Fieldwork: An Anthropological Reader* (2011; co-edited with Jeffrey Sluka) and *Necropolitics: Mass Graves and Exhumations in the Age of Human Rights* (2015; co-edited with Francisco Ferrándiz).

Maria Tapias is a cultural anthropologist interested in the relationships between gender, health and political and economic instability. Her work examines the manifestation of visceral and emotional distress in mothers and infants in the context of Bolivia. Her research interests also include migration and emotions, embodiment and subjectivity among Andean populations and narrative analysis. Her work has been published in journals such as *Medical Anthropology Quarterly*, *Body and Society* and the *Journal of Ethnic and Migration Studies*. She is currently Professor of Anthropology and Associate Dean at Grinnell College, Iowa.

Inger Lise Teig, PhD in Social Anthropology, is associate professor in the Department of Global Health and Primary Health Care, at University of Bergen. Her research interests are organizational ethnography, mental health, critical management, quality of health services, health technology and equity and priority setting in health care. She is in charge of the programme Master in Health Management at the University of Bergen, and holds a position as a senior researcher at International Research Institute of Stavanger (IRIS AS).

Margit Ystanes is postdoctoral fellow at the Department of Social Anthropology, University of Bergen. She holds a PhD from the University of Bergen (2011), with the dissertation *Precarious Trust: Problems of Managing Self and Sociality in Guatemala*. Ystanes' current work critically investigates the use of sporting mega-events as a tool for urban and economic development in Rio de Janeiro. In particular, she focuses on the use of forced removals, and the resistance against them, as well as their impact upon social relationships and stated aims of poverty reduction and urban integration. Among her publications is the co-edited volume (with Vigdis Broch-Due) *Trusting and its Tribulations: Interdisciplinary Engagements with Intimacy, Sociality and Trust* (2016). Her research interests include trust, poverty, development, urbanization, gender and conceptions of nature.

List of Table

CHAPTER 1

Violent Reverberations: An Introduction to Our Trauma Scenarios

Vigdis Broch-Due and Bjørn Enge Bertelsen

The Trauma Conundrum

The concept of 'trauma' weaves together clinical and cultural practices, which immediately shapes it into an attractive object of knowledge for anthropology. Trauma in its contemporary configuration embraces a series of social phenomena of different content, complexity and scale, thus posing analytical challenges on both epistemological and existential levels. Most significantly, the specific culture that 'trauma' grows out of is a generic Western modernity, and the wide array of ideas, practices and controversies the condition trails clearly reflect this grounding in a post-enlightenment milieu. While the etymology of 'trauma' dates back to antiquity simply denoting a wound on the skin, its significance and great potential for shapeshifting first emerged with the frantic pace of modernity across Europe and the USA during the nineteenth and twentieth centuries. Indeed the expansion of trauma into all walks of life and its new psychological mooring in the mind would be impossible without

V. Broch-Due (✉)
Centre for Advanced Study (CAS), Oslo, Norway
Department of Social Anthropology, University of Bergen, Norway

B.E. Bertelsen
Department of Social Anthropology, University of Bergen, Norway

V. Broch-Due, B.E. Bertelsen (eds.), *Violent Reverberations*,
DOI 10.1007/978-3-319-39049-9_1

modernity, not only intellectually but also technologically and politically. Trauma-writ-large tracks together with the industrialization of violence, and they are both characterized by a speedy and spectacular visibility of a modern make. These blown-up versions, however, side-track the slower modes of atrocities and suffering seeping through marginalized spaces, which typically remain out of sight of global attention. As will become evident reading this volume, 'trauma' always speaks its historical moment and cultural modulation and invokes different temporalities and modalities.

And yet, this very *specificity* of trauma discourse has currently been swept aside in public imagination and replaced with a standardized repertoire made for global consumption of trauma victims, symptoms, sufferings, forms of authorized memorialization and medicalized therapy. In this thinly conceived universal semiotics of trauma, speech overshadows enactment. The general motion is toward 'breaking the wall of silence' by downplaying the performative, visceral and embodied memory of violence, which has of course been the standard response ever since the Cartesian gesture developed away from the body and toward the mind. This Western technology of the self travels along well-trodden trajectories imprinted during a long imperial history, seeking to colonize the mind of the 'other' through a vocabulary stretching from 'pacify', 'civilize', 'christianize', 'modernize'—all modulations of a shared desire of Western powers to create a new and more fit personhood out of diverse masses of poor, primitives and heathens, both in the slum of the metropolis and abroad in the (post)colonies. This request for 'personal development' has all along been part and parcel of a more general charter to transform the world according to Western military, economic and political interests. While the focus in the past was on the 'primitive' subject and what was deemed as outdated livelihoods, hygiene, beliefs and governance, the attention has now moved on to the interior of the 'suffering' subject in need of cure.

Such a subtle shift from a patronizing to a pathologizing attitude is simultaneously a turning inward from the social to the individual, thus making a generous space for the traumatic to flourish. During new waves of globalization occurring in the twenty-first century, trauma has crafted itself onto an ever-expanding apparatus of interventionist agendas and standardized programs in the name of development and human rights (or war reparations), which are aimed at the alleviation of poverty and suffering worldwide. A whole trauma industry has grown up in the wake of these intimate intrusions in the name of the 'the good'; a host of pharmaceuticals, therapists, talk shows, self-help manuals, tribunals, memorials and tailored tourist packages have capitalized on the resource avenues opened up in the wasteland of violence and pain. Judith Kay Nelson (2013:19) succinctly sums up its planetary ubiquity:

> [t]here is trauma of all kinds—war, violent crime, oppression, political repression, natural disasters—both down the street and around the world, and with today's media coverage and global accessibility, increasingly there is little difference between the two locations.

Trauma theory has become a universalizing force classifying and regulating the diverse lived experience of violence, suffering and commemoration. 'Trauma' has thus inserted itself into the most distant communities on the globe where many locals have been coached to 'walk-the-walk and talk-the-talk' as words have it, but not without ambiguity and contradictory effects as this volume succinctly demonstrates. From different ethnographical perspectives, all of our chapters call for renewed attention to the particular limits of universalizing axiomatic language and interpretative frames. Interventions in the name of 'trauma' share with all similar interventions, such as 'poverty', 'governance' or 'climate', that they are formulated through Western lenses. When exported to foreign places, they thus show a high propensity of clashing with localized ideas and practices, thereby producing a host of unintended consequences and hybrid forms. Together, the contributions of this volume analyze the multiple articulations of the local and global arenas in an effort to understand how specific trauma thinking, prescriptions and politics have shaped local conditions, and how the 'target' groups' understandings of their own world in turn have (re)shaped dominant trauma scripts and vested them with new meanings, imaginaries, bodily practices and material implications.

It is precisely in these peripheral and marginal settings—not so much in terms of geography but of semiotics and the somatic—that the paradoxical nature of 'trauma' as a generic phenomenon comes into full play. This is because the accuracy of any violent act is always ensnared in error as it were; there can simply be no direct and unmediated recall. Bombarded with an immense amount of stimuli from the exterior and interior world, human perception and recollection has by necessity to pick out, condense and re-present physical and somatic experiences, relying on encryption, distortion and censorship as well as the filtering of language, sensorium and social expectations. The blow is mediated by memory, and memory is mediated by what is meaningful in 'word' and 'flesh' within the cultural context where the violent act occurs. And yet, there is always a limit to meaning in any signification system, a navel of sorts, a liminal point that cannot be interpreted and where meaning simply fails. Here we are at the enigma of trauma; for despite being deeply embodied, it remains essentially elusive, and this ephemeral quality is precisely what allows trauma to reverberate so violently and widely. However, the experiential effects of trauma differ cross-culturally not solely across bodies and minds but also with the workings of time, memory, narration and re-enactment.

The Pace of Violence

To pay attention to the temporal dimension of violence is crucial in order to appreciate why trauma may simmer in the deep structures of the body and only surface in the subject with time passing, sometimes even lingering on for generations to come. We live in an era that privileges the immediate and spectacular—military attacks, explosions, earthquakes, beheadings, torturing, mutilations—all of which produce visually attention-grabbing fatalities that can be easily captured through the camera lenses and widely publicized in an instant on the Web. In the coverage of the perpetually ongoing wars that are fought at the edges of Euro-American states, predominantly in the Middle East and Africa, the spectacularization of violence waged against enemies is typically cast as necessary to safeguard the civilizational integrity of the Western world (Badiou 2012; Zagato 2015; Zulaika 2009). In her book *Regarding the Pain of Others* (2003), Susan Sontag argues that insofar that the photography freezes the viscerally ineradicable impact of a transgressive act, the image side-tracks not only the complex causes of violence but also the full extent of its causalities, whether swift or protracted. This fetishism of the *present* erases from public consciousness other temporalities of violence and suffering, thus making it harder to grasp trauma in its many modalities.

Coining the term 'slow violence', Rob Nixon alerts us to 'a violence that is neither spectacular nor instantaneous, but rather incremental and accretive, its calamitous repercussions playing out across a range of temporal scales' (2011:2). Using environmental degradations as his prime example in the forms of toxic drift, oil spills, ravaged habitats, land mines, genetic mutation, greenhouse gasses and such like, Nixon reworks the earlier notion of 'structural violence'. This concept was once defined by Johan Galtung as the massive chain of causes that may materialize in acts of personal violence but which also constitute violence in itself, such as economic inequality, political oppression, unequal morbidity, racism and sexism, just to mention a few debilitating conditions. These forms of muted violence at work in multiple, differential fields may each be imperceptible and piecemeal, but through accumulation over time, often push those subjected into marginalization and poverty. While Galtung (1969) was of the opinion that 'structural violence is silent, it does not show—it is essentially static, it *is* the tranquil waters (1969:170)', Nixon, in contrast, chooses to foreground 'questions of time, movement, and change, however gradual (p. 4)'. In other words, we are confronted by a *production* of violence as a multiplicity that, by definition, is sensitive to process, context and form as also argued by the contributors to the volume *Violence and Belonging* (Broch-Due 2005).

In our context, this emphasis on the *temporal dynamics* of violence is especially pertinent for certain modalities of trauma that continue to move through tissue, blood, bones and minds of those afflicted. A prime example is the nightmares haunting combatants after the arena of war itself has ended, later showing up as the diagnoses of 'shell-shock' or post-traumatic stress disorder (PTSD). Thinking of violence as accumulative is also useful in comprehending the less spectacular, but sometimes equally devastating, events that take place behind closed doors experienced by victims of domestic abuse, which is often a long-drawn and incremental harming. Most succinctly, the notion of slow violence helps us to theorize better forms of collective trauma, such as the Holocaust, where the perpetrators not only built up its terror exponentially against Jews for decades before the genocide but also where the originary trauma continues to be passed on down the generations and embodied in new forms. Last, but not the least, if we think trauma through both time and space, we get a vista into landscapes of destructions located on the opaque periphery—ghetto, slum, island, savannah, desert, tropical forest, 'poor nation', 'third world'—that remain outside the orbit of concern and compensation from the privileged center (see Chap. 6).

The reason why Nixon wants us to focus more scholarly attention on 'the temporalities of place' is because slow violence works silently, insidiously and out of sight, creating milieus fertile of fear and trauma. Among those particularly hard hit are marginal groups whose very existence is being threatened, their environs turned into wastelands, their livelihoods destroyed by external forces slowly eating themselves into the backbone of society—such as toxic pollution, deforestation, protracted wars or the gradual appropriation of large tracts of land. The resulting dislocation may take the shape of being either pushed out of place altogether or forced to remain in place but inhabiting the crust of a soil that rots and erodes under one's feet, gradually turning into a barren expanse of pure ruination. The ensuing trauma of witnessing a whole life world unravelling, sometimes built over centuries, is a collective form of suffering which remains lodged deep in memory over generations. This volume exemplifies numerous such cases.

Since anthropology feeds on being sensitive to both culture and context, it is perhaps unsurprising that seminal contributions from within the discipline are embedded in the theoretical terrain framed by both 'structural' and 'slow' violence. One example here of an early intervention into the debate of violence as a compound phenomenon is Judith Zur's (1998) empathic account of how Guatemalan indigenous women faced multiple forms of marginalization following sustained periods of violence. Zur's book brought to the table a focus on the historical context and the violently transformative role of war—to societies, to gender relations and to cultural horizons (see also Broch-Due 2005). Furthermore, Valentine Daniel (1996) has written eloquently about the inexpressibility of pain, terror and torture, showing how such transgressive acts are felt at the limits of the personal, violating both the physical and social skin. Because of this, he argues, practices memorializing violent and traumatic events may be tightly constrained by the social conventions set out by the culture in question.

Similar sensitivities to practices of violence and the legacies of trauma, however conceived and problematized, have been treated by anthropologists concerned with various forms of intergenerational transmission of violence and trauma (see, e.g., Feuchtwang 2011; Argenti and Schramm 2010), the longue durée impact of colonial violence on formations of memory and lingering trauma (see, e.g., Bertelsen 2016; Nelson 2009; Argenti 2007; Cole 2001), the ways in which trauma-inducing violence is entrenched in the domain of the colloquial and everyday lives (see, e.g., Das 2007; Das et al. 2000), the tensions between ethical, political and cultural forms of representation and enactment of trauma (see, e.g., Maček 2014; Kwon 2006, 2008; Daniel 1996; Felman 2002; Scheper-Hughes 2002; Honwana 1999) and, lastly, various forms of productive engagements between anthropology, on the one hand, and various strands of psychology, psychoanalysis, psychiatry and the therapeutic sciences, on the other (see, e.g., Hunt 2010; Mollica 2006; Antze and Lambek 1996; Lambek 1996).

In a critical assessment, Lester (2013) points out that anthropologists have been very successful at establishing a 'view from afar' on trauma and scrutinizing its institutional, political and strategic dimensions but losing sight of the ongoing suffering of people. Lester's plea is for an approach to trauma that takes in the relational aspect to world-making (and breaking) that is entailed by experiencing trauma where '[w]e glimpse the edge of our very being, and we feel our ontological aloneness' (2013:754).

While this volume continues the established anthropological focus on the myriad causes and effects of violence, our contributors also respond to this existential plea by binding together the biographical and the social. Our combination of large-scale contextual frames with an intimate frame that focuses on embodiment and emotions allows for a more nuanced analysis of the social, political and personal factors differentially shaping the experiences of violence and trauma. Poverty, too, is incorporated, permeating experience in the form of stigma, psychosomatic ailments and sometimes trauma. While technocratic poverty definitions tend to privilege the purely economic, enumerated in the 'x dollars a day' imagery, being 'poor' cross-culturally and ethnographically is a condition signifying a wide range of physical states, emotions and disabilities, which are embodied and expressed on the skin and clothing, as well as through a whole ledger of material objects and structures (Broch-Due 1995). In other words, through an acculturated physiology and sensorium individuals live harm and marginalization in multiple ways; sometimes the violence is so insidious or chronic that it permeates the whole social milieu, turning it into a *habitus* in the famous terms of Bourdieu (see Chaps. 4 and 9).

Trauma Modalities

Pain and suffering are clearly integral to the human condition and surely have caused neurons firing in the brain, tears breaking and bones aching all back down the evolutionary chain of hominids. Beyond this basic neurobiological substratum, however, trauma and its many configurations are profoundly historical, social and cultural phenomena. Although felt individually, trauma is essentially produced *intersubjectively*—it either strikes in the tense relations between the self and the social or sweeps many selves up in a shared experience of loss and violence, sometimes stretching across generations and deep down through the layers of social memory. Given that such diverse collectives are themselves specific in performance, language and meaning, there is simply no uniform experience, emotion or enactment unvarying through time and space which we could objectively denote as 'trauma'. Likewise, there is no single type or temporality of violent event, no fixed threshold of stress, which inevitably qualifies as traumatic, and there is no single therapeutic regimen capable of healing all trauma across communities and throughout history. Even within a Western compass, many critics have pointed to the serious limitation of conventional trauma talk to account for the varied experiences of actual patients, as well as the many flaws in the factual clinical evidence brought to bear on its too expansive theorizing (McNally 2003).

This volume adds to this critique by deconstructing the dominant tenet of mainstream trauma theory of dealing with suffering *singularities*—whether individuals or uniformly shaped communities—often envisioned on paper as repositories of PTSD or other forms of trauma. Our chapters also make a concerted plea for a more profound sensitivity to context. In their important contribution to the field of violence and trauma, Panter-Brick and Eggerman (2012) deploy the term 'resilience' in the context of Afghanistan. The authors underline the key role played by 'culture' in appreciating in situ social and psychological dynamics of violent conflict and post-conflict turmoil. While the editors are hesitant in using the term 'resilience', belonging as it does to a universalizing glossary which might even be depoliticizing in its aspirational orientation (see also Scheper-Hughes 2008 for a critical review), we think they make a crucial point in emphasizing the ways in which existing socio-cultural orders impact greatly on what they see as 'dynamics of resilience' and what is often too easily glossed as trauma.

Acknowledging such intersubjective, cross-cultural variation in trauma experiences and that events producing incapacitation in one context may be a charter for resistance and renewal in yet another is of course the bedrock of the discipline from which the contributors to this volume speak. Anthropology has met many cultures and compared pain and distress across them. It is precisely from this ethnographical angle that we can fruitfully contribute to the cross-disciplinary conversation about the many modalities of trauma. Anthropologists are positioned betwixt and between social worlds, which allows scholars to use one worldview as a window onto another. Grand sprawling discourses like 'trauma' and 'trust' invite an analysis that employs a double perspective; on the one hand a deep immersion in the 'ontology' of specific cultures, but also the ability to step outside local contexts to occupy an epistemological position employing a critical outsider's point of view and a comparative glance across trauma scenarios, past and present ones.

Such a heightened reflexivity is vital in order to counteract the urge to mimetic simplification within some quarters of anthropology itself. Having been born out of a reaction to the civilizing impulse of European colonialism, the discipline became famous for turning the imperial stance on its head by featuring Western discourses and practices as invariably destructive, while any native discourses and practices were by definition appropriate to their common good. This brand of simplification was common when difference and otherness were on the agenda—the times of the 'savage slot' as coined by in Trouillot ([1991] 2003). This longing for the exotic stance was compromised and left vacant with the wave of post-modernism and, along with the construction of 'the empire of trauma' as explored by Fassin and Rechtman (2009), has now settled on the 'suffering subject', as recently argued by Joel Robbins (2013). Nancy Scheper-Hughes fleshes out this alarmist stance with the declaration that in the postcolonial world,

> … a history of social suffering and woundedness, especially a history of racial discrimination, leads to a vulnerability to mass violence. A kind of collective posttraumatic stress disorder may predispose certain 'wounded' populations to a hypervigilance that can lead to another cycle of 'self-defensive' mass killings and genocide. (2002: 368; for a related argument, see Robben and Suárez-Orozco 2000)

Perhaps such sweeping generalizations are what have given a new push to the theoretical pendulum letting it swing back yet again to the 'savage slot' in some corners of the discipline. This is exemplified by the so-called ontological turn in anthropology whose proponents now insist on a new brand of 'radical alterity' to the extent that humankind is no longer divided by different cultures but by 'different natures' (cf. Henare et al., 2007). We may note with interest that as the pace of globalization dramatically speeds up so too does the dramatic rhetoric of opposing parties in anthropology when they address the conundrum of sameness and difference across humanity.

This volume resists such mimetic play and argues that the dual perspectives of ontology and epistemology are more analytically productive when exploring the myriad and contradictory effects on interventions in the name of scarcity and strain. Western trained humanitarians and local communities alike may be conscious of the manifestations of poverty and suffering in their midst, but their definitions of misery may collide. For example, while Western-inspired developers see the reduction of mobile cattle herds and moves toward sedentarization as the ways to prosperity on the dry East African savannah, pastoralists themselves perceive the lack of livestock as the very definition of poverty itself, and not only because cultivation is more hazardous than herding in these harsh surroundings. For without cattle, a person's ability to make the necessary social and symbolic pathways in the pastoral world is curtailed. With the ensuing loss of respect and even identity, such a person is frequently sloughed off from the pastoral community altogether and thus pushed into a liminal and traumatic existence (Broch-Due 1999).

Focusing on differences in trauma definitions, Kidron (Chap. 3) demonstrates in a comparison that even if the Jewish Israeli paradigm of trauma emphasizes the significance of remembrance in contrast to the valorization of presentism among Buddhist Cambodian, they both share a gesture toward the merit of silence, which goes against the grain of Eurocentric therapeutic regimes that insist on the universal value of confessional modes (see also Chap. 7). This certainly does not settle the score against the relevance of the spoken in other cultural contexts, as succinctly analyzed by Bertelsen (Chap. 8) showing the significance of speech in working through the terrible effects of slow violence among victims of the civil war in Mozambique.

The crucial point here is that whether those brought to the encounter as 'insiders' or 'outsiders' agree or disagree, the terms around which the dissenting parties choose to describe and articulate their attitudes to impoverishment and agony will always remain incomplete and refractory. On the basis of their specific cultural logic and perceptual filters each party will obscure some of the material, subjective, social and historical processes that lead to marginalization and trauma, while highlighting others. Such divergent and partial perspectives bring us to the realization that globalized and local models each come to the problem of poverty and suffering with its specific ideological bias. This is not to say that destitution and distress are merely matters of divergent ideas, but that 'even where the social manifestations are blatantly evident and concrete, the meanings and interpretations are inevitably culturally and conceptually mediated' (Broch-Due and Anderson 1999:31). In spite of the best intentions of aid workers and foreign therapists, and whether their diagnosis is empirically right or wrong, globalizing forces are shaped and played out locally in unpredictable ways.

This proliferation of unintended consequences is precisely because most people do not just humbly receive aid, subjugate to terror, and remain mute in the face of crushing power; they rather profoundly act and react. They may scream, kick, protest, disagree, laugh, mimic, and ironize, deploying the emotional register, etiquettes, and expectations that are available to them within the cultural context in which they are forged as subjects (Chap. 10). Since both poverty and trauma are deeply embedded in politics and social action, the rather limited conventional trauma repertoire of pain, guilt, and shame is poorly equipped to comprehend such complexity and subtlety of response.

And it is exactly concerning the crucial issue of human *agency* that our authors depart from most trauma talk. As repeatedly argued by anthropologists since the 1980s, the dominant development discourse is premised on a notion of hierarchical differentiation where the 'underdeveloped' and the 'marginalized' are cast as bereft of opportunities (for such critique, see Yarrow and Venkatesan 2012). While dominant scripts for alleviating suffering, whether in the form of poverty or trauma, construct those afflicted as a passive mass, as if waiting to be 'lifted out of poverty' as the terminology goes, or as patients in need of treatment, this volume highlights instead the many creative ways people faced with personal and social crises struggle to transform their situation into something more comprehensible and manageable. This volume thus makes a plea for the need to mobilize classical anthropological theories such as rites of passage, liminality and the carnivalesque in order to make a more penetrating and performative analysis of trauma, violence and pain cross-culturally.

The Western Trauma Script

All our contributors engage with different cultural aspects of the dominant Western trauma discourse as a measure against which they argue their own ethnographic cases. We have already touched upon several specific traits of the current 'ontology' of trauma of a Western bent, but the most essential element is an epistemological individualism, which constructs the trauma victim in the shape of a universal subject equipped with an emotional structure where any social molding is stripped down to the bare bone, so to speak. While clearly not a social theory, this cultural paradigm of trauma parses down the subject into an atom in the shape of a patient, isolated from the milieu of significant others (Chap. 5). The trauma patient is either left frozen in time perpetually re-living the original trauma or encouraged to speak out from the void of amnesia with the aid of the therapist and the promise of relief. These options constitute the two camps of Western trauma theory, the 'harder' scientific position against a 'softer' psychological position; both concerned with the individual patient. The concept of trauma itself hovers over the pages fiercely exchanged between these intellectual factions like a disembodied trope devoid of extra-textual context.

The continual disagreement seems even to boil down to their own drawing of the contours of trauma too widely, folding in everything from the bourgeoisie sexual hysterics confessing on Freud's couch in late nineteenth-century Vienna, soldiers trapped in the trenches on the Western Front in 1916, and Jewish Holocaust survivors living today in Israel or the USA. Trauma experiences are, thus, created as the same, regardless of historical period and causes of pain. Thus, in dominant Western diagnosis, trauma appears context free as if childhood rape and shelling of soldiers are essentially the same infliction on the psyche and body, as if blunt violence in the public domain is the same as intimate violence in the family. While these cultural renditions of trauma and memory are a-historical, abstracting and atomizing devices, they also remove agency from those afflicted along with the specificity of their suffering.

And yet the trauma debacle raises intriguing questions about our ownership of our experiences and this puzzle has invigorated academic debates in the seminar rooms of the Humanities during the past decades. 'Trauma' has become a rising star in theorizing about the subject, representation, memory and mediation, lending the term 'trauma' a scope which outstrips its standard diagnosis whether in the camp of neuroscience or psychoanalysis (Chap. 2). For the literary scholar Shoshana Felman, trauma expresses 'an essential dimension of human and historical experience, and a new type of understanding of historical causality and temporality' (2002:171). In *Trauma: Explorations in Memory* (1995) her colleague Cathy Caruth takes up this problem of temporality since traumatic experiences fracture the very experience of time for the person to whom they 'happen':

> The pathology cannot be defined either by the event itself—which may or may not be catastrophic, and may not traumatize everyone equally—nor can it be defined in terms of a distortion of the event, achieving its haunting power as a result of distorting personal significances attached to it. The pathology consists, rather, solely in the *structure of experience or reception*: the event is not assimilated or experienced fully at the time, but only belatedly, in its repeated possession of the one who experiences it. To be traumatized is precisely to be possessed by an image or event. (1995: 4–5, our italics)

Clearly, Caruth is taking the cue from neuroscience rather than psychoanalysis, continuing her engagement with trauma as *Unclaimed Experience* (1996) by turning the scholarly attention from interiority to exteriority. Trauma becomes a trope for the pathology of a particular historical period, notably the twentieth and twenty-first centuries' spectacular atrocities screened through the testimonies of Holocaust survivors who bear witness on behalf of the victims to whom the event simply cannot be processed.

This interweaving of trauma and temporality, of subject and history, is what gives 'trauma theory' its philosophical force: it threatens the epistemological status, and the evidential and ethical value, of recollected and recounted memories. In this expanded version, trauma cuts across the personal and the political, thus entering the public domain where it creates similar amnesia in social memory as in subjective memory. It is inspired by Hannah Arendt's analysis of twentieth-century political discourse as a perpetual machinery for the production of lies which results less in the repression of reality than to replace it altogether by the erasure of memory. Just as the traumatized subject comes into being by forgetting, history seems to come into being by means of its ongoing disremembering and destruction. Recently, there has been a call to extend the horizon and include colonial traumas into the curriculum of novels that are typically mined for trauma traces. In *Multidirectional Memory: Remembering the Holocaust in the Age of Decolonization* (2009), Michael Rothberg responds to this plea by juxtaposing studies of Holocaust, slavery and postcolonial readings. While the editors as social anthropologists welcome this turn to the wider context of history and politics, 'trauma theory' in the humanities remains very much within the Western circuits of conceptions and concern.

Curiously, Western trauma models of whatever cut share an obsession with suffering-writ-large, and therefore tend to stick their patient permanently into the pain slot, seemingly ignoring that real subjects may flitter across the whole emotional register, oscillating between pain and pleasure. In contrast, this volume argues that the transformative potential of human agency and empathy rests precisely on the subjects' ability of playing with all emotions both in recollection and healing, words and acts, as so powerfully evoked in our essays.

Let us outline with some rough brush strokes how our individual chapters engage critically with the cultural theories coming out of the Western trauma scenario as a device to give more nuanced pictures of the complexities and subtleties involved in trauma scenarios across the world.

Trauma and Modalities of Modernity

The ways in which the terms of trauma came to stalk the scene of Western societies during the last centuries are illustrative of the point of its profoundly cultural situatedness. Most poignantly, trauma developed as the sickly underbelly of a new optimistic era putting high scores on progress, freedom and rational thought. Coming out of the age of revolutions on both continents a series of new constitutions were in the making, enshrining in print civil rights and gestures toward democracy, albeit it would take considerable time before women and the working class were included in the constituency of the free and the responsible. Huge developments in infrastructure, such as the railway, the steamship and the telegraph, reordered temporal and spatial structures, both socially and subjectively, thus creating new modes of experiences of scale and connectivity. Charles Darwin similarly upended the intellectual landscape with the publication of *The Origin of the Species* (1859), which removed God from the equation and argued instead that nature was the product of chance collisions and incremental changes through billions of years. Similar ideas were already in circulation for Karl Marx, and Frederick Engels inserted the Darwinian notion of competition for survival on the very first page of the *Communist Manifesto* (1848), declaring, 'The history of all hitherto existing society is the history of class struggles.' The move from the social to the self happened with *The Interpretation of Dreams* (1900), where Sigmund Freud managed to forge into theory the poetic wisdom of the troubling and darker sides of the psyche dating back to antiquity and the Greek tragedies. By carefully analyzing dreams, Freud explained exactly how these currents are forged and encrypted and how they are subject to distortion and censorship. He highlighted how the meaning of desires and wishes is formed and shaped by language, but also where meaning ends because all dreams throw up a point of resistance that simply cannot be interpreted.

The question of 'non-meaning' has ever since enlivened the trauma debacle (Chap. 2). At the time it was first received, however, it reinforced the cultural repertoire of doubt, worry and anxiety, which became an undercurrent reaction to all the proclaimed confidence of modernization across both sides of the Atlantic. For, the huge advances in technology during the nineteenth and twentieth centuries resulted in the industrialization of the war machinery causing huge levels of causalities. New forms of slow violence followed on the heel of colonization and resource exploitation in foreign lands. The decimation of entire cohorts of young men in protracted wars, and a new form of reporting about the atrocities committed against indigenous populations in the colonies by Western profiteers, helped to produce a new sensitivity to the suffering of those others living far beyond the edges of own communities, gradually building the 'empire of trauma' in a Western image. All our case studies are lodged onto the ledger of modernity, although the face of trauma they display and the specific articulation with value systems sometimes foreign to the Western conventions turn our volume into a comparison between many modalities of modernity and marginalization.

This close connection between trauma and modernity of a Western brand is the topic of Broch-Due's opening chapter following this general introduction. Broch-Due embarks on a genealogical mapping of the very term 'trauma'—an undertaking that takes in scholarly histories and conventions from a range of disciplines: from its etymological origins in medical practices and the philosophy of Greek medicine to more modern usages in psychoanalysis and neuroscience. Broch-Due demonstrates the changing nature and usage of the term. She points out that a double origin of the term developed from a corporeal imprint of a 'wound' to become a metaphor where both the body and the mind were constructed as surfaces of signification. In the process, being 'wounded' became stretched from skin to soul. Hovering over the traumatic impact has been the whole question of memory and theories of signification. In excavating modern and classical antecedents to the construction of trauma and the various mind-body configurations that are involved, Broch-Due assesses the impact of interdisciplinary scholarships as diverse as Didier Fassin, Thomas Laquer, Francis O'Gorman, Elaine Showalter, Ian Hacking, Sigmund Freud, Jacques Derrida, Ruth Leys, Silvan Tomkins, Emily Martin, Arnold Van Gennep—to name a few. Crucially, she underlines how the term trauma is continuously produced anew as a vibrant and powerful gestalt, being sandwiched between the domains of the bodily, the social, the self and the sign. These domains are themselves invested with cultural meanings that must be framed locally—and which effectively also constitute the ontological coordinates of worlds. She ends her essay by suggesting that vintage concepts in anthropology like 'liminality' and 'rites of passage' may have an untapped analytical potential which can push a theorizing more sensitive to the diverse experiences of trauma.

Luckily, the contexts under study here vary greatly and they all in complementary ways respond to Broch-Due's call for a renewed attention to the dynamics of relationality, ontology and world-making in trauma analysis. From the temporal fallout from civil war contexts of Mozambique to the managerialism of Norwegian psychiatric hospitals, from the role of laughter in ludic rituals in Chios to the politics of guilt in post-authoritarian Argentina, the volume embraces a range of dynamics that eclipse visions of the singular individual confronting her/his unique trauma in a contextless void. So, in what ways, more precisely, do these texts address and thematize trauma?

In Robben's chapter on contemporary Argentina, ghosts from the authoritarian and violent past of that country are shown to manifest themselves in several ways—some spectral and some material. For one, Robben shows us how what he terms social trauma and collective guilt are imbricated in a context of increasing court cases against those that perpetrated violence during the former violent Argentinian regime. An argument is made that with the weighing on an even scale of social trauma and collective guilt—the latter fueled by demands still persistently made by human rights groups despite the court cases—this produces a complicated situation in terms of overall psychosocial healing.

Taking his point of departure from research on *longue durée* transmissions of trauma and violence on the Greek island of Chios as well as in the Grasslands of Cameroon, Argenti is concerned with the nature of traumatic memory itself and the role that laughter plays in memorialization. Specifically, he critiques the implicit atomizing impetus in much Western-oriented trauma thinking and shows, ethnographically, historically and theoretically, how generative and fundamental the role of ritual laughter is in confronting the presence of violence formally past but still present. Informing his highly original comparison of Cameroonian masked rituals and Chiosian carnivalesque playfulness are key questions regarding the universal or non-universal suffering human subject—as well as their respective collectivities.

A subject of much anthropological (and other) critique of trauma thinking as well as the template of PTSD (see, e.g., also Young 1997 [1995]), the role of speech is the focus of Bertelsen's contribution to the volume. Drawing on ethnographic material from rural and peri-urban Mozambique in the aftermath of civil war (see also Bertelsen 2016), Bertelsen shows how the spoken—speech genres in their Bakhtinian sense—are crucial vehicles for addressing and working with lingering violence. Crucially he underlines how such speech genres not only re-inscribe meaning to violence but also reveal the fundamentally social nature of narrative truth—also in relation to trauma.

Astrinaki's contribution orients the reader toward the impact of structural and economic ruptures and turmoil through exploring the crisis of contemporary Greek society. Mapping the macro-political environs and what she sees as the attack on the social order as well as the Greek state from the dominant European and global economic forces introducing a violent restructuring of society, Astrinaki points to generalized senses of disempowerment and political non-engagement in the population at large. She sees such sense as the result of affective violence and as, effectively, constituting a 'traumatropic' political technology that thoroughly and violently reshapes the political order, political subjectivities and senses of self.

The long-term and changing legacies of large-scale violence are addressed in Carol Kidron's chapter through a daring comparison between the descendants of Jewish Israeli and Cambodian genocidal contexts. Kidron takes her cue from the debate between those that ascribe a universal semiotics or grammar to genocide, on the one hand, and those that underline how such an ascription may silence, eclipse or reconfigure in unhelpful ways particular idioms and cosmologies of suffering. Arguing against what she sees as a reductionist and pathologizing tendency in some interventionist practices, through a rich presentation and comparison between, especially, the Cambodian and Jewish Israeli familial spheres, she shows that these may be seen as non-singular sites of intergenerational transmission that harbor future-oriented as well as past-oriented moral orientations that are irreducible to templates of victimization, erasure or generalized vulnerability.

Norwegian and, more broadly, Western hegemonic notions of ontological security are addressed by Teig in this volume. Taking as her point of departure the debate on psychiatry in the aftermath of the act of terror in Norway on 22 July 2011 in which a total of 77 people were killed by right-wing terrorist Anders Behring Breivik, Teig examines the framework of 'psychiatrisation'—both within the legal framework of courts as well as a concrete institution in Bergen, Norway—to argue for the changing and mass-mediated role that the notion of 'risk' plays in insulating society against trauma potentially inflicted on it by psychiatric patients. Crucially, Teig argues for a correlation between a pronounced and increasing managerialism at psychiatric wards, society's obsession with risk and the consequent reductive framing of psychiatric patients as harboring solely the capacity for trauma-inducing violence.

In her chapter, Ystanes examines the social body of the Guatemalan society and how everyday life is shaped by not only past political violence and war-related atrocities but also the dangers seen to be lurking under the surface that sometimes explode in acts of violence. Exploring political fear of violence in both domestic and public domains, Ystanes shows how the formation of fear is conditioned by sustained impunity of past violence, ongoing inequalities and societal dynamics exposing politically engaged subjects to the very real risk of being subjected to violence. In a sense Ystanes shows us how trauma-inducing dynamics may be endemic to the political order and how fear, far from being a constitutive feature of singular personhood, must be seen as an effect of such continuously induced political order.

Bolivians in Bolivia as well as in Spain form the point of departure for Tapias in her chapter, analyzing how the monotone insistence on therapeutic talk following traumatic incidents may be detrimental to our understanding of the complexities of such rupturing effects on human lives. Instead, Tapias makes a careful analysis of the practices of silences and non-disclosure associated with the familial lives of migrants distributed across vast physical as well as social and semiotic spaces. As Tapias shows, informed by Andean views of silence as expressing a healthy self, there is a grammar to the communication and non-communication of suffering, hardships and violence between migrant individuals and communities in Spain and their relatives in Bolivia. Thus, for Tapias the management of selective disclosure and carefully chosen silences express deliberately chosen strategies to deal with trauma and suffering, rather than indicating being immobilized by these.

Taken together, the contributions, of which we have given mere snippets above, move the analysis further on many analytical scores; in terms of memory, agency, acculturated physiologies and psychologies, signification and performativity. They powerfully show us how humanity lives, conceptualizes and responds to ordeal in a highly diverse manner. The violence that reverberates so widely and diversely, producing suffering and trauma in its wake, comes out of a modernity in the plural that has a capacity both for spectacular forms of impact and the more creeping forms of damage. Whatever major form, violence, trauma and marginalization show up locally in many modulations.

References

Antze, Paul, and Michael Lambek, eds. 1996. *Tense Past. Cultural Essays in Trauma and Memory.* London: Routledge.

Argenti, Nicolas. 2007. *Intestines of the State.* In *Youth, Violence, and Belated Histories in the Cameroon Grassfields.* Chicago, IL: University of Chicago Press.

Argenti, Nicolas, and Katharina Schramm, eds. 2010. *Remembering Violence. Anthropological Perspectives on Intergenerational Transmission.* New York: Berghahn Books.

Badiou, Alain. 2012. *The Rebirth of History.* London: Verso.

Bertelsen, Bjørn Enge. 2016. *Violent Becomings: State Formation, Sociality, and Power in Mozambique.* New York: Berghahn Books.

Broch-Due, V. 1995. *The 'Poor' and the 'Primitive'. Discursive and Social Transformations, Occasional Paper Series, No 5, Poverty & Prosperity.* Uppsala: The Nordic Africa Institute.

———. 1999. Remembered Cattle, Forgotten People: The Morality of Exchange and the Exclusion of the Turkana Poor. In *The Poor are Not Us: Poverty and Pastoralism in Eastern Africa*, eds. David M. Anderson and Vigids Broch-Due, 50–88. Oxford and Athens, OH: James Curry and Ohio University Press.

———, ed. 2005. *Violence and Belonging: The Quest for Identity in Post Colonial Africa.* London: Routledge.

Caruth, C. 1995. *Trauma: Explorations in Memory.* Baltimore, MD: Johns Hopkins University Press.

———. 1996. *Unclaimed Experience: Trauma, Narrative and History.* Baltimore, MD: Johns Hopkins University Press.

Cole, Jennifer. 2001. *Forget Colonialism? Sacrifice and the Art of Memory in Madagascar.* Berkeley: University of California Press.

Daniel, E. Valentine. 1996. *Charred Lullabies: Chapters in an Anthropography of Violence.* Princeton, NJ: Princeton University Press.

Das, Veena. 2007. *Life and Words. Violence and the Descent into the Ordinary.* Berkeley: University of California Press.

Das, Veena, Arthur Kleinman, Mamphela Ramphele, and Pamela Reynolds, eds. 2000. *Violence and Subjectivity.* Berkeley: University of California Press.

Fassin, Didier, and Richard Rechtman. 2009 [2007]. *The Empire of Trauma. An Inquiry into the Condition of Victimhood.* Trans. Rachel Gomme. Princeton, NJ: Princeton University Press.

Felman, Shoshana. 2002. *The Juridical Unconscious: Trials and Traumas in the Twentieth Century.* Boston, MA: Harvard University Press.

Feuchtwang, Stephan. 2011. *After the Event: The Transmission of Grievous Loss in Germany, China and Taiwan.* Oxford: Berghahn Books.

Galtung, Johan. 1969. Violence, Peace, and Peace Research. *Journal of Peace Research* 6(3): 167–191.

Henare, Amiria, Martin Holbraad, and Sari Wastell. 2007. *Thinking Through Things: Theorizing Artefacts Ethnographically*. New York: Routledge.
Honwana, Alcinda Manuel. 1999. Appeasing the Spirits. Healing Strategies in Postwar Southern Mozambique. In *Religion, Health and Suffering*, eds. John R. Hinnels and Roy Porter, 237–255. London: Kegan Paul International.
Hunt, Nigel C. 2010. *Memory, War and Trauma*. Cambridge: Cambridge University Press.
Kwon, Heonik. 2006. *After the Massacre: Commemoration and Consolation in Ha My and My Lai*. Berkeley: University of California Press.
———. 2008. *Ghosts of War in Vietnam*. Cambridge: Cambridge University Press.
Lambek, Michael. 1996. The Past Imperfect. Remembering as Moral Practice. In *Tense Past. Cultural Essays in Trauma and Memory*, eds. Paul Antze and Michael Lambek, 235–254. New York: Routledge.
Lester, Rebecca. 2013. Back from the Edge of Existence: A Critical Anthropology of Trauma. *Transcultural Psychiatry* 50(5): 753–762.
Maček, Ivana. 2014. *Engaging Violence. Trauma, Memory and Representation*. London: Routledge.
McNally, R.J. 2003. *Remembering Trauma*. Cambridge, MA: Belknap/Harvard University Press.
Mollica, Richard. 2006. *Healing Invisible Wounds. Paths to Pope and Recovery in a Violent World*. Orlando, FL: Harcourt.
Nelson, Diane M. 2009. *Reckoning. The Ends of War in Guatemala*. Durham, NC: Duke University Press.
Nelson, Judith Kay. 2013. Grief and Loss in an Age of Global Trauma: Protest and Despair Versus Attachment and Reorganization. *Contemporary Clinical Practice*: 19–27. doi:10.1007/978-1-4614-4124-3_3.
Nixon, Rob. 2011. *Slow Violence and the Environmentalism of the Poor*. Cambridge, MA: Harvard University Press.
Panter-Brick, Catherine, and Mark Eggerman. 2012. Understanding Culture, Resilience, and Mental Health: The Production of Hope. In *The Social Ecology of Resilience*. ed. M. Ungar, 369–386. New York: Springer.
Robben, Antonius C.G.M., and Marcelo M. Suárez-Orozco. 2000. *Cultures under Siege. Collective Violence and Trauma*. Cambridge: Cambridge University Press.
Robbins, Joel. 2013. Beyond the Suffering Subject: Toward an Anthropology of the Good. *Journal of the Royal Anthropological Institute* 19: 447–462.
Rothberg, Michael. 2009. *Multidirectional Memory: Remembering the Holocaust in the Age of Decolonization*. Stanford, CA: Stanford University Press.
Scheper-Hughes, Nancy. 2002. Coming to Our Senses. Anthropology and Genocide. In *Annihilating Difference: The Anthropology of Genocide*, ed. Alexander L. Hinton, 348–381. Berkeley: University of California Press.
———. 2008. A Talent for Life. Reflections on Human Vulnerability and Resilience. *Ethnos* 73(1): 25–56.

Trouillot, Michel-Rolph. [1991] 2003. Anthropology and the Savage Slot: The Poetics and Politics of Otherness. In *Global Transformations: Anthropology and the Modern World*, ed. Michel-Rolph Trouillot, 7–28. New York: Palgrave Macmillan.

Vigdis Broch-Due, and Anderson, David, eds. 1999. *The Poor Are Not Us: Poverty and Pastoralism in Eastern Africa*. Oxford: James Curry.

Yarrow, Thomas, and Soumhya Venkatesan, eds. 2012. *Differentiating Development: Beyond an Anthropology of Critique*. Oxford: Berghahn Books.

Young, Allan. 1997 [1995]. *The Harmony of Illusions: Inventing Post-Traumatic Stress Disorder*. Princeton, NJ: Princeton University Press.

Zagato, Alessandro, ed. 2015. *The Event of Charlie Hebdo. Imaginaries of Freedom and Control*. New York: Berghahn Books.

Zulaika, Joseba. 2009. *Terrorism. The Self-Fulfilling Prophecy*. Chicago, IL: University of Chicago Press.

Zur, Judith N. 1998. *Violent Memories. Mayan War Widows in Guatemala*. Boulder, CO: Westview Press.

CHAPTER 2

Trauma, Violence, Memory: Reflections on the Bodily, the Self, the Sign, and the Social

Vigdis Broch-Due

'Only that which does not cease to hurt remains in memory.'
Friedrich Nietzsche, *On the Genealogy of Morals* (1887)

'Trauma' is the buzzword of our time, delivering 120 million Google results in less than a second. 'Trauma' is clearly a hungry concept consuming some aspects of almost everybody's experience in its wake, whether in the capacity of sufferers, witnesses, or spectators. 'Trauma' spans many trajectories and biographies; it crosses generations and filters into the social memory and historiography of communities and nations. 'Trauma' is culturally twinned with modernity and tensely situated at the heart of Western theories of the subject and signification processes.

'Trauma' started out its etymological existence quite modestly in Greek antiquity as being merely a physical wound—an exterior sign of the infliction of painful injury piercing the skin and affecting the whole organ-

V. Broch-Due (✉)
Centre for Advanced Study (CAS), Oslo, Norway
Department of Social Anthropology, University of Bergen, Norway

V. Broch-Due, B.E. Bertelsen (eds.), *Violent Reverberations*,
DOI 10.1007/978-3-319-39049-9_2

ism. This hurt on the outside is still with us in modern hospitals that are equipped with 'trauma surgeons' or 'trauma wards', but this is hardly the sense that has made trauma talk so resonant and pervasive today. For we are not confronted with a renaissance of a rather morbid interest in physical wounds per se but with an expansion of new meanings that emerged in the late nineteenth century when 'trauma' wedged its wound into the human psyche. Trauma was no longer the visible imprint of a blow to the body but surfaced virtually and violently in the mind as a 'thorn in the spirit', as phrased by the nineteenth-century philosopher and psychologist William James. His contemporary, Sigmund Freud, based his whole psychoanalysis on the fragmenting effects of psychic trauma stemming from any unspeakable or inassimilable experience. As so aptly pointed out by Laplanche and Pontalis, 'In adopting the term of trauma, psychoanalysis carries the three ideas implicit in it over on to the psychical level: the idea of a violent shock, the idea of a wound and the idea of consequences affecting the whole organization' (1973:465). In the nineteenth and twentieth centuries, these expanding mental wounds were still understood to be somatically present in the victims by such symptoms as hysteria, paralysis, flashbacks, sleeplessness, fatigue, tremors, heartbeat, and so on.

But today symptoms are no longer required to be reckoned as traumatized. The 'condition of victimhood' has moved beyond the body and crafted itself onto organized assemblages democratically available to everyone according to the historian Thomas Laqueur (2010). He is showing us how disparate phenomena of 'bygone times' are equally supposed to have lodged a 'thorn in the spirit', whether in the form of a community's history of upheaval, or simply in the course of any normal childhood where parents are held by certain psychologists to be inflicting varying degrees of permanent psychic scarring on their children. The problem with such sprawling usage of trauma, warns Laqueur, is that once the term magnifies into the psychic and metaphorical trace of all pasts in anyone's present, more of a victim's life is obliterated rather than recovered. To this erasure of the complexity of the personal, we might also add that the new 'empire of trauma' simultaneously obscures the contour of the social, in particular the complexity of the space of the inter-subjective, the in between subjects, which can only be addressed in its cultural specificity.

In other words, 'trauma' has become a generic condition of global reach. Conceptually, it belongs among what the anthropologist Clifford Geertz pertinently coined 'thin description' (1973). For it is precisely due to its very elusiveness as an expression that 'trauma' now manages to model both self and the social in minimal, sometimes even measurable terms and, thus, can travel light and confidently across cultural and historical boundaries. Through their endless replications across discursive registers, thin descriptions often assume a taken-for-grantedness that escapes critical scrutiny and specificity. For terms like 'trauma' in their thinnest rendition appear context-free and common-sensical and, for their audiences, deceptively freed from the contamination of authorship, agency, and social context. However, the moment they move out of generic comportment and become firmly situated in social reality, 'thin' descriptions rapidly 'thicken', becoming both politicized and contentious. Trauma is a telling case, and it is to its trajectories and controversies we now turn.

Trauma and Suffering Writ Large

Historical consideration of the two grand concepts that trauma draws close to its condition in Western thought, notably 'body' and 'mind', shows these too to be malleable, sometimes analytically aligned and sometimes being set apart. The corporal and the cognitive domains of human embodiment each trails a constellation of meanings in which particular concepts cluster, often temporarily, before moving on to inform other constellations, discourses, and practices. The clustering concepts around the triad—trauma/body/mind—concern questions of emotions, memory, imagination, and subjectivity—each of which straddles and infiltrates the physical and the psychic in diverse ways, and each has an intimate bearing both on understanding the self and on the social.

Before tracing the body-mind discourse through different times and spatial frames, it is important to remind ourselves that the distinctions we make when we interpret the world are those possible within the pool of social knowledge available at any one time or place. New scientific discoveries and new ways of organizing society change the topology of the known and establish new modes of experience and explanation. In this process, social constructs powerfully at work in the conceptualization of how trauma bridges or breaks the relationship between body and mind—notably gender, class, race, origins—are constantly being fleshed out anew within different and sometimes competing discourses. Since I am offering a critical reading of the tracings of trauma in flesh and thought from an anthropological perspective, I will be concerned less with chronology and more with the *structural repetitions* that have characterized successive theorizations. For throughout the journey of trauma from skin to soul and beyond into the social, certain theoretical and empirical complications and tensions surface recurrently at different historical moments and in different social contexts. As Michel Foucault observes in his essay '*Nietzsche, Genealogy, History*', genealogy 'operates on a field of entangled and confused parchments that have been scratched over and recopied many times' (1977:140).

Let us start out with a summary of the main points in some recent publications about the genealogies of trauma in the Foucaultian tradition and their critiques. *The Empire of Trauma* (2009), written jointly by an anthropologist and a psychiatrist, focuses on shifting 'political uses of trauma' over time. The casts of the drama are various kinds of professional communities who, through their daily routines, the standards of their profession, and their interactions with the state and with clients, build the platform for certain subject positions like 'trauma victim' or 'homosexual', which those communities then regulate by keeping their definitional contours in shape, compassionately or not so, as the case may be. For the work of governance, according to Fassin and Rechtman, is not so much through the intervention of laws but rather through the 'production of truth'. What counts is not whether someone actually is a victim of trauma but how the criteria for deciding who is a victim come into being and who then manages these measures. This process of determining how truth and falsehood are regulated and brought to bear on the identities of selves to the extent that the self incorporates the disciplinary stitches that define a given identity is what Foucault calls 'governmentality'. It is precisely through this lens the authors of the 'empire of Trauma' view how the category of the psychic wound is shaped through debates about the moral legitimacy of victims.

Once the category of trauma was established in the 1880s in the form of post-traumatic stress disorder at the heal of wars and disasters, the initial focus for inquiry was on the numbers afflicted; the puzzle being why only a few of those exposed to a given violent or stressful event developed symptoms. The suspicion was that those afflicted were of a weak constitution and character. Although the French authors themselves do not spend much ink on elaborating the larger social context involved here, for our purpose it is still useful to remind ourselves that this was the time when theories of eugenics flourished. Central to this interest in the generation of bodies was the notion that the poor, women, and other degenerates carried inferior bloodlines that made them more susceptible, both in their flesh and mind, to nerve-racking actions. Since soldiers from the lower classes were more likely than their officers to swell the ranks of those pushed first into the firing lines, they were overrepresented among the afflicted. The focus on the idea of degeneracy rather than class turned these men in distress into suspects, who either were seen as prone to faking their symptoms to get compensation or were deemed downright unpatriotic. Thus morality could, in a circular fashion, be directly read from pedigrees; the better-off through their better breeding had, by definition, higher moral standards and resilience against injury than those of inferior bloodlines.

A century later, the inquiry into the damaging experiences of war had been turned into an ethical question when the experiences of what the trauma patients had witnessed and endured were put onto the agenda. Now doctors pondered how they could draw on individual cases to develop therapies to help those who suffered from similar experiences, thus creating a moral equalizer across communities of sufferers. According to Fassim and Rechtman, the violence of unprecedented scale that surfaced with the Holocaust was a turning point, after which the burden was lifted from the sufferer of torture and abuse and landed closer at home to the perpetrator.

This epistemic shift was also helped by the newfound influence of psychoanalysis in the aftermath of the Second World War, due to its emphasis on confession, which suited the attention paid to experience in this historical period. However, the talking cure has presently lost its power with the resurgence of neuroscience as the dominant discourse. In this newfound pure medicalized version, trauma is lodged as a deep wound in the primitive parts of the brain detectable not through the words of the patient but by EEG scanning. Under the cool blue rays of the machine, morality does no longer enter into things, neither for those responsible for the hurt of others nor for those being hurt, they share in the victimhood of flashbacks and blocked affect. In other words, the trauma victim in the neurological scenario would be no more or less culpable than the victim of a lightning strike or gunshot. We are now at a curious turning point where trauma seems to be leaving behind its presence as 'thorn in the soul' and is travelling back to lodge itself as 'thorn in the flesh'—trauma has still not made the full circle back and re-emerged entirely of the exterior, but as we shall explore later in this chapter, it has started to resurface by touching the skin and spreading across surfaces as a wound in the whole signification system, as it were.

The larger point of the *Empire of Trauma* book is that the technology of questioning produces certain facts while sidelining or silencing others. If the question is posed, as it once was, primarily as a problem of regularity, then investigators will focus on the vulnerability of victims; if it is posed in terms of what has been witnessed by the afflicted, attention turns to the event. No clinical advance can explain the historical shift from one mode of inquiry to the other: the framing of the question about trauma has little if anything to do with substantive knowledge of psychology, psychiatry, or neurology. It does have a great deal to do with what Foucault called 'the production of truth', with the way these disciplines can be mobilized for novel purposes.

The gist of the analysis thus concerns the construction—not the reality—of trauma in the different areas of mental health and the ensuing political implications for assigning who can or cannot claim the rights of victimhood. Ethnographically it deals with three new professional arenas for the production of such 'truths'. 'Psychiatric victimology', developed in Toulouse after an explosion at a chemical plant, validates victim status and focuses on reparation; 'humanitarian psychiatry' draws attention to the causes of suffering among Palestinians in the Occupied Territories and in Israel; 'the psycho-traumatology of exile' concerns the persecution of refugees seeking asylum in an unwelcoming country, France. Together, these movements represent a radical shift in the 'anthropological significance' of victimhood, from a world in which victims were suspect, to one in which 'their suffering, no longer contested, testifies to an experience that excites sympathy and merits compensation'. To this we may add that the trend in contemporary crime fiction, emulating the success of *Gone Girl* (2012) by Gillian Flynn, is to turn the female victim of abuse into a virtual heroine, the plot being narrated by her broken voice through voids in her memory. Through such discursive shifts from blaming to glorifying victims, where the moral first was gradually woven densely into the medical only to slip away from it entirely, a conceptual 'empire' is being built from the grounds of trauma, turning the 'traumatized' into a 'floating signifier' that denotes any number of ills which have little in common other than a name.

In his scholarship, the historian Thomas Laqueur takes another tack in the genealogy of human suffering and its memorialization. Not only is he highly critical of the notion that the attention to the 'psychic wound' is the driving force, but he also disagrees about the chronology, dating the newfound historical sensitivity back to the bloody battlefield of the American civil war which blew up in 1861 (2008). Why this location is of great importance as an engine in the construction of a 'trauma empire', as it were, is precisely because this civil war was among the earliest true industrial wars. Railroads, the telegraph, steamships, and mass-produced weapons were employed extensively. The mobilization of civilian factories, mines, shipyards, banks, transportation, and food supplies all foreshadowed World War I. It remains the deadliest war in American history with a high number of causalities among civilians and soldiers alike resulting in an unprecedented intensity of grief experienced on a large scale. There had of course been massacres, mass killings, and atrocities committed on American soil and beyond before this event—the decimation of native communities throughout colonization is a case in point.

What made the civil war a turning point in public recognition was foremost advances in technology of communication and arithmetical accounting, which greatly helped to deliver the required 'space-time compression', as theorized by the geographer David Harvey (1969). An avalanche of statistics translated thousands of killing scenes into a numeric entity, which, along with the corpses interred in a new grid of cemeteries, delivered the dead as a standardized category of the civil war causalities, both producing new forms of visibility. In her eloquent account of these events, Drew Gilpin Faust (2008) argues that 'this republic of suffering' is precisely predicated on mass literacy, on the telegraphs and postal service that deliver letters and communiqués, on advanced print technology that spews out daily newspapers and pamphlets, on the capturing of the image of loved ones through photography and the preservation of their voices through recording, and on the popularity of the domestic novel and the magazine story that conjured up intimate plots of loss and commemoration in the minds of an expanding readership.

Through the ways in which these media helped create an 'imagined community' as coined by Benedict Anderson (1983), they made an egalitarian response to death possible on a massive scale. In other words, the novelty of the cultural infrastructure made the death of individuals matter through the ways it connected the lives and deaths of those on the battlefield to the lives of those at home. Faust demonstrates how these intimate connections, mostly through letters, generated the demand for a good death, a remembered death, a celebrated death imaginable to ordinary people. Material inscriptions in the forms of photographs and letters constituted the enterprise of identifying, accounting, and numbering, and were deposited in archives conserved for posterity. In short, not only was the whole modern machinery of memory for the first time almost universally available in this war, but it also embraced ordinary people—men, women, and children—regarded as having lived meaningful lives and thus deserved to be remembered by the living. This technology of connectivity, visibility, outreach, and recounting on a large scale is the broader context of death and trauma during the nineteenth- and twentieth-century Western world. These tangible underpinnings of trauma as a social phenomenon—of mortar, steel, paper, and electric waves—are sidetracked in the account of Fassin and Rectman.

This new type of expansive sociality built by technological advances and grounding the 'republic of suffering' triggered, as an unintended effect, a new *sensitivity* that the pain of others is a matter of social concern, creating what the philosopher Avishai Margalit (2004) has called the 'ethics of memory', positing a public duty of commemoration. The core of this dictum concerns the belief that communities are woven together in a thick web of shared memories and obligations to remember bygone acts and those actors putting themselves in harm's way for the common good.

In his *LRB* review of the *Empire of Trauma*, Thomas Laqueur argues succinctly that this collective motion to the social obligations of remembrance surrounding suffering and injury is what has driven its expansion, not the attention to psychic wounds or changing beliefs about death and dying. More significant is the proliferation in collective memory sedimented in memorials, penned in memoirs and protocols, and voiced in truth and reconciliation commissions. These practices and tribunals are aimed at the mastery of a past in the interests of the future. In order to get a better grasp on how such collective acts grow out of a vast range of imperatives, Laqueur argues, 'Maurice Halbwachs, one of Durkheim's protégés, is more important than Freud ... there is no evidence that the category of trauma played a substantial role in it' (2010:23).

While it is clearly the case that a myriad of social factors far removed from the famous Freudian couch contributed greatly to scale up both collective memory and concern for others, the emotional economy still played into the complexity, but maybe less as full-fledged 'trauma' and more in its paler and more widespread twin of 'worry'. This is because the technological advancement during the nineteenth and twentieth centuries totally reorganized Western societies fracturing older forms of sociality and experience. Travelling with train instead of carriage involved a new experience of time, space, and speed, which created dizziness and disorientation in passengers unfamiliar with such transport. Indeed, the great number of fatalities on railway tracks and construction sites erecting new factories and urban housing were among the first recognized trauma victims. To this we may add the two state-sponsored wars and the huge increase in soldiers being stuck for months in the trenches. The arrival of modernity was fraught with ambivalence; on the one hand, there was a triumphant belief in progress, industry, profit, and consumer culture, counteracted by a ruination of lives and the fissuring of small worlds. In the cracks and liminal zones between new and old seeped in a sentiment of endless circular and inconsolable fretting to the extent that the renowned US Senator George Walton declared that worry was 'the disease of the age' discoloring the banner of pure optimism.

The literary scholar Francis O'Gorman (2012) has traced the genealogy of worrying back to the Victorian times, pointing out that its verbal form suggests the problem starts outside the mind and comes at one 'like a wasp at a picnic'. Etymologically, the term 'worry' began as a physical harassment, referring to a chocking of bones in dogs or humans. Most telling, roughly at the same time in Western history as 'trauma' went mental, 'worry' too quit the body and leapt into the mind, where it creates constant unease by goading the subject to speculate about things large and small that might never happen. O'Gorman goes on to argue that as early twentieth century grew more familiar with the indulgence and the fear of this new mental experience of 'what if', it became a sign for the difficulty of 'ordinary' existence and the interpretive struggle of what modern human beings were to be, or not. Worry inscribed itself into the seminal novels of James Joyce, T.S. Elliot, and Virginia Wolfe, making itself known through the interior, fragmented monologues and cyclical, diurnal plotlines that have become the hallmark of high modernist esthetics. The author likens the ways worry has continued to colonize Western minds to a virtual 'metaphysical calamity' simply because the secular subject has renounced the belief that the gods control human destiny. As 'moderners', we are called upon to make existential choices that promise to propel us ahead, but many experience instead a feeling of being dejected, disappointed, left at the end of the day ruminating over what went wrong and whom to blame. What characterizes worry even more than the circularity of thought and language trapped in repetition is the very lack of *proportions* of the problem festering in the mind. This, I shall argue, means that 'trauma' in its expansive form can be read as worry in disguise, and thus being a conduct for the worrier turned 'victim'.

In another critical take on victimization witnessed in the tremendous growth of a 'survivor culture', Elaine Showalter claims that a popular way in which 'we construct a past as a collective' is fueled with blame, vengeful litigation, and conspiracy theories. In *Hystories* (1998), she takes to task the 'trauma survival movement' inspired by Jeffrey M. Masson's *The Assault on Truth* (1984), where he argued that experiences of abuse surfacing in therapy were 'recovered memory' and thus real, and should not, as had become the more prevalent interpretation, be seen as mere figments of imagination produced by therapists in susceptible patients. Showalter favors the latter version asserting that the huge increase in testimonies is the effect of unconscious fears and anxiety, which are attributed to trauma-inducing external causes of dubious realities. As indicated by the play of the book title, hysterics are not relics from Victorian attics but alive, well, and massively recruiting troubled individuals from all walks of life and all over the world. Hysteria has moved out of the clinic to insert itself into the popular narrative or 'hystory', feeding plotlines inspired by a host of psychosomatic ailments, traversing a diverse terrain sweeping up recovered memory of childhood abuse, Myalgic Encephalomyelitis (ME), Gulf War syndrome, multiple personality disorder, to alien abduction, and the list could be extended endlessly.

What is specifically significant in our context is the emphasis put on the role of *mediation* as the means to make the proliferation of anxiety possible. The cultural infrastructure in the twenty-first century has become more sophisticated than the previous centuries, including electronic communication such as the web, where the speed and spread through social media make an escalation of 'hystories' possible on an unprecedented scale. The 'imagined community' of subscribers probably share less than what sets them apart in everyday life, but thin descriptions always have a huge public attraction for those who yearn for purity and simplicity.

Whether we are confronted with an 'empire of trauma', a 'republic of suffering', or a 'community of memorialization', 'the festering of worries' or simply 'hystories' might come down to theoretical inkling and taste of analysis. But all these genealogies help us to understand why compassion for those afflicted by violence and loss has become a global sentiment exported across continents by a host of international organizations and media of communication. On the productive side of the equation, trauma (and suffering) in the generic has its advantages not only by erecting a platform for witnessing, from where people can acquire their status as victims and find treatment for their suffering, but also by creating new paths for exposing the reality of persecution and prejudice, as well as providing a tool in political struggles for recognition and compensation. On the negative side of the equation, the vast expansion of a generic trauma is trailing conspiracy and paranoia, which may easily pit one collective against another, causing even more violence and misery. But most problematic, this gesture toward the generic is erasing as much as it recovers of both situated selves and the social. We need to downsize to the personal and inter-subjective domain and take another track in the circuit of trauma that concerns itself more directly with the controversies surrounding the mindful body and the construction of the subject.

Technologies of the Subject: Freudian Perspectives

The genealogy of the modern subject in the nineteenth and twentieth centuries is embedded in those concerning trauma, suffering, and memories and thus belongs to the same broad historical canvas. Let me give a very rudimentary summary, first of the significance of the broader political economy, which takes up the thread from Laqueur about the particular role of new technologies in shaping experience. We learn from Foucault (1980) that nineteenth-century Europe was like a huge 'workshop' in which power and knowledge were melted together by new types of micro-technologies. This new 'power/knowledge regime' was a response to the problems of population management. It helped the state to organize its citizens so they could be seen and known, and thus controlled. These institutional procedures combined new sites—like prisons, factories, hospitals, and schools—with new disciplinary practices—surveillance, observations, and classification—with new kinds of scientific knowledge and specialization—in criminology, economy, medicine, demography, pedagogy, and psychology.

Foucault calls this new visibility the 'gaze' which is of two kinds: First, synoptic visibility which helped to divide people into ranked groups and spaces. And second, the individualizing visibility that aimed at detailed case studies of persons, their different habits, and histories. In the second half of the nineteenth century, the need for population planning to improve public health, housing, and productivity shifted the attention to reproduction and the family. Sex and sexuality became the objects for medical investigation. The inquiry was soon re-focused to one of sexual difference, of the male and the female. The study of the sexed body was combined with the study of the mind. The gaze, therefore, had to be combined with the technology of confession which could access the deeper recesses of the mind, and this produced new knowledge and power.

The technology of 'seeing' and 'studying' and 'speaking out' was much more productive and penetrating than earlier forms of power. It changed people's ideas about themselves and the world by focusing not on their beliefs but on their behavior. Foucault dramatizes this point by saying that power is in our bodies, not in our heads. By this statement he wishes to stress that the new power/knowledge regime took hold of its objects at the deepest levels—in their daily activities, movements, gestures, and desires. This is precisely what is entailed by the theory of 'governmentality' as employed by Fassin and Rechtman in setting up the 'empire of trauma'. Another obvious example of such a discourse is psychoanalysis, to which we now turn.

Psychoanalysis is obsessed with bodily differences (Freud, 1953–1974). Freud's theory of the construction of sexuality and the production of the Unconscious centers on what he coins the 'Oedipus complex'. This most elemental, erotic, and jealous family drama involves the triangle of father, mother, and the male child. It is a powerful play of bits of bodies that stand as parts for two gendered and different wholes, male and female. It goes as follows: After having identified himself with his mother in a symbiotic unity, the little boy realizes that his mother lacks a penis, that she may after all be different from him. He catches a glimpse of his parents in an intimate act that seems to him as charged with paternal violence. He is excluded: he is not, after all, the center of the universe. Nothing is secure anymore.

This terrible insight and the trauma of coming to terms with it pose the following primary problems: How will he be able to continue enjoying the pleasures he gets from his own body? Will he lose his mother's love? Does his father's love matter to him? Or is father's power in a patriarchal society more desirable than mother's love? During the passage through these difficult moments the boy moves beyond the pleasure principle and into the reality principle. As a reward for accepting the phallic law and repressing his desire for the mother into the deep soils of the mind, he discovers and secures his own separate subjectivity and sexuality. The woman, however, gets more and more mysterious and dissolves into 'otherness' and 'darkness'.

One notes the crucial part played by the activity of seeing in the Oedipus drama. The act, witnessed in secret by the child, is staged close-up where the visual signifiers of sexual differences and sexuality in the Freudian scenario, notably the male and female genitals, are brought into an unequal interplay. Apparently psychoanalysis shares with the technologies of power at the time what Foucault calls the privilege of the eye—the gaze—as a guarantor for truth and knowledge. In his text on '*The Uncanny*', Freud himself theorizes the gaze as a phallic activity and in his interpretation of the Oedipus myth he equates the fear of blindness with the fear of castration. Thus the story of Oedipus weaves the inscription of violence into the representation of gender, making 'trauma' the technique instituting sexual difference itself.

For Freud, the basic fact of sexual difference is that the male has an obvious sex organ, and the female has not; when he looks at the woman, Freud apparently sees nothing. When Freud seeks to throw some light on the contours of femininity, he must get the concealed and mysterious woman to confess. For Freud, this lack of male attributes complicates the passage of the girl through the Oedipal crisis. For prior to this stage, Freud claims that the baby girl is the same as the baby boy. In the phallic stage, the little girl suddenly sees her clitoris as an inferior penis and then decides that she has already been castrated. This penis envy makes it hard for the girl to replace the mother with the father as object of desire and to develop a fully 'mature' femininity. While the controversial theory bars the woman from developing her subjectivity, it bolsters up the male psyche. Read as a projection of the male fear of castration, 'woman' is man's negative or mirror image. In sum, 'woman' is 'the Other'—cast as the object for male desire and male gaze.

These psychic processes in psychoanalytical accounts make several cultural specific claims. The development of the individual self is seen as part of a process by which we separate ourselves from others through the technology of sexual differences. The idea is that an insufficiently separated self is an undeveloped self. Moreover, the Oedipus scenario posits a split between nature and culture—read and represented by the two domains of the psyche. In Freudian terms, this split is a gendered one; the unconscious is a feminized and savage space reigned by repressed and chaotic instincts, while the conscious and the cultural order is controlled by masculine images.

Yet the boundary is permeable. Freud found the path by resolving a puzzle, notably the remarkable preference that dreams exhibit for 'unimportant details of wakening life'. He discovered that the detail served as a displacement for the deeper pulses of the mind. Displacement is a sort of strategy devised by the unconscious to evade censorship. The detail becomes a camouflage allowing repressed contents to surface in the consciousness of the confessing patient. By the same token, the detail serves as a metonymy, allowing the therapist to trace it back to the hidden whole it represents.

Most telling, as Naomi Schor demonstrates, the detail participates in a larger semantic network. On the one side, the detail is allied with the decorative and the decadent—both are linked with femininity in Western aesthetics. On the other side, the detail is allied with the trivial events of the everyday, rooted in the domestic sphere of social life run by women. Thus, the detail is lashed into the hierarchy of sexual difference: the detail is doubly gendered as feminine—and as such, the detail becomes the highway to the unconscious (Schor 1987:4).

Not only does trauma take center stage in Freud's theory about the formation of the unconscious, trauma is also highly gendered carrying a heavy feminine surplus most evident in the hysteric patient. From the symptoms of bourgeoisie women flocking into his surgery, Freud was first of the opinion that 'hysterics suffer mainly from reminiscences'—notably fragmented details of bygone events so disturbing that they were suppressed (Decker, 1991). These tangles of memories kept a link to real experiences although in a twisted, embellished, and transformed form. In his revised writings of the psychogenesis of hysteria, however, Freud erased memory from his explanation, replacing it with fantasy and its origins in the deep pulses of desires and anxieties of the unconscious. Trauma was thereby dislodged from its social mooring in inter-subjective relations that were themselves served by memory's complex ties to external events and settled instead firmly on the singular subject. This move from memory to imagination, from the social to the self, had huge implications not only for the theories of trauma to come, but foreshadowed tremors in the whole signification system itself. It paved the way for Jacques Lacan's rewriting of Freud's focus on the fragmentation of the mind, which is a crucial issue in order to understand better the physic trauma debacle to which we shall turn in the next section.

Here is a brief summary: Lacan translates the Freudian principles of pleasure and reality with two other terms: The Imaginary and The Symbolic Order. The move from the one stage to the other goes as follows: A new-born baby experiences its body in bits. Around the age of six months, the baby moves into the Imaginary stage and manages to bind together the bits into a unified body-image. The child has still no sense of a separate self—it merges with the surroundings and mirrors itself in the mother. The triangulation of this structure occurs when the father breaks up the dyadic unity. By giving up the claim to an imaginary identity with the mother and the world, the child enters the Symbolic Order of language and social institutions represented by the Law of the Father. The

Oedipus crisis comes to signify separation and speech to the child but also lack and loss. The child who learns to say 'I am' and separate this statement from 'you are'—is in fact saying 'I am he who has lost something' or 'I am that which I am not'. With this rewriting, Lacan wants to stress that the speaking subject only comes into being by repressing the desire for the maternal body.

In other words, the move from the Imaginary to the Symbolic Order creates a space for the unconscious. For the phallus that guards the symbolic is also the sign of lack—the repressed desire for symbiotic unity with the mother and the world. When the unconscious moves in place in Lacan's theory, a bar is driven between the signifier and signified. The work of the sign has no longer a reference to the real and cannot, as Freud claimed, be recovered in dreams. This is because the repressed meanings of the unconscious live a restless life in their own form of language. For the unconscious desire—with which we invest the objects in the symbolic order—moves endlessly from object to object or from signifier to signifier, without ever being satisfied. There is simply no proper substitute that can be that primary desire which has been lost forever (Lacan 1977).

What Can Be Remembered or Not—The Trauma Puzzle

Whether in agreement or in opposition, the trauma debate weaves itself from Freudian theories of subjectivity and the formation of memories. The complex plasticity of remembrance is made up of acute remembering and endless forgetting, of recollections sensorial triggered by smell, taste, touch, sound, sight, as well as short-term and long-term memorialization of ideas, events, routines, and temporal and spatial structures, often incorporated. This implies that processes of remembering deploy many temporalities, circular, linear and juxtapositions, or mélanges of these. Memories, past and present ones, may sit side by side depending on their emotional sway; memories stir and impact one another, playing tricks with the real when subject to reflection. Everyday life involves making sense of fragmentary memories. These pieces of remembrance are filtered through sensorium, self-image, and language, thus always culturally mediated.

When memories are shaped into stories and shared with others their comprehensibility depends on the context of experience, as well as the conventions of syntax and meaning of the specific language in question. Thus, memories take on a cultural flavor that through the act of telling archive a wholeness and structure far beyond the memory fragments of the mind. Indeed, after repeated telling, the story begins to supplant the images of the original memories (Hustvedt 2012). The problem with the trauma debacle is that it concerns ***damaged*** memories trailing disassociate states and dangerous repressed stuff that struggle to break into language. These fragile memories remain potential stories in need of rescue by somebody else, which makes them even more susceptible to manipulation than normal memories. This potential malleability makes the vexed tension between memory and fantasy, between sign and referent, between recall and chronology even more precarious.

In *Rewriting the Soul* (1995), Ian Hacking takes us directly to the historical scenario where trauma made the final leap from the exterior to the interior, from 'skin to soul' so to speak, by focusing on the so-called sciences of memory dating back to the 1870s. The emergent discipline of psychology was equipped with the enigmatic dictum that 'what has been forgotten is what forms our character, our personality, our soul'. This absence of memory was particularly seen as acute in pathological states such as 'multiple personality'—a diagnosis based on childhood trauma so severe that the patient can only cope by disassociation, letting one alter ego (or more) experience it for them. Hacking's main interest is not to subject this multiplicity disorder to a 'reality check'. Rather, he deploys the diagnostic system as a window into the emergent techniques to 'scientize the soul' employed by French positivism. He argues that the whole paraphernalia of tests, inferences, facts, and treatment are mutually consistent and self-confirming, calibrated not to any independent standard but to the judgments of a movement within psychiatry. It is thus another version of the ways in which actors within a new discipline convene in 'creating the object of which it speaks'—to paraphrase Foucault.

Whatever the case, from a slightly different angle the puzzle of multiplicity and amnesia can be read as a metaphysical grapple with the body/mind problem in the form of personal identity: Can multiple selves with multiple minds share one body? Or, do the multiple alters just represent the same embodied person and self in different guises? We see here a foreshadowing of the inquiry riddling the theories of signification, notably whether there is a relation between sign and referent or only free-floating signs? A middle ground can be found in Lacan's notion of multiple subject positions and Goffman's role-playing, but as we shall return to in a moment, Derrida later upended this grounding to set the sign free ranging.

In *Trauma: A Genealogy* (2000), Ruth Leys traverses much the same historical terrain as Fassim, Rechtman, and Hacking but focuses her attention firmly on the reality of individual trauma and what has been deemed a proper treatment to it. She takes up the thread from Freud's exploration of childhood sexual trauma and his discovery of the traumatic origin of hysteria, following the evolving debate through the series of world wars and the associated atrocities of the Holocaust, through Vietnam and up to the present. These were significant events where the same unresolved problem about human memory and its vagaries re-emerged episodically in scholarly debate only with minor twists and turns. Her interest is in a Foucaultian methodology of teasing out how *recurrent traces* are recombined, rather than applying his theory of 'governmentality' in the veins of the previous authors reviewed.

The vexed questions throughout her examination are these: Are memories of trauma reliable? Do traumatic memories have a purchase on the real or are they fabrications of a neurotic mind? Does a patient under hypnosis re-experience the original event or recall it? Is the goal of treatment to remember the traumatic event or to forget? Do recollections rest in the patient's experience, or are they the effect of suggestions by the therapist, or do patient and therapist both engage in creation of memory? Are there cultures and milieus of trauma? If so does this collective dimension erase the distinction between perpetrators and victims?

The provisional answers to these fundamental questions about processes of remembering and forgetting, all of which have significant social, political, and legal implications, depend on which side of the table you are seated when playing the memory game. Leys found a fixed double structure inscribed in the trauma scenario throughout time when accounting for the effects of shock on the experiences of trauma victims, notably the oscillation between the 'mimetic' and the 'anti-mimetic' positions. We may add that some critics have pointed out that Leys ignores the 'middle ground' where psychoanalytic and neuroscience approaches overlap in more nuanced theorizing around the body, sensorium and locomotion (Micale 2000, McNally 2003, Kolk 1994, Ogden et al. 2007). While I do agree with this claim, let us tease out her main argument because it helps us to get a better grip on the problem of memory.

The mimetic position constructs the trauma victim as suffering from a severe imitation of the other leading to an immersion so profound as to collapse any distinction between the traumatized victim and the aggressor. This psychic experience shatters the cognitive-perceptual capacities of the victim and, in consequence, makes the traumatic event inaccessible to recollection. The traumatized is like the hypnotized, being so swept up by the spell of the hypnotist's orchestration of tricks as to blindly imitate them in the form of a compulsive repetition or acting out. Amnesia, the seal of a traumatic shock, is thus analogous to a post-hypnotic forgetting. Given the premise of uncontrollable identification and merging with others, doubts about the credibility of the testimony always linger under the surface of the mimetic model. This raises the question of the sufferer's susceptibility to hypnotic suggestions from the therapist and even to the suspicion of a fabrication of false memories. The victims' inability to sever the unconscious obsession with the aggressors makes them somewhat complicit in the violence directed against them.

The 'anti-mimetic' model also concerns imitation but understands what is involved starkly differently. Here the victims are portrayed as yielding imitatively to the enemy but still quite capable of retaining a strict distinction between the boundaries of ego and those of the aggressor or external event. The victim remains a spectator, who can see and represent to herself what is happening. Whatever the damage done to the psychical integrity of the victim, recovery is possible, although the process of healing may be long and arduous. The anti-mimetic model is compatible with, and often gives way to, the idea that trauma is a purely external event that befalls the passive subject and thus uncontaminated by any dimension of fiction or fantasy.

Focusing on the fluctuation between these two extreme positions, Ruth Leys tells a fascinating story of a gradual shift in trauma studies away from psychodynamic theories that emphasized the subject's uncontrollable mimetic identification with the aggressor toward anti-psychoanalytic understandings of purely external stressors and traumatic images as the causes of trauma. The question of survivors' guilt in the advent of Holocaust was what tipped the pendulum in favor of the 'anti-mimetic' version.

Victims of the Nazi camps reported feeling guilty for having survived when so many others died, a confession that resulted in the coining of the so-called 'survivor syndrome' by post-war psychoanalysts. The whole notion of guilt hinges on the subject's unconscious identification with the other and is incomprehensible without a psychoanalytic understanding of subjectivity. But in the heated climate of the post-war era many psychiatrists and philosophers interpreted guilt more literally and in a pre-Freudian manner. Critics felt it was morally preposterous to claim that the survivors were somewhat complicit in their own abuse, being scapegoated and accused of colluding with power. In place of survivors' guilt, critics, such as Terrence Des Pres (1976), emphasized the role played in the victim's survival by social bonding, mutual care, and outright resistance. If identification did take place in the camps, the critics contained, the imitation did not take the form of an unconscious identification with the perpetrators, but of a conscious and strategic mimicry undertaken by prisoners and those in the resistance to secure positions of influence in the camps and to assist other prisoners. Lost in the moral equation was the subtler psychoanalytic insight that we may all desire things in our unconscious that we would find morally disgusting in our waking lives, but fantasizing does not necessarily make us complicit with evil. However, the dispute reminds us about a larger point, namely, the recurrent tension between explanations of trauma based in the self as opposed to the social.

In the neuroscientific model of trauma that during the last decade has taken the lead, however, sociality was of little concern. Also made irrelevant was much of the psychic structure built by psychoanalysis, such as the tense relationship between the conscious and unconscious strata of the mind, and the ways in which remembering and forgetting straddled both these strata. For no longer was trauma believed to be lodged in the mind but rather in the more primitive parts of the brain, and thus etched into flesh. For the non-cognitive model assumes that the traumatic flashback or memory is a literal reproduction of the entire event imprinted on the brain, thus belonging to a system of traumatic memory different from that of ordinary memory. As such it is cut off or dissociated from ordinary recollection, symbolization, and meaning. Brain research explains this splitting of the circuits of memory by claiming that the emotion of an event is stored separately (in the amygdala) from the recollection of the event itself (in the hippocampus). Moreover, traumatic memories are physiologically different from the regular memories, which are supported more by the sensorium. A traumatic experience, in contrast, is escorted by a surge of adrenal stress hormones that actually increases the strength of the memory. Thus, each time the event is recalled, a renewed rush of epinephrine and cortisol reinforces the event's emotional impact and its ease of recall. In other words, each time you remember something awful, the memory and its associated distress are strengthened. The trauma is re-created and enhanced with every recollection. If these studies are to be believed, confronting or working through disturbing, repressed memories, or post-traumatic stress, would continually reinforce the damage, while not thinking about it actually weakens the unbearable memory. This position is of course antithetical to the presumed catharsis effects inherent in the talking cure proffered by traditional psychoanalysis.

Whatever the case, let us tease out the major points in the twentieth century's controversy about personal memory. The 'mimetic' stance considers memory as inherently unreliably subject to physical and cultural influences, a claim refuted by the 'anti-mimetic' stance which rather regards memory as infallibly impressed in the library of our brains. The cognitive and psychodynamic schools continue to claim that recollection is reconstructive, a dynamic mixture of recorded past experience continually reassembled according to past events and present information, and conventionalized to make sense of current cultural and personal contexts. The neuroscientist of the purist brand, in contrast, insists that memory is authentic, a perfectly preserved neuronal record of every experience retained in the brain. The debate between recovered and false memory recycles the same old argument: either we remember everything accurately and it can be retrieved, or our so-called memories are highly malleable and we are inclined to remember according to our own and others' expectations.

Paradoxically this standstill among trauma specialists in the clinics and laboratories has greatly revitalized the seminar rooms of the Humanities, conveniently located outside the orbit of trauma victims and thus uncontaminated by the messy lives of real patients. The conundrum of whether or not memory can conjure traces of the violent impact has given rise to a whole 'Trauma Theory'—in capital letters, initiated during the 1990s by the works of Shoshana Felman, Cathy Caruth, and Dori Laub. Until this moment, the Freudian idea of the unconscious had animated the theorizing in art, literature, and film studies, providing a rich source for interpreting the symbolic nature of sculptures, paint, texts, and movies. For not only was the aesthetic a domain shot through with suppressed desires, fantasies, and traces seeping up from the depth of imagination but also being the very stuff from which the sublime itself has been spun. Whether the taste was in structuralism or post-structuralism, the unconscious is porous and could be pushed in both directions. Apparently not any longer for 'trauma theory' sought to substitute the bedrock of psychoanalysis with insights from neuroscience and a gesture toward exteriority at the expense of interiority.

Most dramatically, memory severed its ties with unresolved conflict and repression and became a mere reflection of brain functioning also in its humanist guise. This flattened the constitution of the subject into a simple division between a conscious mind normally capable of processing experience and, in traumatized selves, a dissociated and pathological section of the mind from which shocking past experiences cannot be accessed. Thus, in sharp contrast to theories founded on the subject constituted by desire, and that insist on the conventional, mediated, illusory, deferred, or imaginary status of the relation between any representation and the 'real', trauma theory claims that there is an absence of such traces turning the phenomenon of trauma into 'an event without a witness' as Felman and Laub elucidate in *Testimony: Crises of Witnessing in Literature, Psychoanalysis and History* (1992). The victim can simply not bear witness, argues Caruth in *Unclaimed Experience: Trauma, Narrative and History* (1996), due to the incomprehensible nature of the violent event which is dissociated.

While thus being a subject constituted by *forgetting*, the trauma victim can come to acknowledge that there are gaps in recollection with the help of a listener. This foregrounds a model of inter-subjectivity built in the space between witness and testifier enabling that which cannot be known to start being witnessed and thus socially processed. As powerfully captured in the book titles, 'trauma theory' shifted the attention in the humanities from the inner lives of subjective minds to the social cooperation between subjects in memory making, and the attention to the wider historical context that produced the traumatic event. Inspired by a close reading of the narratives of Holocaust survivors, the *witness* on the page replaced the victim in the blood as the node of a theorizing that promised not only to elucidate the condition of trauma but also to reform the entire theory of representation (Radstone 2001). It is, explains the film critic Thomas Elsaesser in a special issue of the journal *Screen*, 'not so much a theory of recovered memory as (...) one of *recovered referentiality*' (2001:201, my italics), conjuring the imprint on the brain of the violent event in its actuality, as suggested by some neuroscientists.

This new twist in the problem of representation continues the Freudian tradition of placing trauma at the heart of theorizing, although moving the scenario from the bedroom to the violent street where it became alleviated as the new sublime. The whole question of mediation, however, was put in suspense by trauma theory awaiting the final blow in seminars across the humanities where new additions to theories of signification will soon rip apart any notion of *representation*, as we shall now scrutinize.

From Guilt to Shame: The Affective Turn

In her recent book *From Guilt to Shame: Auschwitz and After*, Ruth Leys argues that the very rejection of survivor guilt has given rise gives rise to a culture wide preoccupation with shame as 'a dominant emotional reference in the West' (2007:4). She portrays this shift 'from guilt to shame' in alarmist terms as a shift 'away from questions of human agency' (150), leading to 'an impulse to displace questions about our moral responsibility for what we do in favor of more ethically neutral or different questions about our personal attributes'. For those who are less familiar with the theoretical 'war on trauma' it might seem rather surprising that these two negative emotions intrinsic to all human experience, notably guilt and shame, are powerful enough in their supposed difference as to stand in as part-for-whole relations to fiercely opposing philosophical schools of thought not only about the source of feelings but the very heart of subjectivity itself. We already have gotten the inkling that guilt plays an important role in psychoanalysis and helps form the bond with the other—as when someone drawn into the maelstrom of anxiety momentarily identifying with the powerful simply because of a secret wish to be moved out of a place of abject powerlessness. In other words, *guilt* emerges in a relationship of *similarity* to another and concerns your reflection on an action, either real or imagined, but what about shame? *Shame*, in contrast, surfaces as an awareness of your *differentness* from others, as a question not of action but of *identity* and personal experience unique to the self. And although shame is usually considered a negative experience, it is also understood to be a more positive emotion than guilt because it holds out the possibility of change; shame carries a potential, it is *anti-mimetic*. In an interview, Ruth Leys explains the difference as follows:

> Whereas the actual or fantasized acts that produce guilty feelings in principle can't be undone, feelings of shame that may be felt as highly negative nevertheless concern aspects of selfhood that are imagined to be amenable to change or correction. I may be ashamed of my identity as 'queer' but I can also learn to take 'pride' in it, or I can decide to change whatever aspect of my identity embarrasses me (2011).

The evocation of the 'queer' identity is not co-incidental since the 'shame' read as *affect* is central in queer theory as formulated by the literary critique Eve Kosofsky Sedgwick (2003) in opposition to the psychoanalytic account of the formation of the subject in language with its rather limited cast of gendered positions as either 'man' or 'woman'. Queer theory as cultural critique has thus found a rather strange bedfellow in neuroscience and anti-cognitive positions on trauma dynamics precisely because they help to move the circuits of feeling down below the cognitive mind to the primitive brain and, thus, into sheer embodiment. Many prominent philosophers and literary scholars like Sedgwick, Giorgio Agamben, Gilles Delueze, and such like are turning their backs on psychoanalytic accounts of feeling and emotions in favor of the evolutionary approach associated with neuroscience. In the scientific paradigm of brain research, like the work of Silvan Tomkins and Demos (1995), affects are discrete, genetically hard-wired programs in the brain that are triggered by a tripwire for an inbuilt physiological-behavioral response that can be discharged in a self-rewarding or self-punishing manner independent of any object whatsoever. In other words, cultural theory and neuroscience share the belief that affects are fundamentally independent of intention and meaning because they are material processes of the body. In short, what they share is a commitment to the idea that there is a radical separation between the affect system, on the one hand, and intention or meaning or cognition, on the other.

Affect is a matter of automatic responses that are held to occur below the threshold of consciousness and cognition and to be rooted entirely in the body. They share a commitment to the idea that there is a 'gap' between the subject's affects and his or her appraisal of the affective situation, such that cognition or thinking comes 'too late' for intention, belief, or meaning to play the role in action and behavior that is usually accorded to them. Material-corporeal-affective programs or dispositions that are independent of the mind determine action and behavior. Such an imprint in flesh is the main tenet in anti-mimetic trauma theories. Moreover, the delayed response has empirically been detected in the laboratories where experimental trials have been conducted on individuals wired to brain scans. To really appreciate why this tiny 'gap' in time between stimulus and response has recently become so attractive to theorists of a post-structural bend, we need to recall the theory of Derrida.

Derrida was dissatisfied with Lacan's phallus imaginary explained earlier because it comes too close to the notion of the fixed sign—the master word—which is always present to itself and which deconstruction wished to expel. To ensure the truly open-ended play of signifiers, Derrida introduces the concept of *différance* (1981). In this concept, meaning is still produced through difference, but this meaning is not fixed, but moves instead in an endless process of deferral that stretches toward empty horizons. The effect of representation may temporarily arrest meaning, but the meaning becomes redefined when it is reinscribed in another discursive context.

Since it is impossible to write completely outside a representational system in order to communicate, Derrida reverts to the corporal domain to flesh out his model. Indeed, he too takes the interior of the female body as the point of departure for the pure play of signifiers. For Derrida speaks from the position of the *hymen*, which in French signifies both the vaginal membrane and marriage. At the same time, therefore, hymen means both virginity and consummation, both purity and impurity, inside and outside, self and other. The meaning—a singular and stable meaning—is simply impossible to fix. Hymen both joins opposites and keeps them apart. What is important is the in-between-ness the way it sows confusion. In Timothy Yates' words: 'The rule of the hymen takes over from the functions of the phallus, complicates them by becoming that into which semen is spilt, and which can advance only in the plural' (1991:236).

With this bodily metaphor Derrida wishes to remind us that while semen comes in millions only one manages to fertilize the egg, if any at all. Semantics and semen are inter-linked by Derrida, His version of textuality and meaning-making invokes a sowing that does not fertilize, of seed spilled in vain. In Spivak's words—'an emission that cannot return to the origin in the father' (Spivak 1976, cited in Yates, ibid.). The effect for Derrida is to install man within woman and to see the sexes as versions of an 'archi-woman'. The imaginary female body only functions as an object—a container—the territory in which the war of signifiers is waged. Like Lacan, Derrida reverts to biology and myth, reinstating sexual difference as nature, as origin of the symbolic. Thus, the body—whether masculine or feminine—is as much imbricated in the matrices of power in the post-structural theory of Derrida. The way Derrida takes the hymen as figure for the text, the undecidability of meaning in any reading or writing, is an example of what Teresa de Lauretis calls the 'violence of rhetoric' (1987:175)

Whatever the case, with the help of the more neutral discourse of neuroscience affect theory has helped to parch down the free play of signifiers beyond any entrapments in flesh to an 'ontological' concern with people's corporeal-affective experiences as they ripple through various forms of 'assemblages' and 'rhizomes' in the post-human terms of Deleuze and

Guattari in their seminal publications with such telling titles as *Anti-Oedipus* (1972) and *A Thousand Plateaus: Capitalism and Schizophrenia* (1980).

The historian Ruth Leys shares with the anthropologist Emily Martin (2013) serious concern with the affective turn in social theory because it comes with a disinterest in the cognitive content. Affect theory erases the subjective intention, meaning, and memorialization of experiences whether these are acts of terror, turbulent events, articles, debates, films, or any other representations. Rather affect scholars turn their attention to the emotional effect on the body of the spectator or victim, regardless of their cultural signification. The whole point of the general turn to affect among recent cultural critics is to shift focus from the level of political debate or ideology to the level of the person's subliminal or sub-personal material-affective responses, where, it is held, political influences do their real work. For Ruth Leys (2011) this turn away from the insights of psychoanalysis and human subjectivity and intentionality to a post-human world is ethically problematic; for Emily Martin it is also ethnographically problematic, simply because affective theory tends to produce very 'thin' descriptions.

According to Martin, in the humanities affect theory is employed to align phenomena that are simply not commensurable; one cannot explain social relationships, places, practices, and institutions that have an independent material existence in time and space by means of brain scans. This is a fallacy of conflating divergent scales but also of not realizing that the emotional apparatus of selves is constrained by the social. Affect theory's trust in the trait of potentiality seems so desirable precisely because it implies creativity, openness, and infinite possibility unconstrained by social conventions. As a more robust replacement for this rather impossible and imaginary potentiality, Emily Martin ends her essay by suggesting that in the ethnographic method lies another kind of potentiality: notably 'to examine the ontological position that comparison between two social worlds opens up. One key to what is unique about the ethnographic move is that it allows us to see an ordinary, everyday, natural setting in its context but from a certain point of view' (2013:152).

For ethnography shares with psychoanalytical accounts that focus on meaning and intentionality, a need to provide thick descriptions of life experiences in more or less naturalistic settings, an exercise which is both time-consuming, energetic, and requires empathy and social skills. Affect assessments can be accomplished either in the laboratory by reading brain scans as those tested are presented with images and other stimuli or by sitting at your desk in the philosophy department with the occasional walkabout to feeling the pulse of cities. If not combined with other approaches to the self, the social, memory, imagination, and trauma, the turn to affect obviates the need to worry about collecting detailed reports from the subject as to what she or he is actually feeling, the effects on sociality, and social memory.

Mimesis, Violence, and Liminality

In my introductory essay in *Violence and Belonging* (2005), I reflected on the formative power of violence as a transitional experience in biographies, communities, and cosmologies, arguing that classical theories about taboos, rites of passage, and sacrifice are closer to psychoanalytic approaches to subject formation than has commonly been accredited. Let me pick up the thread here and explore what purchase liminal experiences can have on the analysis of trauma.

Physical violence figures prominently in several transformative occasions that some anthropologists label merely 'symbolic'. It is inflicted on the subjects' bodies in intimate, tangible, and often, extremely painful ways. Specific agents are ritually authorized and empowered by the social collective to perform the transformation visually and viscerally in human flesh. The technologies of violence employed range from etching wounds and tattoos on the skin of the initiands, or cutting and reshaping their genitals. In the comparative annals of initiation customs, there is a long list of such ordeals that novices are required to tolerate while in the liminal phase. They are deprived of food, sleep, and company; they are forced to do strenuous tasks or endure uncomfortable body postures; they are often humiliated and alarmed. While the severity of suffering inflicted on the subjects of ritual initiation varies greatly, the violent form it takes almost everywhere is clearly significant for shaping the experience of those subjected to it and spectators alike. For out of the bodily pain and torments endured during the liminal phase, the novice is reborn at the end of the ritual a different person, formed by the ritual experience and equipped with a new status, knowledge, and roles. Rites of passage—birth, initiation, marriage, and death—are occasions on which the biography of individuals is woven into that of the community. Rites of passage are thus occasions where people 'perform operations on their identities' to paraphrase Marylyn Strathern (1988). Rites of passage are an expression of the community's desire to put everybody and everything in place. They work on the novice's deep-seated desire to reach a new, perhaps more empowered, status; they are thus about positioning and repositioning and the urge to situate oneself within the social whole.

In transitional rituals the wound on the skin produces a wound in the soul—but rather than causing traumatic dissociation, the pain endured powerfully *enacts the new subject into being*. From this we can draw a simple but significant point also for this volume: severe pain obviously affects the subject, but not all pain and suffering are traumatic, however severe. I believe that in order to keep its analytical force, the concept of trauma therefore has to be clearly delineated. Trauma, I shall argue, is brought into being when the bond between the self and the social is severed, when there is no *culturally acceptable framework of meaning* that can make sense of terrifying experiences.

As a complicating starting point, there is simply no fixed definition of unspeakable acts universally applicable. The case stories contained within the ethnographic annals of anthropology clearly attest to a cultural relativism in what is deemed abhorrent and acceptable. For example, while the headhunting practiced until quite recently among some Melanesian tribes was said to generate a sort of euphoria in both the perpetrator and the community (Rosaldo 2000), it generates horror and disgust when images of these same acts of violence are broadcast from the killing fields of the Middle East. Despite such plasticity in cultural values, what clearly *is* a universal human condition is the deep drive and desire to belong, to be part of an *inter-subjective* collective where different selves are molded together through act, flesh, affect, feeling, and words; making it possible to mirror and model one another in a shared flow of experiences and meaning. When the incorporated topology of the social world cracks open, the self is lost in a maelstrom of confusion, terror, and incomprehension as it is thrown into the chaos of trauma. Traumatic violence does not create meaning, it shatters it.

The importance of the social in the creation of the self is integral to the classical theory of Arnold Van Gennep (1909), *Rites de Passage*, which, he pointed out, typically has a tripartite structure: a phase of separation, followed by a phase of muddled liminality, and finally a phase of reincorporation. The smooth flow of time is fragmented into a sequence of discrete moments separated from one another by 'gaps' and punctuation marks—so to speak. The middle phase of marginality—the Latin *limen* meaning a 'threshold' or boundary—is a sort of fertile chaos of both becoming and loss thus full of ambiguity, fluidity, and uncertainty. What Victor Turner (1995) called 'dominant symbols', which are highly evocative, emotional, multi-vocal, multi-layered and condensed, typically control this 'betwixt and between' stage and, aligned with scripts of ceremonial performance, combine to effect ritual transformation. Thus the ideological and sensory power of these dramatic symbols forces the self, with encouragement of the spectators, to move on to the next stage in the sequence, eventually leading to social integration and renewed stability for both subject and collective.

But what if that anxiety of the *limen* leaves the marginalized subject dangling in chaos and turns the liminal into a condition of being, even stigma, rather than becoming? What if the liminal is trapped between different sets of role expectations, different forms of sociality, and different social orders? What if the liminal is neither traditional nor tightly scripted but a permanent flux of conflicting expectation and values where uncertainty prevails and perpetual instability is the order of the day? What if the liminal becomes the real borderline between life and death? By entertaining these out of sync conditions we can see the contours of the liminal as trauma; as haunting experiences that cannot be culturally incorporated, but remain unspeakable and inchoate in the deeper layers of the mindful body as dissociated states and somatic ailments.

Let me briefly sketch out an ethnographic scenario from Northern Kenya consisting of endemic violence between ethnic groups but where the dynamics of overlapping warscapes of regional scale and military complexity have created new configurations of pain and trauma in victims and perpetrators alike. In order to appreciate why violent acts can produce very different emotional effects in those subjected to them, we need to resist the urge to treat violence as an essence but rather examine carefully the contexts for its application. Violent action must be understood as a set of cultural practices and forms whose meanings can only be made sense of through an understanding of the wider political and economic context of the society within which violence appears, evolves, and achieves its effects (Broch-Due 2005).

Cattle raiding among pastoralists in the region are endemic and violent, often leading to death and destruction. However, it occurs within very different frames of meaning and registers of emotion. Traditionally it rested on a notion of generative violence that carries in its heart a *positive valuation* of the 'other', the foreign cattle, wives, and children that were the traditional targets for organized raiding among Nilotic warriors. These captives were typically incorporated into the family and clan of the captors, embodying a generative vitality that nourished the conquering community. Calves and children are not only the reproductive locus of pastoralists' communities, but the foundation for wealth production: economic, political, and social. Working capital here is embodied more than monetary. Among the elderly segment of my interviewees I was surprised to find how common it was to have been born into one ethnic group, fostered in another, and later married into a yet different group. The practice of exogamy clearly aided this remarkable fluidity of ethnic identities in individual biographies, but it was not reproduced in younger segments of the population despite the continuation of inter-marriage between certain ethnicities, such as Turkana and Samburu. One obvious reason for the decline in child and bride capture is the presence of the state, but it also reflects a dramatic change in patterns of violence during recent decades, a pattern in which people are simply killed during raids rather than captured.

Taking life certainly happened back in the 1980s, particularly between male enemies. Killers would etch tattoos deep into their skin as a permanent mark of their fame and bravery. However, it was very inauspicious to kill women and children and in the rare cases where this happened, huge compensation payments of cattle had to be paid. Anybody who had taken another's life in combat had to go through a lengthy purification ritual in which the perpetrator had to spend a liminal period in solitary confinement outside the camp. He would be wearing strips of white skin reflecting his deeds, had dietary restrictions, and had to perform other uncomfortable cleansing acts before he was finally allowed back into the community through a rite of reincorporation in which his mother would demarcate a path by throwing water on the ground which 'led' him back into her house, where she would feed him milk from her decorated leather container. This is only a summary description of a very rich and textured ritual—spatially, temporally, and symbolically (Broch-Due 1990). The main point is that its evocative force is precisely that the distress, discomfort, and pain involved in the liminal phase led the killer into a new subject position with an acute awareness of Turkana visions of life and death. In these cases killing did not produce trauma because the experience could be culturally incorporated.

Today, these values linked to regenerative violence are breaking down and gradually being replaced by a more destructive violence based in a *negative valuation* of 'the other', which in the most extreme form is characteristic of the warfare orchestrated by modern states and other militarized agencies whose violence is merely instrumental (Hutchinson 1996).

During the last two decades, ethnic boundaries have solidified, finishing a process that started during the colonial era when the British sought to get rid of pastoralists' nomadic fluidity by fixing them in 'tribes' and 'territories' that could be demarcated and controlled. Political and economic forces beyond the unruly pastoralist belt of Northern Kenya are driving this 'purification' of ethnic identity. The savannah, once seen as relatively worthless brush hinterland, has, in the age of safari tourism, become extraordinarily valuable; even more so as new commercial niches are opened up by eco-friendly, high-market operations. These are often tied up with private conservancies, many of them based on converted settler ranches run by white Kenyans, with funding from global consortia. As the savannahs are swallowed by tourist enterprises, pastoralists are being squeezed together on ever-shrinking pastureland and forced to fight between themselves for what remains of the commons, further essentializing their identities and territorial boundaries in the process. Since ethnicity has become the deciding factor in granting access to state resources, development revenues, and business possibilities, it has become saturated with the most brutal politics. The extreme violence surrounding land disputes today is due in many instances to tribal militias who, over the years, have turned into a kind of rural mafia, extorting money from villagers, raiding farms and cattle camps, burning houses, and striking deals with local politicians. Minority ethnicities have come under constant threat of eviction and expulsion in areas they traditionally ranged with their livestock but where they are now regarded as 'intruders' and 'foreigners' by the new re-colonizing regimes struggling to 'put everybody in their place' (Broch-Due 2000, 2005).

These chaotic processes produce extreme levels of uncertainty not only about identities and resource flows but also about the very survival of self and community in the face of escalating violence. On the ground this translates into several 'warscapes' (Nordstrom 1997) each with its own distinctive profile of recruitment, operational dynamic, and looting, sometimes overlapping, sometimes colliding. This diversity, where pockets of more traditional devices of meaningful response to violence exist among modern forms of brutalization and militarization, creates a virtual 'field laboratory' for the study of trauma in the form of *cultural disintegration*, currently experienced by many victims and perpetrators. What has become clear through my recent research project is that a new site of traumatic liminality has opened up in the cracks and fault lines between competing value systems and forms of sociality, fracturing these different universes of meaning and practice. It is a contact zone marred by conflict with dynamic akin to what Gregory Bateson once coined 'schismogenesis' (1935).

I want to continue by focusing on the perpetrators of this new violence, usually young men. The gendering is significant because these pastoralist societies are traditionally organized through age-groups and generation systems, which have always been the bedrock of defense and attack. The purification ritual for killers outlined above is a cultural recognition of the ambiguity inscribed in the roles of warriors who protect life by securing a generative potential but also shed blood and destroy life. But now elders can no longer condone the indiscriminate killing that has become the trend even in more localized raiding. A growing number of young people are trapped between the pastoral life worlds of their parents and the small savannah towns where tourists pass through and schools install in them so-called modern values. This opens up new horizons of expectations, which they rarely can satisfy materially, but which motivate many to participate in cattle raids for profit in which killing has become the order of the day. Thus, new cohorts of warriors now being initiated during school holidays, still through spectacular ceremonies, find themselves caught in a 'betwixt and between' state in which their mothers and elders simply refuse to participate in purification rituals for those who have participated in acts of violence where women and children have been slain or mutilated. My interviews among this specific group of men who reluctantly admit to having committed horrendous acts are characterized by incoherent gaps in their narratives and complaints about nightmares, flashbacks, trembling, and even being followed when awake by a terrifying 'twin ghost'—a kind of dark double—all classical symptoms of dissociation and trauma. Many try to drown out these psychosomatic ailments with alcohol and drugs but with only temporary relief.

In sharp contrast, the interviews with yet another group of perpetrators who had completely severed ties with their parents' communities did not show up any traumatic testimonies but voiced rather frank and unfeeling accounts of their destructive acts, often denigrating the victims of their violence. These men had become totally assimilated into town life and a more militarized form of violence. They saw themselves not as warriors, whom they ridiculed as dressed up in 'feather and beads', but as modern soldiers wearing uniform-like clothes, even if most could only afford T-shirts and trainers. They emulated the army, both the national and the British, both of which happen to have their training ground in the area. Many had secured employment in the barracks where they could observe the military in operation, read their manuals and listen to their exploits.

This formative experience in a form of numb and valueless violence has subsequently led to car thefts, hijackings, elephant poaching and other criminal activities that they carry out apparently without any emotional squeamishness. They too were big consumers of drugs and alcohol, which probably played their part in numbing their responses. They showed no psychosomatic signs of trauma and had no problems in talking about their brutal actions.

I have focused here on the changing modalities of masculinity to highlight my point about the social complexity involved even in such peripheral places as Northern Kenya where competing value systems collide, tearing holes in the cultural fabric around core questions of life and death, thereby generating traumatic experience. The significance of cultural dissociation where painful experience simply cannot be integrated within dominant cultural frames is also very evident in the experience of many victims of contemporary violence (Broch-Due 2005).

However, when the liminal is folded back into the tripartite structure of rites of passage—as a *becoming*—it can also be a stage for the healing of traumatic experiences. And it is exactly as performative acts working on the body of the afflicted that the liminal achieves its reconstructive work on broken selves. Turkana ritual dramaturgy literally returns the subject back to an embryonic position during the liminal stage; the novice lays curled together, covered by a cow skin which imitates the membrane of the womb. While nobody can actually remember intrauterine life or early infancy, traces of that floating, fragmentary, and unformed corporeal world remain within our psychic structure and return to haunt the subject at critical moments. Under the supervision of a ritual expert (always a maternal clan woman), the novice has to reenact birthing, crawling, standing up, and walking, accompanied by being fed the appropriate food for each stage, until the grand finale is reached when the subject has to gaze down into a special leather container with liquid butter which both in name and meaning signifies wisdom. By crossing this threshold the novice is enacted into a new subject position where the fragmented bits are put together in a new mature form, as it were (Broch-Due 1990).

Anthropological theories of the liminal provide a crucial model which not only is more sensitive to the diverse ethnographic spectrum of trauma scenarios and their histories but might also be able to bridge psychoanalysis and neuroscience, ending the schism between 'mimetic' and 'anti-mimetic' approaches.

Some Final Reflections

My own journey into the landscape of trauma theory and the problems of memory, imagination, subjectivity, and emotion it touches upon, I must admit, has left me with a feeling of being trapped in a sort of scholarly warscape in which one is forced to camp with one army or the other, no fraternizing with the enemy allowed. In this chapter I have tried to trace some of the discursive shifts in the controversies that have gone on historically around the notion of trauma in Western analytical traditions. The condition of trauma has been shunted from discourse to discourse in various attempts to defuse its explosive potential. It has been re-described in terms that relate it to 'natural' conditions, 'cultural' conditions, 'pathological' conditions, 'mental' conditions, and many others. The impetus for each discursive shift comes from historically specific struggles over the interpretation of the concept of trauma in its previous discursive site. As a result of such struggles of trauma's relations to mind and body, to silence and speech, to memory and forgetting, to self and sociality, trauma is now moved on to a new site where it has inscribed itself in a vocabulary of affect and the 'post-human' where it has already become the focus of new interpretative struggles. My own addition to this extensive list is the 'liminal'.

Behind all the shifts in definitions and interventions we can see the contours of something that seems to be at the core of all trauma discourses, a constant feature behind the endlessly transforming face of trauma: it brings a whole emotional and moral universe into play. The apparently unavoidable moral overtones of trauma are typically mobilized in situations where the whole notion of sociality, personally and politically, is being encouraged, challenged, negotiated, or negated. At the core of these situations are primary questions of power, subjectivity, and remembrance. Ideas of origin, gender, and race, both as social relations and as symbolic resource, are heavily implicated in any configuration of trauma, violence, memory, and personhood. Its genealogy reveals poignantly the ways in which very fundamental ethical questions are formulated in and through the discourse and treatment of trauma. In sum, we need to attend not only to wounds to the skin and the soul but also to the forms of sociality that produce them, and, finally, to the signifying system through which we represent and understand these wounds and sufferings.

References

Anderson, B. 1983. *Imagined Communities: Reflections on the Origin and Spread of Nationalism*. London: Verso.

Bateson, G. 1935. Culture Contact and Schismogenesis. *Man* 35: 178–183.

Broch-Due, V. 1990. The Bodies Within the Body: Journeys in Turkana Thought and Practice. Dr. Philos. Dissertation, University of Bergen, Norway.

———. 2005. *Violence and Belonging: The Quest for Identity in Post Colonial Africa*. London: Routledge.

Caruth, C. 1996. *Unclaimed Experience: Trauma, Narrative and History*. Baltimore, MD: Johns Hopkins University Press.

Decker, H.S. 1991. *Dora, Freud, and Vienna 1900*. New York: The Free Press.

Deleuze, G., and Guattari, F. 1972 (2004). *Anti-Oedipus*. London and New York: Continuum.

———. 1980. *A Thousand Plateaus*. Minneapolis: University of Minnesota Press.

Derrida, J. 1981. *Dissemination*. Chicago, IL: The University of Chicago Press.

Des Pres, T. 1976. *The Survivor: An Anatomy of Life in the Death Camps*. Oxford: Oxford University Press.

Fassin, D., and R. Rechtman. 2009. *The Empire of Trauma: An Inquiry into the Condition of Victimhood*. Princeton, NJ: Princeton University Press.

Faust, D.G. 2008. *This Republic of Suffering: Death and the American Civil War*. New York: Knops.

Felman, S., and D. Laub. 1992. *Testimony: Crises of Witnessing in Literature, Psychoanalysis and History*. New York: Routledge.

Foucault, M. 1977. Nietzsche, Genealogy, History. In *Language, Counter-Memory, Practice: Selected Essays and Interviews*, ed. D.F. Bouchard. Ithaca, NY: Cornell University Press.

———. 1980. *Power/Knowledge: Selected Interviews and Other Writings, 1972–1977*. London: The Harvester Press.

Freud, S. 1953–1974. *The Standard Edition of the Complete Psychological Works of Sigmund Freud*. Vols. II, VII. London: Hogarth Press and the Institute of Psycho-Analysis.

Geertz, G. 1973. Thick Description: Toward an Interpretive Theory of Culture. In *The Interpretation of Cultures: Selected Essays*. New York: Basic Books.

Hacking, I. 1995. *Rewriting the Soul: Multiple Personality and the Sciences of Memory*. Princeton, NJ: Princeton University Press.

Halbwachs, M. 1992. *On Collective Memory*. Chicago: University of Chicago Press.

Harvey, D. 1969. *Explanation in Geography*. London/New York: Edward Arnold/St. Martin's Press.

Hustvedt, S. 2012. *Living, Thinking, Looking*. London: Sceptre.

Hutchinson, S. 1996. *Nuer Dilemmas: Coping with Money, War, and the State.* Berkeley: University of California Press.
Kolk, B. van der. 1994. The Body Keeps the Score: Memory & the Evolving Psychobiology of Post Traumatic Stress. *Harvard Review of Psychiatry* 5: 253–265.
Lacan, J. 1977. *Écrits: A Selection.* Trans. A. Sheridan. New York: W.W. Norton.
Laplanche, J., and J.-B. Pontalis. 1973. *The Language of Psychoanalysis.* London: The Hogarth Press.
Laqueur, T. 2008. Among the Graves. *London Reviews of Books* 30(24): 18.
——— 2010. We Are All Victims Now. *London Reviews of Books* 32(13): 19–23.
de Lauretis, T. 1987. *Technologies of Gender. Essays on Theory, Film, and Fiction.* Bloomington: Indiana University Press.
Leys, R. 2000. *Trauma: A Genealogy.* Chicago, IL: University of Chicago Press.
———. 2007. *From Guilt to Shame: Auschwitz and After.* Princeton, NJ: Princeton University Press.
———. 2011. The Turn to Affect: A Critique. *Critical Inquiry* 37(3): 434–472.
Margalit, A. 2004. *The Ethics of Memory.* Cambridge: Harvard University Press.
Martin, E. 2013. The Potentiality of Ethnography and the Limits of Affect Theory. *Current Anthropology* 54(S7): 149–158.
McNally, R.J. 2003. *Remembering Trauma.* Cambridge, MA: Belknap/Harvard University Press.
Micale, M. S. 2000. We Cannot Stress Enough. *Times Literary Supplement*, 27 October.
Nordstrom, C. 1997. *A Different Kind of War Story.* Philadelphia: University of Pennsylvania Press.
O'Gorman, F. 2012. Modernism, T.S. Eliot, and the 'age of worry'. *Textual Practice* 26(6): 1001–1019.
Ogden, P., et al., eds. 2007. *Trauma and the Body: A Sensorimotor Approach to Psychotherapy*, Norton Series on Interpersonal Neurobiology. New York: W.W Norton.
Radstone, S. 2001 (ed.), 'Special Debate: Trauma and Screen Studies', *Screen* 42:2 (Summer) 188–216.
Rosaldo, R. 2000. Of Headhunters and Soldiers: Separating Cultural and Ethical Relativism. *Issues in Ethics*, 11(1). The Markkula Center for Applied Ethics.
Schor, N. 1987. *Reading in Detail: Aesthetics and the Feminine.* New York: Methuen.
Sedgwick, E.K. 2003. Shame, Theatricality, Queer Performativity: Henry James's The Art of the Novel. In *Touching Feeling: Affect, Pedagogy, Performativity*, Series Q. Durham, NC: Duke University Press.
Showalter, E. 1998. *Hystories: Hysterical Epidemics and Modern Culture.* New York: Colombia University Press.

Spivak, G. 1976. *Of Grammatology (translation, with a critical introduction, of Derrida's text)*. Baltimore, MD: Johns Hopkins University Press.
Strathern, M. 1988. *The Gender of the Gift. Problems with Women and Problems with Society in Melanesia*. Berkeley: University of California Press.
Tomkins, S., and V. Demos. 1995. *Exploring Affect: The Selected Writings of Silvan S Tomkins*. Cambridge: Cambridge University Press.
Turner, V. 1995. *The Ritual Process: Structure and Anti-structure*. New York: Aldine de Gruyter.
Van Gennep, A. 1960 [1909]. *The Rites of Passage*. London: Routledge and Kegan.
Yates, T. 1991. Jacques Derrida: There is Nothing Outside the Text. In *Reading Material Culture: Structuralism, Hermeneutics and Post-Structuralism*, ed. C. Tilley. London: Routledge.

CHAPTER 3

Universalizing Trauma Descendant Legacies: A Comparative Study of Jewish-Israeli and Cambodian Genocide Descendant Legacies

Carol A. Kidron

According to critical scholarship (Fassin 2009; Pupavac 2006), international agents of memory, be they mental health practitioners, international NGO workers, or genocide scholars, have globally disseminated a Euro-Western model of trauma-related victimhood (Young 1995). In order to explore the potential tension between the universal semiotics of genocide suffering and divergent particular genocide legacies, an ethnographic comparative study of the lived experience of familial genocide legacies of Israeli Holocaust descendants and Cambodian genocide descendants is presented. It will be asserted that culturally specific Jewish-Israeli and Buddhist Cambodian paradigms and practices of memory deviate from the globally disseminated reductionist profile of the pathologized and enlisted trauma descendant and therefore problematize therapeutic and socio-political interventionist practices that 'treat' genocide legacies as universal.

C.A. Kidron (✉)
Department of Anthropology, University of Haifa, Haifa, Israel

V. Broch-Due, B.E. Bertelsen (eds.), *Violent Reverberations*,
DOI 10.1007/978-3-319-39049-9_3

Trauma Theory and the Emergence of Universal Axioms of Suffering

According to psychological research, trauma survivors may suffer from a multitude of emotional and behavioral symptoms diagnosed as post-traumatic stress disorder (PTSD) (DSM IV 1994). In studies of Holocaust victims, the disorder was found to impair survivor/veteran parenting, whereby the effects of PTSD may potentially be transmitted to their children (Barocas and Barocas 1973). Although non-clinical findings have failed to show evidence of psychopathology, both clinical and non-clinical studies have found that descendants of Holocaust victims and Vietnam veterans may suffer from maladaptive behavioral patterns and a damaged sense of self (Sagi-Schwartz et al. 2003; Zilberfein 1995). According to the logic of the PTSD paradigm, if left untreated, the long-term psychosocial effects of survivor and/or shell shock trauma could be transmitted from generation to generation. A familial 'wall of silence' is said to often shroud the history of parental suffering in oppressive silence. The metaphor of the 'wall of silence' signifies the absence and erasure of the genocidal past (Bar-On 1992). At once pathologizing and eliding the possibility of the lived experience of silently inscribed and embodied forms of presence of the past, the majority of scholars of memory, mental health practitioners and humanitarian workers worldwide have encouraged trauma survivors and their descendants to give voice to their repressed and silenced past of personal suffering and/or familial maladaptive relations (Kidron 2009). Talk therapy in therapeutic settings and public forms of testimony and commemoration aim to liberate the silenced past, put forth as not only individually healing but also socio-politically redemptive for the collective (Herman 1992; Leys 2000).

Intergenerational Transmission of the Burden of Memory

According to the Holocaust scholarship, as Holocaust survivors are thought to repress their traumatic pasts and often resist testimonial voice, descendants have taken it upon themselves to work through the silenced past and act as surrogates for their parents, testifying to their own childhood memories in the shadow of genocidal suffering or to their recollections of fragmentary accounts of genocide suffering (Danieli 1998). The scholarship has traced the descendants' transition from silence to voice in Israel and around the world, documenting multiple forms of representation ranging from political activism challenging the silencing of survivors in national hegemonic narratives, therapeutic practices, heritage tourism, the documentation of the parental tale or artistic representation of the traumatic past (Feldman 2008; Kidron 2010b). As in the case of the descendant's psychosocial profile, the scholarship rarely questions core scholarly axioms, namely, that descendants wish to seek out the survivor tale and undertake public forms of representation and that they would experience commemoration as liberating.

Universalizing the PTSD Construct

The above axiomatic assumptions pertaining to Holocaust descendants have been globally circulated via trauma brokers, museologists and genocide scholars, ultimately engineering a globalized 'ideal type' genocide descendant profile (Altounian 1999; Ida and Young 2003). Cambodian genocidal trauma has attracted extensive scholarly attention (Kinzie et al. 1984) with research focusing both on first- and second-generation traumatization (Huang 1998; Rousseau et al. 1999; Rubin and Rhodes 2005). These studies conclude that survivors of the Cambodian genocide continue to suffer from PTSD-related emotional scars and somatized bodily distress while their children—be they in Cambodia, or Cambodian-American, Canadian or Australian young adults—have been found to exhibit increased symptomology causally related to their parents' traumatic experience (Stevens 2001). According to Rubin and Rhodes, as witnesses of their parents' traumatic fragmentary narrative re-enactments, descendants mirror parental PTSD and ultimately suffer from their own intrusive memories of parental trauma (Rubin and Rhodes 2005). Although the above studies emerge from totally diverse socio-cultural and national contexts, these studies utilize standardized psychological models and measures focusing solely on interfamily psychosocial dynamics. We may ask, do Cambodian youth perceive themselves as suffering from the scars of transmitted PTSD? Do they wish to work through and articulate the familial past, or does Cambodian culture present alternative meaning systems which differentially make sense of genocide memory and constitute different forms of familial interaction and intergenerational transmission of the past?

Enlisting the Wounded Genocide Witness

Building upon the axioms of trauma theory, yet concerned with the macro processes of the politics of silenced or curtailed collective memory, culture studies and human rights discourse also call for the voicing of silenced narratives of victimization and subjugation (Alexander (2004; Munyas 2008). From this perspective, the narrativization of survivor and descendant legacies facilitates the civic and moral act of public testimony (McKinney 2007). As genocide historians have asserted, pathos-filled and cathartic testimonies at 'truth tribunals' not only document the violent past and contribute to the collective stock of memory but ideally facilitate restitution, reconciliation and coexistence (Kiernan 1996). Scholars of ethnicity and immigrant studies promote the working through of Cambodian Diasporas and public testimony to the genocide past.

Whereas the therapeutic discourse locates descendant genocide legacies as silenced and trapped in the psychic recesses of the traumatized self or in the fractured intergenerational channels of communication in maladaptive family systems, humanitarian regimes position genocide memory as trapped within the politically victimized, subjugated and thereby disempowered and silenced self and family. Both the therapeutic and humanitarian moral economies share in common the foundational grammar of expert intervention in private familial lived experiences of the past and the engineering of public vocal displays of personal and familial narratives of suffering. In this way the individual victim, descendant and family unit are discursively fashioned as perpetually vulnerable and dependent upon collective, national or global forces to enable the liberation of their silent voices in a redemptive public sphere.

However, do descendants wish to access verbal accounts of their legacies and publicly commemorate violent histories or are there other channels of 'remembrance', other forms of silent transmission of the past interwoven in the social milieu of everyday familial life (Halbwachs 1980)? When globally exporting Eurocentric models of traumatic suffering and resistant testimonial voice to victims around the world, to what degree has interventionist discourse and practice taken culture-specific conceptions of suffering, healing and memory work into account (Hayden 2007)? Has Eurocentric psychosocial and politicized memory work weakened the survivor's link to traditional culture-specific and familial forms of healing and remembrance (Rousseau et al. 2001)?

Anthropology's holistic perspective and methodology enable a grounded and culturally sensitive exploration of the descendant's phenomenological experience of trauma-related wellness, illness or resilience and acceptance or resistance to public forms of memory work (Lambek and Antze 1996), allowing descendants to articulate their 'lived experience' of suffering and voice. There have, however, been few attempts to apply this approach to genocide descendant experience. The sub-field of the anthropology of genocide has presented a culture-sensitive portrayal of the impact of trauma and alternative forms of commemoration (Hinton 2004; Argenti and Schramm 2010). Nevertheless, the ethnographic moral/political mission liberating victims from the 'shadows of silence' has often elided the way apolitical everyday taken for granted practices are sustained and transmitted to create the lived presence of the past.

Exploring the 'every day lived presence' of the Holocaust past, I undertook an ethnographic study of Holocaust descendants in Israel entailing 75 interviews with second and third generation descendants and participant observation at multiple meso-public sites of memory. Contrary to the literature (and vocal descendants in Israeli literary circles and popular culture), the majority rejected or critiqued the pathologizing construct of PTSD, although many did feel they were emotionally impacted by the Holocaust past. While asserting that survivors, the third generation and other non-survivors must participate in all important commemorative projects, they themselves expressed little or no desire to participate in collective monumental commemoration as carriers of Holocaust memory. Instead, they presented accounts of (a) the silent non-pathological presence of the past in embodied person-person and person-object interaction in the everyday life of the family and fragmentary tales of survival that transmitted an enriching genocide-related meaning world; (b) they also depicted survivor-specific non-monumental communal practices of Holocaust memory in voluntary meso-public organizations that simulated intimate family silent memory (Kidron 2005, 2010b). The minority who chose to participate in monumental forms of commemoration refer to Jewish paradigms of memory to account for their obligation to act as public carriers of memory and described themselves as suffering from transmitted PTSD.

We might ask do descendants in other cultural/socio-political contexts accept the pathologizing construct? Do they retain alternative culture-specific responses to traumatic suffering, other forms of remembering or forgetting? Have activists successfully recruited descendants to communal or national organizations where they are providing testimony to their own or their parent's past? If not, how may we explain differential legacies and responses that challenge the 'universal semiotics of suffering' (Fassin 2009)?

The Comparative Case Study and Methodology

Building on the above study of Israeli Holocaust descendants, two comparative ethnographic studies of descendant genocidal legacies were undertaken: one of Cambodian-Canadian descendants (2005–2006, 2011) (Kidron 2010a, 2012) and the other of Cambodian descendants living in Cambodia. The present study will compare the findings pertaining to Israeli Holocaust descendants to data accessed in Cambodia in 2013. I conducted 55 interviews with children of Holocaust survivors. Accessing the sample using a snow-ball method, Israeli descendant respondents ranged in age between 35 and 55, with equal gender representation.[1] In-depth interviews were conducted using a semi-structured and thematic format. Interviewees were asked open-ended questions about themselves and their families, allowing them to narrate and present the self as they saw fit. The great majority were born in Israel, to survivor parents who had immigrated to Israel from Europe in the late 1940s and 1950s after surviving Nazi extermination camps, forced labor camps, ghetto incarceration or extended periods of hiding. After an initial period of economic hardship, the majority achieved middle- to upper-middle-class status and the majority of descendants had some form of higher education.

Research in Cambodia in 2010 and 2013 entailed 50 in-depth ethnographic interviews with Cambodian descendants, between the ages of 17 and 33, as well as 20 interviews with Khmer genocide survivors. A good number of these respondents officiated as Khmer Buddhist monks, nuns and funerary priests. Participant observation was also undertaken at national urban and communal sites of commemoration and at Theravada Buddhist 'wats' (temples). Interviews were also undertaken with agents of genocide memory including NGO officials, local genocide scholars and mental health practitioners.

Descendant respondents' parents had survived genocidal conditions of forced migration, forced labor, near starvation and the loss of loved ones. The great majority of the descendants' families are still experiencing extreme economic hardship, many still living in poor urban neighborhoods or the rural countryside, although the descendant generation has benefitted from recent educational and economic opportunities. Approximately 35 percent of the descendants had attended or are attending a vocational school, a community college or university.

The cross-cultural comparative study is challenging as it entails such extremely different socio-eco-political contexts. The Israeli legacy of the Holocaust involves the German Other as perpetrator while vocal national commemoration in the Israeli State is undertaken by a relatively privileged Jewish majority. In contrast, the Cambodian descendant faces the more recent and ambiguous legacy of what has been most problematically termed 'auto-genocide' still very much in the grips of post-genocide recovery.[2] Descendants in Cambodia experience this very different socio-political reality characterized by the scars of French colonialism and feared subjugation by neighboring Vietnam, tense coexistence with Khmer Rouge perpetrators and their descendants, and until recently, collective silence regarding the genocide past (Ledgerwood et al. 1994). Narratives of victimization and truth tribunals are now beginning to provide nationalist glue in this still conflict ridden society. These important contextual differences most certainly alter particular dialectics between divergent contexts and the culturally framed experience of genocidal legacies. Nevertheless, the present study aims to artificially disentangle the 'threads' of context and culture to examine differential experiences of genocidal legacies. It is precisely a close comparative examination of similarity and difference that may allow for the isolation and analysis of factors uniquely constituting particular trauma descendant legacy.

Silent Traces of the Genocide Past: *Jewish-Israeli Descendants*

Holocaust descendant respondents claimed that due to the silence in their homes, they had little to tell me regarding their parents' past. When asked why they did not break the silence, and ask questions, the great majority of descendants explained that they feared opening up old wounds and hurting their parents. Sylvia explains: 'I think I felt I would hurt them, I didn't think they could take going back *there*. But ... to be honest, it was ... also fear of hearing what they would say or how they would say it … I just wanted to leave it alone.' Descendants would then proceed to tell me who had perished in their families and where their parents had spent the war years. However, they could provide only approximate details of the dates or duration of their incarceration/hiding. When asked them about their experience of familial silence, evocative accounts of the fleeting, yet sorely felt, presence of the past emerged. Rachel recounts:

E: I'm sorry, but I think I don't have much to say, I don't know more than just very basic facts about my parents' experience. You know, they were in Auschwitz, they were liberated and made Aliya [emigrated to Israel]. I don't know … they … we never spoke about it at home. You didn't speak about it … at least not then. There was just silence. (long pause) But you know, *it* was there, all the time, everywhere.
C: What was there?
E: The Holocaust … (pause) it was like a dark cloud hanging over everything.
C: Could you tell me what you mean by a dark cloud?
E: It's hard to describe.
C: Could you maybe tell me what it felt like?
E: I guess it's a mood, or … maybe more … it's hard to put into words.

Rachel accounts for her 'ignorance', pointing to the fact that speech, as a medium of the transmission of knowledge, was not utilized. The phenomenon is contextualized, as she explains silence surrounding the Holocaust was previously normative behavior. After pausing, however, she refers enigmatically to a non-verbal form of presence, as she states 'it' or the Holocaust, was 'everywhere', perhaps foreboding, like a 'dark cloud'. Beyond Rachel's use of the metaphor, it was impossible for her to describe 'in words' what a cloud/Holocaust felt like. Also evoking the complex feeling world constituted by traces of the Holocaust past, Chanit too describes the presence of the Holocaust in her home: It's so very hard to say what it felt like …. I guess you might say it was a kind of echo resonating … all the time. An echo is not a static or continuous sound but it rather undulates, heard one moment and gone the next. The echo cannot transmit a clear content of events, or voices from the past, but rather one is left only with the vague impression of what was and is no longer. Paradoxically, despite their inherent movement, both the cloud and the echo remain present in the home 'all the time'.

The metaphoric descriptions above beg a number of questions. How can the Holocaust be 'present' in the home without speech? Something absent must be signified in order to become present. However, without speech and the knowledge speech entails how is the Holocaust past signified? After a number of 'failed' interviews eliciting only references to domestic silence and the absence of historical knowledge, I experienced a breakthrough with one descendant who recalled her own embodied responses to what she termed the 'presence of the Holocaust' every night when her mother cried in her sleep. In response, I changed my opening question from 'What do you know about your parents' past?' to 'Was the past present in your home?' From that point on, I received hours of accounts of the non-verbal and partially verbal traces of Holocaust presence, including parent-child silent face work, person-object interaction and diverse forms of embodied practices of survival forming a silent matrix of genocide presence interwoven within the everyday domestic life world (Kidron 2009).

For example, when asked about the presence of the Holocaust in the survivor home, Emma recounts her nightly practice of preparing for the Nazis:

E: The one aspect of daily life that I can link to the Holocaust was that every night, at a very young age, maybe 6 or 7, I would prepare my shoes, placing them next to my bed, so that if the Nazis came I would have shoes ready. I would also fold my clothes in a way that would be easy to put on.

C: Do you know where you got this habit?

E: I remember placing the shoes in the center of the floor in front of my bed so that if I had to get up and I had to wear the shoes in a hurry I would be able to. Why were shoes so important? My mother apparently told me how she walked in the snow. I remember her saying how cold it was how she almost froze to death. Now I know it was the Death March. Then it didn't matter what it was, just that it was something terrible. Then I just desperately wanted to have shoes handy ... so that I wouldn't have to walk barefoot in the snow, so I would prepare it in such a way, so that if the Nazis came ... I specifically took the Nazi as the enemy, because it was so terrible. Now it wasn't that my mother sat down and told me what had happened to her. I think I just picked up on all sorts of things that floated in the home.

C: I don't really understand how you can pick up on things without being told?

E: I remember bits of a story I heard about how shoes were really important like how someone got so hungry that they cooked their shoes and ate the leather. So I didn't make it up, my imagination was not that developed, I guess I just put things together.

Emma phenomenologically experiences the presence of the Holocaust in the silent 'micro-moments and micro-acts' of daily life (Bakhtin 1981). The habitual practice of preparing for bed and laying out one's clothes become shaped by association with the distant conditions of the Holocaust death world. For the seven-year-old Emma, shoes were not merely another piece of attire but an essential tool of survival, which, if carefully prepared in advance, would allow her to walk in the freezing snow.

Verbal Fragmentary Transmission of Genocidal Past

Descendants recount parents' sporadic fragmentary verbal references to their Holocaust experience. These references took two forms: the first, Holocaust Dicta (Wajnryb 2001:192); and the second, fragmentary 'mythic' tales of survival. Dicta were brief one-sentence references to conditions withstood during the Holocaust, such as cold, hunger, forced labor and the threat of death. The majority of descendants describe hearing dicta in the most mundane moments of daily life, arising when they complained of their own relatively minor hardships eliciting in their parents critical references to their own survivor suffering. As Dan explains, dicta, such as 'You think you're hungry, you don't know what hunger is' were opportunities to access rare bits of descriptive information, embodied sensations and ultimately for moments of empathy. As Dan recounts: 'When they told me I had no idea how hungry one could be, I would try to imagine what it was like not to eat, or to eat so little and to be weak … so I could imagine what it was like to be there … understand how it was for them.'

Almost all Jewish-Israeli descendants interviewed recalled their parents having occasionally and apparently spontaneously recounted a near death experience. These accounts were always brief, and devoid of historical detail. Told with great pathos, in monologue form, they never triggered a dialog with family members nor did they evoke questions.

Beth recounts her father's tale as follows:

B: You know … I remember my father … told us that there was a lake near the ghetto and every day he would escape and swim across the lake and steal food for him and his father and then swim back across the lake, trying to keep the food dry, and sneak back into the ghetto without getting caught. If he were caught, they would have killed him for sure. He would emphasize how difficult it was to swim in the cold water and how he kept going by thinking about how he couldn't let his father down. … he was only 10 years old.

C: Did you ever ask questions or ask for details?

B: No never. He just told his story and that's it. But thinking about my life I realize that I'm swimming that lake too. I've made choices that were wrong, that made my life difficult but I didn't alter my path, no matter what. No matter how hard it was, I always tried not to disappoint anyone, especially family. Even when I should have changed paths, given up, been selfish, I kept swimming along. Just like my father. But now … with my career in shambles … I'm not sure I can make it to the shore this time.

Emphasizing the perseverance required to escape the ghetto, Beth highlights her father's bravery, endurance and commitment to the welfare of his father. Beth does not know which ghetto her father was in. These 'domesticated family myths' function as 'the symbolic coinage of exchange between generations' transmitting key values, beliefs and practices, allowing for a model for personal and familial choices (Bertaux and Thompson 1993:36). As such, Beth 'transposes' the embedded meaning of her father's swim across the lake to her own personal choices and sacrifices.

Silent Traces of the Genocide Past: *Cambodian Descendants*

Cambodian descendants described almost complete silence in their homes surrounding the genocidal past. They had extremely little knowledge of their familial history. When asked to explain why he didn't ask his parents about their genocide experience, Soper responded: 'It's not polite to ask elders too many questions.' Referring to culturally particular parent-child relations, Dorn explains: 'It's not just because of the Pol Pot time. I can't remember having too many conversations with my parents about anything personal. That's the way it is in Cambodia, hierarchy is important and speaking directly about that kind of thing would be disrespectful.'

Although, according to the therapeutic discourse, silence might signify the presence of repressed traumatic memory, according to the above descendants it is culturally normative behavior and not trauma that sustains familial silence. Although few descendants were reflexive regarding the relative value accorded to speech and silence in different cultures, this finding is consistent with Mathews (2000) study concluding that it is considered improper for Asian young people to question elders regarding what might be emotively disturbing.

Approximately 65 percent of the sample asserted that the painful nature of the genocide past could account for familial silence. Pich recounted: 'Why would I want to talk about such terrible things? This time is over and we should talk about the present so we can make a good life for ourselves.' Although at first glance this perspective recalls the Jewish sample's avoidance of speaking with parents about the difficult past, Pich's case above (and others like it) does not seem motivated solely by the desire to protect the survivors from painful references to the past. Rather, Pich's avoidance resonates with a more culture-specific avoidance of disturbing ruminations and interactions as well as culturally particular present and forward-looking perspective. As will be discussed below, the cultural avoidance of speech surrounding emotionally distressing matters is expressed in the Khmer idiom of distress known as 'keut chraen', or 'thinking too much' (Van de Put and Eisenbruch 2002). Ethno-psychological 'treatment' of 'thinking too much' calls for the distraction of the sufferer by talking to them about positive aspects of their lives, so that they not dwell on difficult emotions.

When asking Khmer descendants regarding the possibility of silent traces of the genocide in their childhood homes all respondents were perplexed by the question with many respondents asking 'how could the past be present?' After explaining the question with the help of a diagram depicting the movement of the past via an arrow into the present and future, respondents insisted the past was over. A number of Khmer asked, 'Why would we want something so terrible to be in our present?'

In great contrast to the Israeli descendant sample, only one Cambodian descendant depicted a silent trace of genocidal presence in the form of person-object interaction. Sokun recounted as follows:

> My father could not cremate his brother because he was killed in the Pol Pot time. We don't know where his body is. But he took some of his brother's clothes and the Achar [Buddhist priest] helped him burn it and we use that as ashes of my uncle. We put his ashes in the family stupa [small tower-like monument housing ashes of up to 7 generations of the familial dead]. I was a young child but I remember the sadness of my father in the ceremony. But it is good we have this to help my uncle be reborn. Many people have nothing.

In contrast to the Jewish sample above and in keeping with the aforementioned Khmer normative, respectful and more distant parent-child relations, Sokun does not depict detailed vicarious identification and emotive interaction with his father. He ends his account on a positive note referring to the performance of traditional ancestor worship and the potential of his uncle's rebirth. The absence of (descendant recollections of) painful moments of interaction with the ashes raises questions pertaining to the avoidance of frequent genocidal memory work, post-genocide closure and the valorization of presentism and forward-looking perspectives.

Verbal Fragmentary Transmission of the Genocidal Past

Echoing Holocaust descendants, a majority of Khmer descendant respondents describe fragmentary verbal references to the genocide past. As in the Holocaust case, these references take two forms: short dictum and the longer yet no less fragmentary mythic tales of survival, both embedding explicit moral lessons regarding valorized modes of being. Sarith recalls her mother saying: 'You are spoiled. You don't know what it is to be hungry and to search in the forest to find a root to keep you alive.' Aiming not only to transmit brief glimpses of the death world they experienced, Cambodian parents would primarily use dictum to discipline and educate what they perceived as potentially spoiled or lazy children. Kat recalls his father saying: 'You are disrespectful to me but if you knew how easy it was to lose your family you would not speak to me this way'. In keeping with Holocaust dicta, the great majority of descendants depicted the appreciation of food and family as the central themes of Cambodian parental dicta.

Although far less common than in the Holocaust sample, Cambodian descendants also recall mythic tales of survival embedding moral messages and validated key scenarios of survival. Sotheara recalls:

> 'When my brother and I would complain about the food she prepared for us my mother would tell us how she would work in the rice fields, hungry all day and sneak away to look for food. Many people were so hungry they died when they ate them because they didn't know how to cook them but she did because her grandmother taught her what you can eat in the forest and what you can't. I think she wanted to tell us to appreciate what we have and not complain. But not only that—also to have skills, be resourceful and remember what your elders teach you.'

Echoing the dicta above, the scarcity of food, hunger and the struggle to skillfully survive are the most common themes of Khmer mythic tales of survival. Yet the pedagogic tales designed to educate 'spoiled' children encapsulate additional cautionary components relevant for present life worlds—namely, the importance of heeding one's elders and recalling their mundane lessons. Pheakday recounts:

> My father was a child in the Pol Pot time. Children were taken away from their parents to work carrying fertilizer for the Khmer Rouge. He missed his parents, so he would work very hard so that once a month they would let him visit his parents. Today we have a good life—we can't understand what it is like to be separated from our family. We need to appreciate them and take care of them.'

The above tales transmit lessons pertaining to hard work, responsibility and family solidarity. As Ledgerwood and colleagues (1994) note, family separation during the genocide destabilized the key social unit or heart of Khmer society, while the rehabilitation of psychosocial and moral well-being of family life remains central to post-conflict recovery.

Comparing the above tales to those recounted by the Holocaust sample, both the Jewish and Khmer tales are devoid of historical detail. However, key differences may be isolated. In contrast to the Israeli accounts above, Khmer descendants do not recount any attempts to emplace themselves in the past to vicariously experience the death world, explore the emotional crises of their parents' battle of survival, or even to test their own skills of survival. The tale is primarily an allegory instrumentalized for present-day and future challenges facing the descendant generation and far less a mnemonic tool to re-present the otherwise inaccessible past in its own right. Although these tales most certainly come to frame descendants' moral universe and meaning worlds, they do not appear to act as a narrative bridge to the past, once again highlighting a forward-looking perspective.

Legacies of Post-Traumatic Stress

Jewish-Israeli Descendants

When asked about their parents' mental health, the great majority of the Holocaust descendant sample stated that their parents did suffer from symptoms of post-trauma; however, 80 percent of this sample insisted that considering the intensity of their suffering, they were highly resilient and did not require therapy. Regarding their own mental health, the great majority of descendants asserted that they were not suffering from the transmitted effects of PTSD. The entire sample showed familiarity with popular cultural literature on transmitted PTSD and approximately 25 percent had experienced some form of short- or long-term psychosocial therapy or support group. Nevertheless, more than half of this 'psychologically sophisticated' sample critiqued the transmitted PTSD construct and the efficacy of therapy as did almost all of those who had not undergone therapy.[3]

However, descendants did claim they were in fact 'srutim', a Hebrew slang expression literally translated as 'scratched'. Although parallel to the English slang 'cracked', it also implies the superficiality of their wound. Descendants explained that these scars were not markers of pathology, or even experienced as distressing, but were relatively benign emotive markers of difference. Hannah recounts: 'There's no point to go to therapy. Of course we're srutim [scratched], how could we grow up with them [survivors] and not be different. But we're not sick, what happened to them just made us more sensitive, to our own pain and to the pain of others.' Echoing Hannah's re-interpretation of descendant transmitted scars as a mode of emotional being rather than as a psychological disorder, Leah adds:

> I have had a very hard life. But I am proud of the fact that I know who I am and have worked on myself, dealing with all my emotional sritot [scratches] and I hope improving myself all the time. But this Holocaust thing … it's just too intense, part of our flesh … you can't really 'cure' it. It will always be there … to remind us of what happened. Carrying it is not only about us and our lives, but about something larger … it's the kind of burden you have to carry.

Leah perceives herself as fulfilling a 'larger' moral mission of collective Holocaust commemoration, by virtue of the emotional burden she carries.

The accounts of the permanence of an emotional wound, and the disinterest in coping skills or disbelief in what Leah terms a 'cure', are conceptualized as a form of descendent commemoration. The 'scratch' appears to be a marker of a particular phenomenological experience incommensurable with the dichotomy of wellness or illness. If cultural meaning worlds differentially frame the moral order pertaining to the value of genocide memory and filial obligations, then descendant 'scratches' or emotive markers, such as recollections of intersubjective moments with traumatized parents, might also be differentially experienced and conceptualized. Moreover, if the markers of emotional difference signify the semiotics of a morally valuable Holocaust presence and not merely a personal form of suffering, then treatment, healing and closure are not only untenable but undesirable. Collective meaning worlds may even be perpetuating individual scars as testimonial badges of honor. Interpreted as such, one cannot 'diagnose' descendants as either solely vulnerable or resilient to distress as they remain both vulnerable to and empowered by the scars of past 'difference' (Kidron 2012).

Cambodian Descendants

As psychological discourse and practice have yet to be widely disseminated in Cambodia, the very great majority of descendants were unfamiliar with the constructs of PTSD and almost none of the descendants had heard of transmitted PTSD. Questions were therefore posed regarding 'emotional well-being' to which the overwhelming response was again that their parents were not emotionally 'sick' or 'unwell'.

However, approximately 70 percent of the sample claimed that their parents experienced bouts of 'occasional sadness' when viewing media references or representations of the Pol Pot time or when hearing stories from other survivors. As Heum recounts, 'sometimes my mother would hear about the tribunal and get very sad. She would remember how she suffered.' When asked how often this sadness occurs and about the trajectory of the experience, the descendant asserts: 'If she does not think too much about the past she does not stay sad very long. Today she has her family, she is not alone, and she has plenty of rice, so she is not sad.' As briefly described above, respondents explained that according to Cambodian worldviews dwelling too much on the past and most especially a difficult or evil past—or Keut Chran literally 'thinking too much'—would be cosmologically, spiritually and physically damaging to the self, the family and the community. Ethnopsychology prescribes the loving attention of family members to distract those dwelling on difficult thoughts. In the case of my respondents they described literally stopping parents from recalling the genocide past by reminding them they are now blessed with all the rice they need and a new family that is safe and working toward a better future.

Cambodian descendants did not unsolicitedly identify their avoidance of ruminations over the difficult past with Buddhist precepts. Nevertheless, both survivors and descendants noted that visits to the local Buddhist Wat, meditation and ancestor veneration and merit exchange were the best cure for 'sadness' and 'too much thinking' about the genocide. When asked why meditation was helpful, Kat, who was waiting to pick his aunt up at the Temple Wat, explained: 'When my aunt sits with the Monk she learns Dhamma and meditates about the correct path, and she stops thinking too much about what happened. She tries to accept what the past brought her and look to her future journey.' When directly asked what Buddhism taught them about the genocide past, approximately 60 percent referred to the beneficial Buddhist lesson of acceptance of one's Karma, the acceptance that suffering is a central component of life, and the attempt to learn from one's past mistakes to make a better future. It appears that Buddhist principles tacitly frame ethnopsychological perspectives on health and well-being.

When asked about the intergenerational transmission of trauma to the descendant generation, Cambodian descendants were unanimously perplexed by the question. When I re-phrased the questions asking if they were 'emotionally sick' or 'emotionally wounded' by their parents' suffering in the Pol Pot time, all descendants interviewed responded that they were not emotionally wounded by the genocide. Khemrack asked 'how could I be hurt if I was not in the Pol Pot time?' When asking them if their parents' 'sadness' made them sad as well, all descendants asserted they were sad to see their parents saddened but that it could not make them sad—again—as they had not been there. Although empathizing with parental suffering, the Khmer respondents do not seem to vicariously identify as do Jewish descendants constituting emotional scars or 'scratches' as commemorative badges of honor (Kidron 2009). Although once again beyond the scope of this chapter, consistent with Canadian-Cambodians, here too the psychological dynamics of intergenerational transmission of distress or disorder via maladaptive parenting may be at odds with Cambodian conceptualizations of parent-child interaction and the potential long-term impact of genocide.

Unlike the Canadian Khmer sample (Kidron 2010a, 2012) descendants in Cambodia once again did not unsolicitedly appeal to Buddhism as a cultural source of emotional resilience or immunity to PTSD. Again, it might be tentatively suggested that in the more homogenous cultural context of Cambodia, as compared to the Western multi-cultural Canadian context, Buddhist meaning worlds may have remained taken for granted frames of experience. Nevertheless, as will be seen below, Buddhist spiritual world views do surface when accounting for Khmer descendant resistance to genocide commemoration in Cambodia.

Genocide Testimony and Commemoration

Jewish-Israeli Descendants

The remembrance and re-enactment of the past are key Jewish cultural tropes (Yerushalmi 1982). Re-enactment takes place via ritual and liturgy where perpetual narration of biblical mythic sequences guarantee that they remain culturally embedded as blueprints for interpretation. The imperative of personal remembrance encompasses the commemoration of communal and personal dead. The individual, perceived as the eternal witness embodying memory, and the community of which he/she is a part loop back to the past in order to make that past present and to create a meaningful 'place' for the events and people on the continuum of history. Filial responsibility to the memory of one's parents and ancestors is of special importance and is deeply embedded in Jewish cosmology and praxis. The individual is also obliged to transmit the past to future generations. However, the Jewish witness need not have been an eye witness to the past, as knowledge of the past is sufficient to require testimony and transmission (Young 1990). These deep structural Jewish paradigms of memory have found intense 'revival' and transposition in the Israeli nation state as State-sponsored memorial sites and ceremonies publicly glorify Holocaust survivors and fallen war heroes, and collectively enlist survivors and bereaved families, and engineer pedagogic pilgrimages to Holocaust death worlds (Feldman 2008). All these forms of memory work function to constitute the moral mission of those citizens prepared to carry the burden of collective and personal memory (Kidron 2009).

In keeping with the above Jewish cultural tropes, the descendant sample unanimously expressed great concern with the future of Holocaust commemoration. Beyond the silent form of embodied-emotive commemoration of the transmitted 'scratches' of the Holocaust past, the majority also recounted partaking in private votive practices of lighting candles in memory of the Holocaust dead and those more religiously observant recounted participating in synagogue-based communal prayers commemorating both family members killed in the Holocaust and communities lost to the genocide (Kidron 2009). However, when asked about the transmission of the Holocaust past to their children, or participation in public forms of commemorative testimony to the past, the majority of descendants explained that they preferred to remain silent and allow survivor grandparents and the education system to transmit personal and collective legacies. Others recounted that after exposure to practices of survival and Holocaust-related meaning worlds in their childhood, their children too would have to 'learn to know and to feel' the wounds of the past 'for all those had died' (Kidron 2009). When further broaching the subject of descendant avoidance of public commemoration, respondents provided two recurring explanations. The first referred to the silent presence of the past in the parental home 'surviving through them in every breath we take'. As walking testament to the Holocaust this would obviate the need for public commemoration. The second expressed concern over the mis-representation of their private memories where historicity would usurp lived memory.

Cambodian Descendants

The Khmer descendant sample expressed disinterest in public national or communal commemoration of the genocide past. Regarding the National Genocide Museum at Tuol Sleng, previously a prison in which thousands of Khmer Rouge victims were tortured and killed, and Cheok Ek, a commemorative site erected at the killing fields and mass graves of thousands of victims, descendants interviewed assert that these sites are of critical importance as they authenticate and document the devastation of the Khmer Rouge period. Descendants also support the recent inclusion of genocide history as part of high school curricula so that future generations will be more knowledgeable about the national catastrophe.

However, despite the above support of national genocide documentation and museological representation, when asked if they had visited these sites or if they will visit them in the near future, the great majority (even those living in the capital in the vicinity of the museums) either said they have not visited these sites or remained non-committal as to planning actual future visits. When pressing the issue, a number of explanations emerged for descendant absence at and indifference to national sites of memory. As Bory explains: 'We need to move on and not to look back. We need to know the history, learn it in school and, yes, sure see those places like Toul Sleng—I do want some time to go and show my children—but that's enough. Cambodia needs now to think about now—and make a better future.' Like Bory, although the majority of descendants interviewed assert national commemoration is of value, they do not feel genocide representation should have an overpowering presence in Cambodian everyday life. As Sokun, an activist in a grassroots Khmer NGO, explains:

> All our generation should know what happened. I'm not saying no to education about genocide. Students must see the killing fields. But we have to take care not to become victims who speak endlessly of suffering. We should become strong from the lesson of our mistakes. I teach the past only to change the future.

In keeping with trauma-related avoidance of 'too much thinking' above, both Bory and Sokun present a future-oriented perspective, narrowing the relevance of memory work to the betterment of present Khmer life and related moral pedagogy. When asked Contia about possible pedagogic trips to monumental and communal sites of memory, she asserts: 'Cambodia should not become one big place of bones, bones everywhere. The government is using this past instead of solving today's problems.' In great contrast to professional agents of memory in Israel, a number of Khmer activists in Cambodia insist on minimizing routine genocide memory work, channeling the moral lessons of the past in the service of a better future. Nor can one ignore the subtle critique of the politicization of genocide memory threatening to transform Cambodia into what Contia terms 'one big place of bones'.

The majority of descendants in Cambodia did not appeal directly to Khmer culture in general or Buddhist precepts in particular to account for their general disinterest in collective commemoration. Once again the homogeneity of the Cambodian society and the taken-for-granted nature of the way Buddhist meaning worlds frame lived experience perhaps obviate the kind of reflexivity born of identity politics in diasporas such as Canada (Kidron 2012). Nevertheless, when directly asked whether Khmer culture and/or Khmer Buddhism could in any way explain their feelings about genocide commemoration, 65 percent of the descendants, many of whom had spent time at Buddhist temples during their youth, evoked the Buddhist forward-looking values pertaining to the acceptance of Karma, and forward-looking perspectives cited above in their responses to the question. Buddhist monks (and veteran monks)—some of whom are engaged in local grassroots NGOs—provided unsolicited responses, tracing the connection between Buddhist perspectives and Cambodian descendant disinterest in collective forms of genocide memory. As Andana explained:

> Buddhism teaches us that the present is the mother of the future. We don't need to look back. We don't forget our family. But we look back to how they died only if we can learn from it. But many times we don't know why someone suffered. If you can't know the Karma—the reason for their fate—no reason to look back to the way they died. We exchange merit for them all the time. But they are part of our present helping us to have luck, health and begin well for the future and we help them to go to their better future—how they died is not important for us now.

Andana's account of the purpose and limits of familial ancestor veneration marginalizes the circumstances of death namely genocide history and commemoration. As long as merit is exchanged, both the living and the dead may continue forward toward their destinies while backward-looking explorations of one's difficult personal (or collective) Karma and fateful death would do nothing to promote successful rebirth and a better future.

Nevertheless, skeletal remains of unidentified genocide victims have been exhumed and housed in semi-monumental communal commemorative 'stupas' (memorial towers traditionally containing only ashes of familial dead) constructed in temple compounds in major towns and villages across Cambodia. Participant observation in the summer of 2010 and 2013 found that villagers did not commemorate the genocide at these sites, nor did they venerate their deceased relatives who perished in the genocide. Instead, relatives were venerated in privately owned and erected family stupas (or in smaller stupas constructed in their yards at home) which contained the ashes of deceased relatives who had died before the genocide or the names or surviving objects of the genocide dead in lieu of their absent remains.

When asking my respondents about prayer or visitation at the above collective communal genocide stupas (displaying mass skeletal remains), the very great majority assert that there is no need for communal sites of genocide commemoration, and that the national sites (Tuol Sleng of Choek Ek) in the capital are sufficient. Asking Pich why she does not venerate the collective Cambodian genocide dead housed in the communal genocide stupa in her village, she responded: 'No skulls—no, no [laughs nervously] I am afraid and don't want to see them.' When asked her why she does not want to see the remains, she states: 'Those skulls, those places are so terrible. Only evil things happened. I don't want to see. But you know, those skulls, those who died a bad death—their spirits—[she laughs] they are still there unhappy how they died. They are dangerous. We don't need to go there.' Echoing Davis' (2008) account of Khmer spirit beliefs and funerary practices, victims who have met an untimely violent death may remain trapped between the realms of the living and the dead unable to begin their journey to rebirth, haunting the living and awaiting their relatives' rituals of veneration/merit exchange. Raising perhaps a more mundane dilemma, approximately half of the survivors interviewed and the great majority of the descendants interviewed asserted that there would be no point to venerate at the collective stupas. As Kat stated: 'there is no way to know if the bones of my father are actually in the [collective] stupa. I asked Kat if when exchanging merit with his father in the family stupa he thinks about the way his father died in the genocide, he responded: 'why would I think of how he died … I just pray to him like to the others.'

Pich's and Kat's disclosure above presents one of the little discussed issues facing the Khmer in the wake of genocide. It would appear that contemporary sites of collective genocide memory in Cambodia designed in keeping with Euro-Western forms of atrocity tourism may be incommensurable with Khmer Buddhist spirit beliefs and rites of ancestor veneration and merit exchange. Not only must all dead be immediately cremated by family members to prevent arousing the anger of the dead relative and future haunting, the ashes must be housed in familial ossuaries or stupas (either in the home or in the local temple compound) and venerated (via all important gifts of food, money and beloved objects) by family members and only by the family, weekly or at the very least on major holidays. Those suffering a violent and untimely death become especially vulnerable to haunting and are all the more in need of familial 'care'. As the mass death of millions in Cambodia has made it impossible to identify and privately cremate the remains of family members, countless souls remain in a spiritual limbo of sorts. Although officials may have undertaken mass Buddhist cremations officiated by funerary priests mandated to cremate the unidentified dead after the genocide, the politics of genocide memory has opted for the expediency of preventing or delaying mass cremation of the dead in favor of the public display of remains in communal stupas, which according to a number of critical Khmer descendants serves to attract the attention of 'atrocity tourists' from around the globe.

When asking descendants about the future of familial genocide memory and the legacies to be transmitted to their children—the third generation—in contrast to Israeli descendants and parallel to Canadian Khmer (Kidron 2012), the great majority of Cambodian descendants insist that although their children must learn the history of this terrible time in school, they do not wish to burden their children with the few painful tales of suffering they heard from their parents. Consistent with the forward-looking themes embedded in the texts above, Sarith asserts, 'I will tell my son and daughter to remember how lucky they are that they have a strong family and they should work hard to make a good life for themselves. But no I don't want to tell them about that terrible time. They will learn in school about the history. It's enough. My parents did not tell me what I did not need to know, my children too only need to know how to be good people, to work hard to learn skills to make a good future for them and for their family.'

Discussion

The comparison of Cambodian and Israeli Holocaust trauma descendant genocidal legacies has highlighted significant differences in the experience of emotional wellness and future trajectory of familial and collective commemoration of the genocide past. Findings pertaining to the culturally specific Cambodian and Jewish-Israeli paradigms and practices of memory problematize the globally disseminated reductionist profile of the pathologized and enlisted trauma descendant and therapeutic socio-political interventionist practices universalizing genocide legacies (Fassin 2009).

Both Israeli and Khmer descendants recount some form of non-pathological presence rather than the absence or erasure of the genocide past in the everyday life world of the survivor home. Genocide presence took two forms—silent embodied presence and verbal fragmentary presence. While both samples depict their respect for survivor silence, differences emerge in the attributed reasons for this choice, with Cambodians appealing to culture-specific interfamilial silence and Israeli-Jews relating to interpersonal concerns for parental well-being. Moreover, the degree and 'content' of the silent presence of genocide in the everyday life worlds of the two samples differ. There was a relative absence of non-verbal embodied traces of the genocide past in the domestic life of the Khmer. In great contrast, Israeli descendants recount a perpetual amorphous sense of genocidal presence, as well as non-verbal mechanisms of intergenerational transmission of the past such as person-object interaction and embodied practices of survival.

However, both Israelis and Khmer recall brief verbal references to the past in the form of dictum and fragmentary mythic tales. These references were seen to embed and transmit key genocide-related personal values and scenarios. Importantly, however, although in both samples dictum and mythic tales provided backward-looking glimpses into the genocidal past, the Jewish-Israeli sample recalled both empathic and vicarious identification with past suffering as well as the present adoption of embedded moral modes of being. In contrast, the Khmer sample pointedly asserted that the sole experience and value of these tales was the adoption of forward-looking moral modes of being. Although the above silent embodied and verbal fragmentary traces of the genocide past are in keeping with Bertelsen's (present volume) reading of the way post-conflict sociality in everyday life 'reshapes meaning in the face of violence's capacity for erasure and inscription', the Israeli and Khmer appear to differentially and selectively utilize, represent and re-inscribe the past as semiotic resource. While Israelis 'put the past to work' in the service of re-presencing the past and shaping one's present in its image, the Khmer appear to enlist the past to re-form the personal and collective present and future. Jewish and Khmer cosmological worldviews (in both cases) and contemporary politics of memory (in the Israeli case) appear to be critical in any attempt to unpack these particular and differential instrumental representations of the past.

Deconstructing the universal semiotics of trauma theory (Fassin 2009), Khmer respondents assert they are not suffering from the intergenerational effects of PTSD, whereas the Israeli sample describes the experience of an emotionally 'inscribed' wound that cannot be healed. Most interestingly, core religious Jewish and Buddhist paradigms of memory may have engendered these very different experiences of what has been conflated in the literature as a potentially universal trauma-related and intergenerationally transmitted experience of distress and suffering. Although psychological literature has in fact turned attention to individual resilience and culture-specific spiritual/cosmological 'protective layers' that buffer the traumatized self, the great majority of academic and popular cultural accounts continue to present trauma victims and their descendants as psychosocially vulnerable, while ignoring more positive characteristics such as forward-looking strength of spirit, human endurance and hope (Eggerman and Panther-Brick 2010) or alternatively the emotively empowering potential of acceptance of a collectively valorized emotional scar of familial suffering. Both the Jewish-Israeli sample and the Cambodian sample have found ways to make the surviving embodied and emotive traces of the genocide past culturally meaningful that resist the pathologization and victimization of therapeutic constructs. The data above allow us to consider the way culture-specific values, practices and modes of being have been erroneously conflated under the rubric of traumatic experience.

Regarding the transmission of genocide memory, in keeping with Broch-Due's reading of the return to the micro-spheres of everyday sociality, the corporeal and the affective (Chap. 2) descendant narratives disclose the way the intersubjective familial sphere appears to covetously sustain private-domestic forms of genocide memory either directly competing with or apathetic to practices in the national and collective sphere. The descendant body, the descendant moral self and the intersubjective space of survivor-descendant-ancestor relations, all dialectically constituted in the survivor private sphere (or at the private familial stupa/ceremony), become the privileged sites of genocide memory. By domesticating genocide memory, intergenerational transmission of genocide-related moral modes commemoratively inscribe both backward-looking and future-oriented moral lessons without recourse to disempowering grammars of erasure, psychosocial vulnerability or victimization.

Rejecting the role of public/collective carriers of future memory, both samples show little interest in providing public testimony to their parents' past and the Khmer even have their doubts regarding the degree to which they will transmit the little historical knowledge they do have to future generations. Once again, culture-specific Jewish and Buddhist/cosmological paradigms emerge as shaping these attitudes. Although Jewish paradigms promote the practice of intergenerational transmission of memory, the Israelis suffice in their existential wound, preferring to relegate the role of transmission to their survivor parents and the education system. Alternatively, the Khmer appeal to Buddhist cosmological principles (albeit often tacit) such as Karmic acceptance and the perpetual familial relations with the dead which constitute forward-looking modes of being and obviate the need for national or communal genocide memory.

As far as the future of public collective memory of the genocide, the samples express key differences regarding the centrality/marginality of genocide memory. Whereas the Israeli sample views the future of public Holocaust remembrance as very important, the Khmer appear indifferent to future public or even communal commemorative projects. Although the Khmer frequently refer to the 'ideoscape' of genocide, namely, the pedagogic ideational lessons learned and transmitted to rehabilitate themselves, their families and Cambodia, in keeping with the idiom of distress 'thinking too much', they selectively remember only empowering forward-looking lessons while strategically 'forgetting' the darker components of genocide history.

Problematizing one of the key axioms of memory studies, newly imposed Khmer collective/communal sites of memory paradoxically do and do not 'relieve viewers of their memory burden' (Young 1993:5; Chap. 4). In keeping with Euro-Western cosmopolitan genocide memory, the Khmer appear to envision monumental sites of memory such as Tuol Sleng as 'divesting themselves of the obligation' to commemorate the genocide obviating for some even the moral necessity of visiting these sites with their children. At the same time, however, ancestor veneration and Buddhist ritual practices in the familial sphere work to restore the cosmological imbalance of countless untimely 'bad deaths' and sustain the perpetual presence of and exchange with relatives who lost their lives in the genocide. It should be noted, however, that in contradistinction to the universal semiotics of global genocide commemoration, it is precisely the function of Buddhist familial and communal ritual ancestor veneration to correct for and thereby marginalize the circumstances of ancestral death and suffering and thereby 'normalize' the genocide dead. Despite the above communal and familial correctives to genocide suffering, Cambodian findings point to the new forms of top-down hegemonic orchestration of collective memory and trauma therapy within local urban and village life and provide an opportunity to capture culture change in the making. It will be interesting to see whether globalizing trauma brokers and interventionist NGOs will tip the balance in favor Euro-Western trauma profiles and/or testimonial voice or if a unique syncretic culture-specific and context-specific 'glocal' form of memory work and therapy will evolve.

The above discussion of trauma and memory work has repeatedly highlighted the constitutive role of particular cultural meaning worlds and moral modes of being in descendant legacies. Despite the extensive ethnographic accounts of culture-bound illnesses, somatization, healing and related belief systems, and cross-cultural studies of collective memory, there have been few attempts to examine the way the above core-cultural conceptualizations of illness and memory work de-legitimize or valorize remembering and forgetting or how and why they constitute unique mechanisms of transmission, be they verbal, embodied or ideational (Hinton 2004). Particular cultural sensibilities are deployed in references to Buddhist acceptance and the Jewish burden of memory. Culture-specific religious, cosmological and spiritual worldviews also shape the very distinct contours of the Jewish and Khmer experience of emotional well-being and moral rectitude. Despite recent forays into the realm of cultural ontologies, alterity in its own right still remains problematic, evoking the scepter of essentialism or anxiety over the elision of macro political, historical or socio-economic interpretations (Abu-Lughod 1991). Socio-political contextual analyses allow for the more comforting route of translation into a universal common language of suffering. Trauma theory is one such universalizing force classifying and regulating the diverse lived experience of suffering. The above findings call for renewed attention to the 'particular' limits of universalizing axiomatic language, where translation of descendant accounts into the universal semiotics of suffering would have ultimately overshadowed subtly unique and multi-faceted responses to genocide.

Notes

1. Similar questions were used with both Holocaust and Cambodian descendants. These questions attempted to elicit responses along the following themes: parental past and present behavior and parent-child relationship; childhood memories of genocide-related dialog or story telling and/or genocide-related practices in the home, past and present 'consumption' of trauma-related discourse and cultural products, participation in genocide-related practices in the public domain and finally envisioned future of commemorative practices.
2. The use of the term genocide to describe the massacre, starvation and expulsion of the victims of the Khmer Rouge is problematic. As outlined by Quigley (2000:6–7), an expert in International Law invited to attend the 1979 trial of Pol Pot and Leng Sary to determine whether they could be tried for the crimes of genocide, the

term genocide was defined by the UN convention for the prevention and punishment of crimes of genocide in 1948. Genocide was defined by the convention as the intention to destroy a whole or part of a national, ethnic, racial or religious group. Quigley (as do Genocide scholars) explains that the controversy has arisen surrounding the use of the term genocide when applied to the case of Cambodia as most of the victims, like the perpetrators, were Khmer—'so there was no racial animus behind the actions'. Only a small minority of the victims could be classified as ethnic, religious or national Other (Chinese, Muslim Cham and Vietnamese) and due to the political nature of Khmer Rouge motives, it is not clear that the perpetrators intended to kill these victims only due to their ethnic/religious status as Other. Nevertheless, Quigley concluded that as the definition of genocide includes intention to kill a whole or part of a group—then the victimization of Khmer intellectuals or religious leaders would be considered a part of a national and ethnic group and would then be consistent with the UN definition. Genocide scholars, including those Khmer scholars working in Cambodia to document the events, have used the term genocide, in some cases for lack of a better word, and in other cases due to the emergent geneology of the term now used to classify a wide array of human loss and suffering. It might be claimed that considering the nature and scale of loss in Cambodia, the use of another term would raise no less difficult questions concerning global hierarchies of suffering.

3. As clarified above, the question posed to the descendants and in the chapter herein is not a diagnostic one as to whether they are or are not suffering from PTSD, but rather if and how the illness construct as cultural construction does or does not meaningfully frame their experience. As seen in the discussion that follows, descendants articulate emotive difference using an alternative cultural idiom, allowing for an analysis of the semiotics of their experience rather than a psychological diagnosis of their mental health.

References

Abu-Lughod, L. 1991. Writing Against Culture. In *Recapturing Anthropology: Working in the Present*, ed. Richard G. Fox, 137–162. Santa Fe: School of American Research Press.

Alexander, J.C. 2004. Toward a Theory of Cultural Trauma. In *Cultural Trauma and Collective Identity*, eds. J.C. Alexander, R. Eyerman, B. Geisen, and P. Sztompka, 1–30. Berkeley: University of California Press.

Altounian, J. 1999. Putting into Words, Putting to Rest and Putting Aside the Ancestors—How an Analysand Who Was Heir to the Armenian Genocide of 1915 Worked Through Mourning. *International Journal of Psycho-Analysis* 80(3): 439–448.

Argenti, N., and C. Schramm, eds. 2010. *Remembering Violence: Anthropological Perspectives on Intergenerational Transmission*. New York: Berghahn Press.

Bakhtin, M. M. 1981. *The Dialogic Imagination*. Trans. C. Emerson and M. Holquist. Austin: University of Texas Press.

Barocas, H.A., and C. Barocas. 1973. Manifestations of Concentration Camp Effects on the Second Generation. *American Journal of Psychiatry* 130(7): 820–821.

Bar-On, D. 1992. Israeli and German Students Encounter the Holocaust Through a Group Process: 'Working Through' and 'Partial Relevance'. *International Journal of Group Tensions* 22(2): 81–118.

Bertaux, D., and P. Thompson. 1993. Introduction. In *Between Generations: Family Models, Myths, and Memories*, eds. D. Bertaux and P. Thompson, 1–12. Oxford: Oxford University Press.

Danieli, Y. 1998. Introduction: History and Conceptual Foundations. In *International Handbook of Multigenerational Legacies of Trauma*, ed. Y. Danieli, 1–17. New York: Plenum Press.

Davis, E.W. 2008. Between Forests and Families: A Remembered Past Life. In *People of Virtue: Reconfiguring Religion, Power and Moral Order in Cambodia*, eds. D. Porter, A. Kent, and D. Chandler, 128–146. Nordic Institute of Asian Studies: Copenhagen.

Diagnostic and Statistical Manual of Mental Disorders: DSM IV. 1994. Washington, DC: American Psychiatric Association.

Eggerman, M.B., and K. Panter-Brick. 2010. Suffering, Hope, and Entrapment: Resilience and Cultural Values in Afghanistan. *Social Science and Medicine* 71: 71–83.

Fassin, D. 2009. Humanitarian Politics of Testimony: Subjectification Through Trauma in the Israeli-Palestinian Conflict. *Cultural Anthropology* 23: 531–558.

Feldman, J. 2008. *Above the Death Pits, Beneath the Flag: Youth Voyages to Holocaust Poland and Israeli National Identity*. New York: Berghahn.

Halbwachs, M. 1980. *The Collective Memory*. New York: Harper Colophon Books.

Hayden, R. 2007. Moral Vision and Impaired Insight. *Current Anthropology* 48: 105–131.

Herman, J.L. 1992. *Trauma and Recovery*. New York: Basic Books.

Hinton, A.L. 2004. *Why Did They Kill: Cambodian in the Shadow of Genocide*. Berkeley: University of California Press.

Huang, L.N. 1998. Southeast Asian Refugee Children and Adolescents. In *Children of Color: Psychological Interventions with Culturally Diverse Youth*, eds. J.T. Gibbs and L.N. Huang, 264–304. San Francisco, CA: Jossey-Bass.

Ida, D., and P. Young. 2003. Southeast Asian Children and Adolescents. In *Children of Color: Psychological Interventions with Culturally Diverse Youth*, eds. J.T. Gibbs and L.N. Huang, 265–295. San Francisco, CA: Jossey-Bass.

Kidron, C. A. 2005. Children of Twilight: Deconstructing the Passage from Silence to Voice of Second and Third Generation Holocaust Descendants Within the Private and Public Spheres in Israel. Ph.D. thesis. Hebrew University, Jerusalem.

———. 2009. Toward an Ethnography of Silence: The Lived Presence of the Past in the Everyday Lives of Holocaust Trauma Descendants in Israel. *Current Anthropology* 50: 5–27.

———. 2010a. Silent Legacies of Trauma: A Comparative Study of Cambodian Canadian and Israeli Holocaust Trauma Descendant Memory Work. In *Remembering Violence: Anthropological Perspectives on Intergenerational Transmission*, eds. N. Argenti and C. Schramm, 185–220. New York: Berghahn Press.

———. 2010b. Embracing the Lived Memory of Genocide: Holocaust Survivor and Descendant Renegade Memory-Work at the House of Being. *American Ethnologist* 37(3): 429–451.

———. 2012. Alterity and the Particular Limits of Universalism: Comparing Jewish-Israeli Holocaust and Canadian-Cambodian Genocide Legacies. *Current Anthropology* 53(6): 723–754.

Kiernan, B. 1996. *The Pol Pot Regime: Race, Power and Genocide in Cambodia Under the Khmer Rouge*. New Haven, CT: Yale University Press.

Kinzie, J.D., R.H. Frederickson, R. Ben, J. Fleck, and W. Karls. 1984. Post-Traumatic Stress Disorder Among Survivors of Cambodian Concentration Camps. *American Journal of Psychiatry* 141(5): 645–650.

Lambek, M., and P. Antze. 1996. Introduction: Forecasting Memory. In *Tense Past: Cultural Essays in Trauma and Memory*, eds. P. Antze and M. Lambek, xi–xxxviii. New York: Routledge.

Ledgerwood, J., M.M. Ebihara, and C. Mortland. 1994. Introduction. In *Cambodian Culture Since 1975: Homeland and Exile*, eds. M.M. Ebihara, C.A. Mortland, and J. Ledgerwood, 1–26. Ithaca, NY: Cornell University Press.

Leys, R. 2000. *Trauma: A Geneology*. Chicago, IL: University of Chicago Press.

Mathews, R. 2000. Cultural Patterns of South Asian and Southeast Asian Americans. *Intervention in School and Clinic* 36: 101–104.

Mckinney, K. 2007. Breaking the 'Conspiracy of Silence': Testimony, Traumatic Memory and Psychotherapy with Survivors of Political Violence. *Ethos* 35: 265–299.

Munyas, B. 2008. Cambodian Youth: Transmitting (his)tories of Genocide to Second and Third Generation in Cambodia. *Journal of Genocide Studies* 10: 413–439.

Pupavac, V. 2006. Humanitarian Politics and the Rise of Disaster Psychology. In *Handbook of International Disaster Psychology*, eds. G. Reyes and G.A. Jacobs, 15–34. Westport, CT: Praeger Publishers.

Quigley, J. 2000. Introduction. In *Genocide in Cambodia: Documents from the Trial of Pol Pot and Leng Say*, eds. H.J. De Nike, J. Quigley, and K.J. Robinson, 1–18. Philadelphia: University of Pennsylvania Press.

Rousseau, C., A. Drapeau, and R. Platt. 1999. Family Trauma and Its Association with Emotional and Behavioral Problems and Social Adjustment in Adolescent Cambodian Refugees. *Child Abuse and Neglect* 23(12): 1263–1273.

Rousseau, C., M. Morales, and P. Foxen. 2001. Going Home: Giving Voice to Memory Strategies of Young Mayan Refugees Who Returned to Guatemala as a Community. *Culture, Medicine and Psychiatry* 25: 135–168.

Rubin, A., and L. Rhodes. 2005. Narrative and the Intergenerational Transmission of Trauma Among Cambodian Refugees. In *Perspectives in Cross-Cultural Psychiatry*, eds. A.M. Georgiopoulos and J.F. Rosenbaum, 157–178. Philadelphia, PA: Lippincott William and Wilkins.

Sagi-Schwartz, A., M.H. van Ijzendoorn, K.E. Grossmann, K. Grossmann, and N. Koren-Karie. 2003. Attachment and Traumatic Stress in Female Holocaust Child Survivors and Their Daughters. *American Journal of Psychiatry* 160(6): 1086–1092.

Stevens, C.A. 2001. Perspectives on the Meaning of Symptoms Among Cambodian Refugees. *Journal of Sociology* 37(1): 81–98.

Van de Put, W.A.C.M., and M. Eisenbruch. 2002. The Cambodian Experience. In *Trauma, War and Violence: Public Mental Health in Socio-Cultural Context*, ed. Joop T.V.M. de Jong, 93–134. Berlin: Springer.

Wajnryb, R. 2001. *The Silence: How Tragedy Shapes Talk.* Crows Nest, Australia: Allen & Unwin.

Yerushalmi, Y.H. 1982. *Zakhor—Jewish History and Jewish Memory.* Seattle: University of Washington Press.

Young, J.E. 1990. *Writing and Rewriting the Holocaust: Narrative and the Consequences of Interpretation.* Bloomington: Indiana University Press.

———. 1993. *The Texture of Memory: Holocaust Memorials and Meaning.* New Haven, CT: Yale University Press.

Young, A. 1995. *Harmony of Illusions: Inventing Post Traumatic Stress Disorder.* Princeton, NJ: Princeton University Press.

Zilberfein, F. 1995. Children of Holocaust Survivors: Separation Obstacles, Attachments and Anxiety. In *A Global Perspective on Working with Holocaust Survivors and the Second Generation*, ed. J. Lemberger, 413–422. Jerusalem: JDC-Brookdale Institute & Amcha.

CHAPTER 4

Social Trauma, National Mourning, and Collective Guilt in Post-Authoritarian Argentina

Antonius C.G.M. Robben

On 16 June 1955, shortly after noontime, naval aircraft took off from Ezeiza airport to Plaza de Mayo in downtown Buenos Aires. The mission was to attack the presidential palace and topple Juan Domingo Perón from power. For days there had been rumors about an upcoming coup d'état, and several naval rebellions had taken place in the early morning hours before the aerial raid. The planes reached Plaza de Mayo air space at 12:30 PM and released their bombs. Twelve persons were killed and fifty-five wounded in a direct hit on the presidential palace, the Casa Rosada, but Perón was unharmed because he had taken refuge in the nearby War Ministry. The devastation on the Plaza de Mayo was great. Civilians died from the shattered glass that fell from buildings surrounding the nation's governmental heart, and from the gunfire by marines advancing toward the square. Bombs also hit a trolley and a school bus. A second air raid at 1:10 PM killed even more people because truck after truck filled with Peronists had arrived to defend their leader. Meanwhile, loyal government

A.C.G.M. Robben (✉)
Utrecht University, Utrecht, The Netherlands

V. Broch-Due, B.E. Bertelsen (eds.), *Violent Reverberations*,
DOI 10.1007/978-3-319-39049-9_4

troops were arriving at the Plaza de Mayo and were attacked by a final aerial assault at 3:30 PM. The coup d'état failed in the end because the army succeeded in quelling the military rebellion. An estimated 350 people were dead and more than 2000 wounded, many of them civilians (Cháves 2005:70–72; Robben 2005a:20).

In his radio address at 6:00 PM that same day, Perón told his supporters to return home in peace and leave the streets to the army, but the traumatic attacks had whetted people's desire for revenge. The metropolitan curia at the Plaza de Mayo went up in flames, and 17 churches were ransacked or set ablaze. In the following days, Perón tried to defuse the volatile political situation that threatened a decline into civil war. In a conciliatory gesture, he gave only mild prison sentences to the military rebels but a new coup was already in the making. Besieged by continuous street protests organized by the political opposition, Perón threatened to unleash his supporters and allow the Peronist union central to organize an armed militia. Privately, however, he feared the destruction he had witnessed in 1939 at the end of Spain's civil war. On 18 September 1955, the Argentine army and navy rose in rebellion. Perón fled to the Paraguayan embassy and abandoned Argentina on 3 October (Potash 1980:189, 200–202; Torre and de Riz 1993:262–263). The Peronist Party was outlawed, and General Lonardi became Argentina's new president but was ousted by hard-liner General Aramburu in January 1956.

The indiscriminate bombing of the Peronist crowd gathered at the Plaza de Mayo set a violence-trauma-violence dynamic in motion that resulted three decades later in a traumatized society. This traumatization cannot be reduced to the June 1955 bombardment or to the various repressive dictatorships that followed, not even to the junta that ordered tens of thousands of disappearances between 1976 and 1983, but Argentina's complex national trauma accumulated during these turbulent decades. Violence did not simply beget more violence, as the spiral of violence notion implies, but violence ensued trauma and trauma led to a violent response. Social trauma does not imply the disempowerment that often occurs through psychic trauma but, on the contrary, can incite people to violence and protest. This violence-trauma-violence dynamic became an overdetermined whole by operating at different linear and non-linear temporalities and different levels of social complexity, namely, the public, political, domestic, and personal domains. The escalating violence and cumulative trauma manifested itself in street crowds, politico-military organizations, families, and the self. These multi-level manifestations of violence and trauma cannot be reduced to one another, but interlinkages make consequences spill over into other domains. For example, the disappearances occurred in the political domain of politico-militaryorganizations, intruded on the lives of searching relatives in the domestic domain, and injured the tortured captives in their personal domain as the self and their political subjectivity were affected deeply.

The trauma concept has been criticized for medicalizing sociopolitical conditions and historical processes while turning political actors into victims and psychiatric patients (Fassin and Rechtman 2009; Kleinman and Kleinman 1991; Kleinman 1999). Social suffering has been offered as an alternative by doing more justice to the political, economic, moral, and institutional forces that cause what are mistakenly diagnosed as individual pathologies. I have retained the term social trauma because the conceptual shift to social suffering involves a relabeling that downplays the diversity of violent experiences among human beings and societies. The concept of social suffering denotes a universal human condition and fails to distinguish between such different phenomena as poverty and genocide. Finally, empirical studies of political violence that take social trauma as their key concept pay as much attention to the complex circumstances of severely afflicted populations as do studies that use suffering as the core concept (Alexander 2012; Hinton and Hinton 2014; Kirmayer et al. 2007; Martín-Baró 1989; Robben and Suárez-Orozco 2000).

How did Argentina come to terms with the social traumas of its divided society, mourn the many losses and violent deaths, mend its social and political gaps, and restore faith and trust in peaceful social and political coexistence? This chapter provides a sociocultural analysis of Argentina's national mourning process, drawing inspiration from a psychological model that conceives of personal mourning as an oscillation between loss-oriented and restoration-oriented coping processes. After describing the cumulative traumatization of Argentine society between 1955 and 1983, I will adapt social psychology's Dual Process Model of Coping with Bereavement (DPM) to a sociocultural frame to analyze Argentina's contested national mourning and its periodic oscillations between loss-oriented and restoration-oriented coping. Elsewhere (Robben 2014), I demonstrated in a comparison of Chile and Argentina that societies may differ in the relative weight of the two coping process. Here, I will argue that Argentina's much greater emphasis on loss, retribution, and accountability than on restoration and reconciliation has resulted in assigning a collective responsibility to the three decades of political violence and traumatization with far-reaching consequences on the psychosocial healing of a bereaved Argentine society as the disappearances are regarded increasingly as genocide.

The Traumatization of Argentine Society

The June 1955 bombardment of the Plaza de Mayo traumatized Peronist crowds by exposing their vulnerability, hurting their identity, and inflicting unacceptable losses. But rather than paralyzing people in fear, as might happen to traumatized individuals, Perón's followers reacted with retaliatory violence immediately after the carnage. Furthermore, a Peronist resistance movement arose among a working class disaffected with the new rulers. Strikes erupted, and sabotage was committed on power stations, factories, and public transport. A military rebellion took place in June 1956 that was harshly repressed. In particular, the summary execution of eight workers at the garbage dump of José León Suárez was a traumatizing event that helped motivate the rise of a Peronist guerrilla insurgency one decade later.

The transition from a military to a civilian government in 1958 did neither lessen state repression nor cease the violence by the disenfranchised Peronist movement. Striking workers occupied in January 1959 the Lisandro de la Torre meatpacking plant to protest its privatization, and were assaulted with Sherman tanks. Street fighting broke out and the Buenos Aires neighborhood of Mataderos was barricaded in an insurrectional atmosphere. Nationwide repression crushed the willingness to strike, and the major labor unions entered into a pact with the government to negotiate labor disputes and earn fringe benefits for their members.

The March 1965 elections finally allowed the Peronist party to return to Congress but the victory was short-lived as in June 1966 the military took control over the government again. Growing opposition to the Onganía dictatorship from an alliance of Peronist workers and students in 1969 culminated in a series of major street protests. A May 1969 urban insurrection in Córdoba galvanized the widespread resentment against authoritarian rule and heralded years of middle-class protest, large street demonstrations, and the emergence of small guerrilla groups. The summary execution of retired Lieutenant-General Aramburu in 1970 by Peronist guerrillas made the Argentine military step up its repression that included torture, disappearances, and the assassination of 16 guerrillas at the Trelew naval prison in 1972. Reminiscent of the massacre of workers at José León Suárez in 1956, the flux of guerrilla recruits increased and the crowd mobilizations continued unabated. Free elections had become inevitable and resulted in a massive victory for the Peronist party in May 1973. Hundreds of imprisoned insurgents were given amnesty. The astonished Argentine military were now convinced that not due process but the physical annihilation of revolutionaries was the only right response to a future resurgence of guerrilla violence.

Perón made his long-awaited return to Argentina on 20 June 1973. What was to be a celebration became a deadly fire-fight between right-wing and left-wing Peronists in the enormous reception crowd gathered at Ezeiza Airport. The plane carrying Perón was forced to land at Morón air force base instead. Perón assumed the presidency in October 1973 but could not reconcile the increasingly violent factionalism within his political movement or halt the renewed attacks on the armed forces by the Marxist People's Revolutionary Army. His death in July 1974 further increased the political violence. Armed violence took the place of the dwindling street crowds that became altogether forbidden in March 1976 when the military assumed power once again. Tens of thousands of disappearances traumatized the guerrilla organizations and the revolutionary left beyond recovery, and inflicted a national trauma on Argentina during years of state terrorism. Growing labor unrest and human rights protests made the Argentine armed forces embark on the disastrous invasion of the Falkland/Malvinas Islands in April 1982 that ended in a humiliating defeat by a British expeditionary force. A transitional military government assumed power in June 1982 to prepare the country for the October 1983 elections that were won by Raúl Alfonsín.

President Alfonsín faced a society that had been traumatized between 1955 and 1983. A complex violence-trauma-violence dynamic had emerged that consisted of two temporalities. Many events occurred during these three decades that were traumatic in the act because of the violence involved, but certain events were also traumatizing in the sense that they had an afterlife that lead to social trauma. Unlike the traumatic violence that was almost a constant in Argentine society whose linear temporality continued to feed the desire for resistance and repression, the traumatizing events existed in a non-linear temporality of extraordinary significance for the people affected. The June 1955 bombardment of Plaza de Mayo, the 1956 massacre at José León Suárez, the 1970 assassination of Lieutenant-General Aramburu, the 1972 Trelew massacre, and the 1973 amnesty of convicted guerrillas were among the traumatizing events that became social traumas because they infused each other with new meaning as enduring social injuries.

The violence-trauma-violence dynamic unfolded on four levels of social complexity, as the overdetermined impact of the disappearances shows. The disappearances had been intended to create fear and uncertainty among the insurgency in the political domain and intimidate relatives into political paralysis. A social trauma had also been generated on the domestic level by the disruption of family life, the shattering of household ties, and the stigmatization of searching members. Parents felt somehow they had failed their children by not having been able to protect them at the moment of abduction, and thus sensed they had violated the basic trust between parent and child. Grandmothers had similar bonds of attachment to their missing grandchildren and hoped to provide them with the trust and protection that they had been unable to give to their disappeared children (Robben 2005b). Finally, many former abducted captives had been traumatized by their torture and disappearance.

In response to the national concern about the predicament of the disappeared, in December 1983 President Alfonsín created the National Commission on Disappeared Persons (CONADEP) to discover whether or not they were alive somewhere. The truth commission concluded after nine months of painstaking investigations that the disappeared were dead and that forensic anthropologists had discovered several mass graves and anonymous burials in cemeteries throughout the country. The refusal of the military to admit to the disappearances and reveal the whereabouts of the assassinated captives would hold Argentine society hostage for decades and hindered the mourning of national losses.

The Dual Process of Mourning Massive Violent Death

The grief work hypothesis of Freud (1968) and Bowlby (1981) has guided most analyses of national mourning. Confronting a loss, rearranging, and eventually severing the affective tie with the deceased have been regarded as most beneficial for bereaved individuals because the healing benefits of psychological avoidance and repression have been shown to wear off quickly (Shear 2010). The grief work hypothesis became criticized during the last few decades by constructivist approaches in social psychology that questioned the assumption that grief aims at undoing the tie between bereaved and deceased. Instead, constructivists argue that mourners can create a biographical narrative that incorporates memories of the dead in their daily lives. Such meaning reconstruction is essential to the grieving process, especially where violent deaths are concerned (Currier et al. 2006; Neimeyer 2001; Robben 2014; Valentine 2006; Walter 1996, 1999).

The DPM, developed by the social psychologists Stroebe and Schut (1999, 2001), applies sense making not only to the losses of bereaved persons but also to their shattered lives through an oscillation between loss-oriented and restoration-oriented coping processes. Mourners attend intermittently to primary losses that revolve around the bond with the deceased (loss orientation) and pay complimentary attention to secondary losses to deal with life's challenges without the deceased (restoration orientation). These two coping strategies do no occupy mourners permanently because the flow of everyday life provides them with rest and distraction. Also, the term restoration does not refer to a desirable outcome of the oscillating mourning process because each of the two coping strategies contains positive and negative affects, dependent on the death's meaning (Stroebe and Schut 1999:214). Mourning, namely, complementary processes of attending to loss and restoration, may thus be beneficial or harmful for the bereaved person (Stroebe and Schut 2001:66–69). The DPM applies to intrapersonal and interpersonal coping, and accommodates gender and cultural differences. The degree of attention to the two coping processes can vary significantly from person to person, between men and women, and from one culture to another (Stroebe and Schut 1999:218–220, 2010).

The DPM has been designed to address psychological processes of personal bereavement but can also be applied to processes of contested social and national mourning developed in previous work (Robben 2014). The model needs to be adapted of course to the collective level where mourning has other social complexities in which not individuals but a group or society as a whole becomes the bereaved party. I draw therefore an analytical distinction between personal, social, and national mourning. Personal mourning refers to the coping of bereaved individuals. Social mourning involves collective processes and occurs among members of a particular social collectivity, such as a political party, labor union, regiment, ethnic group, human rights organization, or religious congregation. National mourning involves the contested coping with individual or massive death by a heterogeneous collection of state institutions and social collectivities, including those with negative, hostile feelings about the dead, because bereaved societies do not constitute a unified whole of equally affected members. On the contrary, bereaved societies are generally highly divided over the dead, and some sectors may even argue that the deceased are not a cause for mourning but for celebration. National mourning does therefore not require a consensus about how to cope with the dead, how loss and restoration orientation are manifested, and how these coping processes relate to one another or which balance should be struck between them. National mourning occasions a politics of oscillation, namely power struggles about how to cope with the losses and address the restorative challenges. Memory struggles are a common manifestation of the politics of mourning because, as in the case of personal mourning, 'meaning reconstruction in response to a loss is the central process in grieving' (Neimeyer 2001:4; Robben 2014:336–337; Stroebe and Schut 2001).

The search for meaning is particularly pronounced where massive violent deaths are concerned, due to the different involvement of victims, perpetrators, survivors, and bystanders. Parallel loss- and restoration-oriented processes compete for national prominence or even hegemony, and may thus coexist within one bereaved society. Governments often play an influential role in channeling or directing national mourning by promoting historical narratives, taking policy measures, and organizing commemorative rituals that are contested by social collectivities (Butler 2004; Holst-Warhaft 2000; Kwon 2006). Power struggles among competing collectivities and state institutions can be disclosed by focusing on the oscillations between rivaling loss- and restoration-orientated practices.

National loss orientation concentrated in Argentina on the predicament of the disappeared, the exhumation of mass graves, the accountability of perpetrators, and the remembrance of the dead and disappeared. National restoration orientation involved the coexistence of former enemies, the memorialization of past political violence, and the reparation and treatment of tens of thousands of survivors, such as bereaved and searching relatives, torture victims, and exilees. Argentina's emphasis on loss orientation, rather than restoration orientation, resulted from institutional pressures, notably by certain governments and the armed forces, and power struggles with and among social collectivities, especially groups of retired military officers and human rights organizations that brought competing meanings, narratives, and memories to the national mourning process. Although lop-sided, competing loss-oriented coping processes oscillated with contentious restoration-oriented coping processes, and vice versa. The armed forces, successive governments, military interest groups, and human rights organizations tried each to enforce a particular combination of loss and restoration orientation. The conflicting political agendas and ensuing power struggles precipitated a contested national mourning that gave more attention to loss- than restoration-oriented coping practices (Robben 2014:337). The emphasis on the national confrontation with the massive losses of the dictatorship has underplayed national efforts to restore and rebuild the bereaved Argentine society as becomes clear from an analysis of the oscillations of national mourning from 1983 onwards.

Retribution and Remembrance in Argentina

Raúl Alfonsín won the October 1983 elections on a message of truth and justice. This call for truth remained urgent when he assumed the presidency in December 1983 because of persistent rumors about disappeared persons who were still being held captive in secret detention centers. Alfonsín appointed a truth commission comprised of known critics of the military dictatorship, and Congress facilitated the investigation by abrogating the amnesty law which the transitional military government had passed to benefit the armed forces and the guerrilla organizations. The findings by the CONADEP commission could now be passed on to criminal court and make good on Alfonsín's electoral promise to hold the military juntas and commanding officers accountable for state terror (Robben 2005a:319–324).

Alfonsín had misgivings about the desire of the human rights movement to put everyone involved in heinous deeds on trial. Concerned about a backlash that might threaten the budding democracy, Alfonsín proposed to prosecute only high-ranking officers who had ordered the systematic human rights violations, while regarding low-ranked troops as having acted under due obedience. He hoped to let bygones be bygones, institutionalize the armed forces into the Argentine state, and achieve social peace (Giussani 1987:238–240; Malamud-Goti 1990). Alfonsín carefully avoided using the term national reconciliation in order not to suggest that the government wanted victims to forgive the perpetrators. The due obedience proposal became the first dispute between the government and a human rights movement supported by broad layers of Argentine society about the national mourning's loss and restoration orientation toward the country's unrecovered dead.

Alfonsín's social peace agenda failed when the CONADEP commission reported in September 1984 that all disappeared should be presumed dead, with the exception of several hundred kidnapped babies given away to childless military couples. The commission had been able to document 8960 disappeared persons but the human rights movement claimed that around 30,000 people had disappeared (CONADEP 1986:447–449). These findings made the human rights organizations unwilling to make amends with the military and they insisted on retributive justice. Their emphasis on further truth finding into the repression maintained society's attention on the dead and disappeared. The majority of the Argentine people supported the human rights movement's demand to abandon the official restoration-oriented policies until past losses had been dealt with properly and exhaustively. The Alfonsín government redefined its restoration-oriented measures through an oscillatory response. The attention to secondary losses became restricted to removing the administrative legacies of the military regime, reinstating the rule of law, and accepting the truth commission's findings that the disappeared were dead and the armed forces and police their executioners.

Most high-ranking officers disputed the CONADEPs underlying historical narrative. They claimed that the Argentine armed forces had legitimately defended national sovereignty against the revolutionary insurgency, and that numerous disappeared were living abroad (Areas 1984:11). Retired officers held religious masses to honor the 508 dead of the armed and security forces who had been killed between 1960 and 1989 (Díaz Bessone 2001) and encouraged civilian solidarity organizations to organize demonstrations in their support. Despite these manifestations of loss orientation, the social mourning process of the bereaved military was much more oriented toward restoration than that of the searching relatives who demanded truth, justice, and active remembrance of the dead and disappeared. In fact, the transitional military government had already set the tone in April 1983 when it advocated a national remembrance of the state's fallen defenders and the reconstruction of a divided Argentine nation: 'Time has come to face the future: it will be necessary to mitigate the wounds that every war produces, confront a new phase with a Christian spirit, and look toward tomorrow in sincere humility' (Marchesi 2005:180). The restoration-oriented memorialization of past violence became articulated through a historical narrative that presented dictatorial rule as a necessary stage of nation-building during a violent political period of Argentine society influenced by the ideological struggles of the Cold War and fanned by international support from the communist world powers to Argentina's revolutionary insurgency (Robben 2011).

The military's persistence in denying their involvement in the disappearances, and the call for retribution by the human rights movement, held the two opposed groups hostage to each other's memory politics and made them pursue different combinations of loss and restoration orientation. National mourning focused primarily on loss orientation toward the assassinated-disappeared because the human rights organizations were far more influential in Argentine society than the military. This loss orientation was directed to a quest for truth, the recovery of the remains of the disappeared, the prosecution of perpetrators, and a continuous remembrance of the dead and disappeared in street protests, testimonies, a noted media presence, and numerous cultural expressions. The less prominent loss orientation of the military became manifested in religious services to honor their dead, memorial plaques on military premises, and frequent calls for the amnesty of the indicted officers.

National mourning consisted in the mid-1980s of multiple oscillations in which the public loss orientation on the disappeared by the human rights movement was most prominent in Argentine society, while the military losses were hardly given any attention in the news media and the public domain. This politics of oscillation demonstrates the analytical advantage of an anthropological translation of the DPM in understanding national mourning and shows also where national mourning and personal mourning differ. Individual mourning implies a personal adjustment, as Stroebe and Schut (2001:60) argue: 'the [DPM] model describes the necessity of oscillation, that is, a regulatory process, for successful outcome rather than claiming that confrontation is adaptive and avoidance of grief is maladaptive.' National bereavement is not a regulatory process that evolves toward a growing adjustment to the primary losses and secondary changes of the bereaved. Society is not an integrated, unified whole but has a social complexity and social disaccords that entail different social mourning processes and different intra-group oscillations that may enter into conflict with one another and the national state about how and when to mourn the dead.

Restoration-oriented processes received less national attention in Argentina than loss orientation. The human rights movement, the political opposition, and many citizens argued that Argentina could attend neither to the legal and financial problems of persons with disappeared breadwinners nor to the transitional problems of the country's budding democracy before relatives could rebury their missing dead, the armed forces had taken responsibility for the disappearances, and the perpetrators had been convicted. The government maintained, however, that the CONADEP truth commission had transformed the disappeared from being alive yet missing into dead yet unaccounted for. They had become mournable victims of state terror, and the government proposed legislation to normalize their legal status and slowly achieve social peace. These issues divided Argentine society for decades on end. They made loss orientation predominant in national mourning, and efforts at restoration orientation less influential.

The dispute about the exhumation of mass graves in the mid-1980s demonstrated clearly the complexity of the reigning loss orientation, even within the same group. Forensic investigations had been undertaken since December 1983 to provide judicial proof to prosecute the military, to end the uncertainty for the searching relatives, allow them to bury their dead, and get on with their lives. By December 1984, a large faction of the Mothers of the Plaza de Mayo became disgruntled about the ongoing exhumations because they failed to reveal the identity of the executioners and did not lead to criminal convictions. This group of searching mothers accused the Argentine government of deliberately trying to induce grief work to create social peace by loosening the affective ties between relatives and exhumed disappeared. The personal mourning and the reburials would allow bereaved relatives to accept the losses, diminish their political activism, and make them more willing to accept the state's restoration-oriented policies (Robben 2005b). Freud's (1968) and Bowlby's (1981) grief work hypothesis was given a political charge, and was employed to interpret personal and social healing as reactionary means to preserve the political status quo. The mothers argued that their children had disappeared for desiring and pursuing fundamental political change. The inconclusive disappearances generated a political agency among the mothers and turned personal losses into their children's spiritual and ideological rebirth. Memorialization in museums and memory places was therefore unacceptable, unlike an active remembrance in marches and protests. In the same vein, economic compensation for having a disappeared relative was refused as hush money. This dispute about loss orientation caused a division in 1986 between the large Mothers of the Plaza de Mayo Association and the considerably smaller Mothers of the Plaza de Mayo Founding Line.

The Founding Line and most other human rights organizations supported the exhumations, accepted reparation payments, and acknowledged grief work as beneficial. These expressions of loss orientation existed alongside those of the Mothers of de Plaza de Mayo Association, and therefore did not involve an oscillation toward restoration orientation. Furthermore, the reburial of exhumed remains might help personal mourning, as the Founding Line mothers readily admitted, but reburials were also political acts that motivated the bereaved to pursue the prosecution of perpetrators with even more resolve.

The demand for accountability was finally honored when the nine junta members, who had ruled Argentina between 1976 and 1982, were facing court in April 1985. But where the human rights movement considered the trial as the beginning of extensive retributive justice, the government saw it as the end game of transitional justice and a final stage toward the normalization of civil-military relations. Defense Minister Raúl Borrás declared even before court proceedings began that 'the country cannot live forever with an open wound. A final full stop has to be put to this' (Areas 1985:8). Legal advisors to Alfonsín had proposed in 1983 that only a small number of commanding officers should be prosecuted to foster social peace but this restoration orientation was faced time and again with strong public opposition from Argentine society. The conviction of five junta members in December 1985, of whom General Videla and Admiral Massera received life sentences, and the acquittal of four others raised hopes among human rights organizations that hundreds of officers would now also face justice. President Alfonsín, however, feared years of trials that would destabilize the budding democracy, and he successfully submitted to Congress the 1986 Final Stop law that placed a statute of limitations on new indictments, and the 1987 Due Obedience law that freed most officers from prosecution (Robben 2005a:331–335).

The meaning of what constituted an indictable loss was changed by the amnesty legislation because the government and the judiciary created a distinction between, on the one hand, human rights violations carried out in the line of duty for which the junta commanders had already been convicted in place of the material offenders, and, on the other hand, violations executed by perpetrators on their own account, in particular the theft of property, rape, and the kidnapping of babies. The assassinated-disappeared had become transformed into negotiable losses by absolving the actual culprits. Society's right of redress was sacrificed to benefit social peace and democratic consolidation. These political decisions were renewed attempts to reach a compromise of conflicting demands about loss and restoration orientation, and achieve a comprehensive national mourning of Argentina's massive losses. The human rights movement organized massive street demonstrations in opposition but this time

President Alfonsín prevailed because of congressional support for his halt to retributive justice.

President Carlos Saúl Menem, Alfonsín's successor, stayed the course on social peace. He pardoned hundreds of military officers and former guerrillas in October 1989, and proposed even to release the convicted junta commanders 'to heal without more ado the bleeding wound of the Argentine body' (Pisani 1990:7). Massive protest marches were organized by the human rights movement, and 63 % of the respondents in a November 1990 opinion poll opposed the anticipated measure (Anonymous 1990). In December 1990, Menem signed the presidential pardon and also implemented reparation payments for the victims of state terrorism so that they could get on with their lives. Former political prisoners received compensation payments in 1992, and the indemnification for a disappeared relative was established in 1994 at $224,000. By 2004, eight thousand claims had been approved.

President Menem's policy shift from a coping orientation on loss to one on restoration was certainly successful. The military had been appeased, many relatives of the disappeared had accepted compensation payments, and the human rights movement was largely silenced as can be inferred from the absence of major street protests during the early 1990s. The human rights movement was swept up in the prevailing mood of the times and shifted from a hitherto dominant loss orientation through active remembrance to a restoration-oriented concern for memorialization. Fearing oblivion, it tried to turn its historical narrative of state terrorism, systematic disappearances, and crimes against humanity into the hegemonic national memory. Unlike remembrance, which is a loss-oriented narrative practice, memorialization is restoration oriented because, as Young (1993:5) has observed about Holocaust memorials: 'For once we assign monumental form to memory, we have to some degree divested ourselves of the obligation to remember. In shouldering the memory work, monuments may relieve viewers of their memory burden.' Memorialization impressed on Argentine society the historical truth of state terror and disappearance, and provided searching relatives with a new identity as bereaved relatives who might not have mourned their personal losses in the absence of identified remains and mortuary rituals but at least had assumed the collective losses and accompanied the oscillations in the social mourning process.

A shock went through Argentine society when in March 1995 retired navy captain Adolfo Francisco Scilingo revealed that he had participated in death flights during which sedated captives were thrown from planes into the South Atlantic Ocean (Verbitsky 1995). The flights had already been mentioned in the truth commission report and former disappeared had testified about their existence but now a perpetrator had confessed to this gruesome practice, and at a time when the public contestation about the past had dwindled. Scilingo's confession brought into the open that the various players of national mourning continued to maintain radically different meanings about these deaths. The bereaved relatives realized that they would never be able to recover the remains of their loved ones. The military considered the dead to be irredeemable subversives who deserved their spiritual fate, while the human rights movement regarded Scilingo's revelations as undeniable proof of state terror and the most persuasive argument for accountability. Argentine society was once again struggling with the national mourning of its massive losses.

Afraid that more perpetrators would come forward and in support of President Menem's threatened social peace agenda, the commanders of the three armed forces admitted in April 1995 to the mistakes of their institutions during the dictatorship. Army Commander Balza was heavily criticized by 70 retired generals who continued to defend the repression. This open conflict among the Argentine military came to a burst in June 1998 when General Balza declared that the armed forces had used a standard operating procedure for separating guerrillas from their children and handing them to childless military couples. The Grandmothers of the Plaza de Mayo had been investigating these child thefts for two decades and helped indict adoptive parents. Balza's declaration implied that these kidnappings could no longer be classified as individual acts beyond due obedience but were an integral part of the criminal plan of abductions and disappearances for which the junta leaders had been convicted. General Videla was arrested on kidnapping charges on 9 June 1998 and extradition requests were issued to detain commanders living abroad.

The public clamor about the missing children upset the government's peace agenda and exposed its reluctance to investigate the whereabouts of its abducted citizens, whether disappeared or kidnapped. Possibly, the consecutive governments feared that an official, proactive search for these children would be a constant reminder of the past's unresolved issues and entail an enduring loss orientation in the public domain. The Alfonsín government did establish a National Genetic Data Bank in May 1987 but the search for the children was entirely left to the Grandmothers of the Plaza de Mayo. Only in December 1998 did the Argentine government provide financial support through the Historical Reparation Fund. By May 2015, 116 children had been located.

Argentina's attention became again focused on its massive deaths by Videla's and Massera's detention on kidnapping charges, and created a favorable political climate for a nationwide memorialization of the past. In July 1998, a Memory Park was founded in Buenos Aires along the banks of the River Plate to create a symbolic connection to the disappeared thrown alive into the Atlantic Ocean during the death flights. The day of the military coup d'état, 24 March, became an official Day of Memory in Buenos Aires in 2001 and a national holiday in 2006. The Buenos Aires city legislature created in December 2002 the Space for Memory Institute (Instituto Espacio para la Memoria) for 'the preservation and transmission of the memory and history' of state terrorism, and to 'promote the strengthening of the democratic system, the consolidation of human rights, and the prevalence of the values of life, liberty, and human dignity' (Careaga 2009:110). By 2009, there were already around 200 memory sites in Buenos Aires city alone as signs of state terror in the public landscape, and dozens have been added since (Memoria Abierta 2009). These sites of memory revealed a restorative coping with the massive disappearances by incorporating the dead and disappeared into people's daily lives.

The enhanced restoration-oriented memorialization oscillated in a reinforcing way with a loss-oriented prosecution of perpetrators. The 1998 arrest of General Videla encouraged the human rights movement to pursue actively the derogation of the amnesty laws and presidential pardons of the late1980s. This initiative caused substantial unrest among the military and made them eager to ease the public call for accountability. Army commander Brinzoni proposed in mid-2000 to organize a round table dialog among members of the armed forces and human rights organizations to resolve the issue of the disappeared and achieve national pacification. Similar talks had begun a year earlier in Chile as a reconciliatory gesture toward the raised animosities because of the October 1998 arrest of former dictator Pinochet in London. But Argentina was not Chile, where consecutive governments had successfully pursued a national reconciliation agenda, despite the opposition of a small human rights movement (Robben 2014). The entire Argentine human rights movement was unwilling to negotiate with the military.

A federal judge declared in March 2001 that the 1986 and 1987 amnesty legislation was unconstitutional, but it required the proactive stance of President Néstor Kirchner, elected in 2003, to accelerate the slow derogation process. Kirchner resurrected Alfonsín's 1983 electoral promise of truth, justice, and normalized civil-military relations in an effort to bring about social peace: 'I want a united Argentina, I want a normal Argentina, and I want us to be a serious country but, furthermore, a more just country' (Kirchner 2003). He made a clean break with the past by retiring the 44 highest-ranked officers, and declaring on 7 July 2003: 'It was painful that we Argentines came face to face, but we must find a point of reunion [*reencuentro*] that helps us overcome this sad history,' and added that 'the reunion cannot come from silence or complicity' (Cibeira 2003). Kirchner meant that social peace could only be achieved through accountability, and placed the military before a difficult choice: either swallow the derogation of amnesties and pardons or be prepared to be extradited to Spain for their involvement in the disappearance of Spanish citizens living in Argentina during the dictatorship. Meanwhile, President Kirchner was able to turn the Supreme Court to his hand by appointing politically loyal judges, and he encouraged Congress to revoke the amnesty legislation. The Supreme Court derogated the amnesty laws in June 2005 and ruled in April 2007 that the presidential pardons had been unconstitutional. In January 2016, 660 defendants had been convicted (many received 25 years to life imprisonment), 60 accused had been acquitted, and 851 accused were still under indictment. There were 58 fugitives from justice (Procuraduría de Crímenes contra la Humanidad 2016:8).

Kirchner's resolve to bring hundreds of perpetrators to justice had surpassed a similar loss orientation of the Alfonsín government by far but, instead of distinguishing degrees of responsibility to avoid tensions in civil-military relations, Kirchner invested in a complementary restoration orientation. He encouraged the memorialization of state terror by steering the course of national mourning toward a more even balance of loss and restoration orientation, combining retributive justice with national memory politics.

Genocide and Collective Guilt

The human rights trials began in 2006. Retired Police Commissioner-General Miguel Osvaldo Etchecolatz was the first to appear in court, and his conviction to life imprisonment for six homicides and eight disappearances reverberated beyond the court room in La Plata when Judge Carlos Alberto Rozanski sentenced him on 19 September 2006 for 'human rights violations committed in the framework of a genocide that had taken place in the Argentine Republic between 1976 and 1983' (Rozanski et al. 2006:101). Rozanski commented later that 'here, a part of a national group was persecuted and annihilated. This defines the genocidal perpetrator: the one who decides to annihilate' (Pertot 2006). His verdict was ratified by the Supreme Court in March 2009.

The term genocide was not undisputed. Judge Martín Lozada (2008:73–75) argued that the legal qualification genocide did not apply because the disappeared had not constituted a clearly defined group and were not assassinated as members of a group but targeted because of individual political convictions. The psychologist Vezzetti (2003:154–164) stated that the Argentine victims were persecuted and killed for what they did and what they thought, while Holocaust victims had been massacred for who they were. Furthermore, whereas the industrial genocide of the Jews rested on a bureaucratic rationality and a banality of evil, as Lozada and Vezzetti argued, Argentina's state terrorism had been inspired by sociopolitical vengeance and ideological volition. The scholarly debate failed to influence the human rights movement because it was eager to prosecute everyone tainted by the dictatorship that could be charged with crimes without a statute of limitations (Robben 2012). Finally, the defense lawyers of the accused Etchecolatz had dismissed the genocide charge, arguing that Argentina had been involved in a war against subversive terrorists who tried to impose a totalitarian regime on Argentina, and that a constitutional government had ordered the armed forces in October 1975 to annihilate the guerrilla insurgency (Ramos Padilla 2006).

Judge Rozanski had based his argumentation on the 1946 United Nations resolution that condemned the destruction of any group as genocide; the 1985 conviction of the five junta commanders for their systematic plan of extermination; a 1998 ruling of Spanish judge Garzón; and the scholarly argument about an Argentine genocide by sociologist Feierstein (Rozanski et al. 2006:88–94). Spanish judge Baltasar Garzón had written a legal opinion in 1998 that genocide had indeed taken place in Argentina when the military decided to eliminate a national group that was contrary to the country's Western, Christian culture (Roht-Arriaza 2005:47). This interpretation was given a conceptual foundation by Argentine scholars. The human rights lawyer Mántaras (2005:68) argued that the Argentine military had organized a genocidal infrastructure to exterminate not a pre-existing but an emerging national group of opponents to their economic plan, while Feierstein (2008:26) compared Nazi Germany and Argentina in terms of ideological, structural, and processual similarities. Both regimes employed genocidal social practices to annihilate particular groups. Argentina's national group consisted of guerrilla combatants and the members of revolutionary social movements (Feierstein 2006:150).

The category shift from state terrorism, the term used most often by the human rights movement, to genocide implied also a change in the loss orientation of national mourning and hindered oscillations with restoration orientation as not the adjustment of Argentine society to its past violent divisions but the focus on the loss of lives stood central in national mourning. The national trauma continued to preoccupy Argentina as genocide became the interpretive frame of memorialization. The public confrontation between proponents and opponents of the military dictatorship hardened, and questions were raised about a collective responsibility for the political violence of the 1970s. Not just the military were held responsible for the regime of torture, disappearance, and assassination but the term genocide implied a complicity of Argentine society as a whole.

This conceptual reframing of past violence and trauma, as well as the explicit comparison with the Holocaust, has been casting collective responsibilities that implicate many Argentines in the dictatorial repression and are complicating psychosocial healing. 'Representations of the past ... structure strategic interaction between adversaries. They open—and foreclose—opportunities for the peaceful resolution of disputes. The menu of choices available to victims and survivors—from reconciliation to revenge—is filtered through representations of the past' (Meierhenrich 2006:320). Genocide makes psychosocial healing much harder than war crimes or even crimes against humanity because an armed conflict between military and insurgents carries a certain war logic missing from the indiscriminate extermination of people. According to Ricoeur (2006:473), 'There is no punishment appropriate for a disproportionate crime. In this sense, a crime of this sort constitutes a de facto instance of the unforgivable.' Whereas state terrorism confined the massive violence to the military and made junta members and commanding officers individually accountable, the term genocide implies the complicity of most Argentines through active support or passive acceptance.

The adoption of the genocide frame by the human rights movement, certain politicians, journalists, lawyers, and judges has been heightening the social tensions in Argentina. In December 2009, legal evidence was stolen from the human rights secretariat of Buenos Aires province. In July 2010, a military solidarity organization posted hundreds of names and addresses of trial witnesses on the Internet, accompanied by the message: 'Know the names of the terrorists and their addresses: They could be your neighbors and teachers and approach you as friends … They live among us.'[1]

In April 2010, Hebe de Bonafini of the Mothers of the Plaza de Mayo Association condemned three newspapers, two publishers, and seven journalists during a political-ethical trial at the Plaza de Mayo for 'having exploited the people, allowing that people were killed and tortured, and that the horror was silenced' (Anonymous 2010). In July, three judges from Mendoza were denounced before a disciplinary tribunal for not having investigated disappearances, assassinations, and denunciations about torture and sexual abuse during the dictatorship. Aside from members of the press and the judiciary, the list of suspects might be extended to building contractors, real estate agents, food suppliers, transportation firms, and other companies as businessmen profited from commercial activities with military administrators at all levels of government. The director of the Cordoban human rights office, Luis Miguel Baronetto, shares this observation: 'The magnitude of the genocide would not have been possible without the approval and applause of hegemonic sectors of Cordoban society: businessmen, members of the judiciary and Church, politicians, academics, and unionists who have not yet been tried or convicted' (Baronetto 2010).

Conclusion

Successive Argentine governments, the armed forces, human rights organizations, and military interest groups have been enwrapped for decades in discursive, political, legal, and memory disputes about how to cope with the massive violent deaths suffered during the 1976–83 dictatorship. Loss orientation prevailed over restoration orientation in the national mourning of Argentine society during 1983–90 and after 1998, whereas multiple efforts were made between 1987 and 1998 to attend to secondary losses. Amnesties, pardons, and due obedience legislation were attempts at social peace that faced strong oppositional forces within Argentine society that opted for truth finding, retributive justice, and active remembrance alongside restoration-oriented memorialization rather than reparations and restorative justice. Retribution has therefore been so tenaciously pursued by Argentine human rights organizations because a legal arbiter weighs the scales of truth and justice, and settles in court what cannot be agreed upon in public. The 2003 Kirchner government understood this contested coping dynamic well and achieved a more balanced loss- and restoration-oriented national mourning by a policy of vigorous prosecution and sustained memorialization. The sentencing of perpetrators for genocide since 2006 has shifted this balance again to loss orientation as a collective guilt descended over Argentine society, demonstrating that trials offer only temporary solutions to deeper political conflicts.

This chapter has argued that the national mourning of tens of thousands of people who were assassinated and disappeared in Argentina during the dictatorship did not only revolve around the meaning, memory, and ties of the dead, as the grief work hypothesis would have it, but that such loss orientation was complemented by a restoration orientation toward the reconstitution of the post-conflict society. I have conceptualized national mourning as a power struggle among governments, human rights organizations, armed forces, bereaved relatives, and military interest groups about the oscillation of loss-oriented and restoration-oriented coping processes.

Argentine national mourning attended between 1983 and 1990 principally to primary losses through exhumations, truth finding, retributive justice, active remembrance, and periods of intense public protests by an active human rights movement. Reconciliatory initiatives by the 1987–1998 governments had mixed success. Adversarial groups refused to enter into dialog, while reparation and memorialization were only slowly accepted. Amnesty laws and presidential pardons had to be tolerated because of the reigning distribution of power in Argentina but were eventually overturned by periodic pressure from human rights organizations. This contestation bore fruit in 1998 with the detention of pardoned military commanders. This chapter has shown that loss and restoration orientation have co-existed in Argentina. Argentina's emphasis on remembrance and retributive justice was interspersed by policies of social peace. The arrest of former junta members Videla and Massera in 1998 caused important shifts toward loss orientation to cope with the primary losses of massive violent death. This seemingly sudden change can be attributed to a politics of oscillation that matured over years of opposition to the dominant distribution of loss and restoration orientation. Argentina's Kirchner government consolidated in 2003 this oscillatory shift with the prosecution of perpetrators. Retributive justice and memorialization became government policies in 2003 and moved toward collective guilt in the mid-2000s because of the adoption of genocide as a competing frame of interpretation next to state terrorism and crimes against humanity. Increasingly more social groups and sectors were blamed for the past violence, and they were held accountable in street protests, publications, films, memory sites, and trials. The accused retaliated with public counterprotests, the intimidation of witnesses, and the theft of legal evidence, and have even been charged with several disappearances. Collective guilt is assuming the place of individual guilt, thus diluting the responsibilities of perpetrators to the entire society and making psychosocial healing a greater challenge.

My analysis does not imply a value judgment about the national mourning of past massive deaths by Argentine society, nor does it draw any conclusion about which measures of loss and restoration are desirable for a post-conflict society. Every society has the sovereign right to judge its past and its perpetrators in the ways it sees fit. But what this analysis of Argentina does indicate is that an overemphasis on restoration-oriented reconciliation hurts people's sense of justice and moral beliefs, while a predominant attention to loss-oriented retribution loses sight of people's inevitable coexistence in a bereaved society.

Acknowledgments I thank Vigdis Broch-Due, Bjørn Enge Bertelsen, and Margit Ystanes for inviting me to the stimulating conference in Bergen. I am indebted to them, and also to Nicolas Argenti and Carol Kidron for their insightful comments.

Note

1. Originally available at: http://presospoliticosargentina-archivo.blogspot.com/2010_07_01_archive.html. Accessed 23 August 2010; hard copy in author's possession.

References

Abierta, Memoria. 2009. *Memorias en la ciudad: Señales del terrorismo de estado en Buenos Aires*. Buenos Aires: EUDEBA.

Alexander, J.C. 2012. *Trauma: A Social Theory*. Cambridge: Polity Press.

Anonymous. 2010a. Bonafini hizo su 'juicio ético' a la prensa a ahora irá por los jueces. *Clarín*, April 30. http://edant.clarin.com/diario/2010/04/30/elpais/p-02189640.html. Accessed 2 August 2016.

———. 2010b. El indulto no tiene hinchada. *Página/12*, November 21.

Areas, T. 1984. El shock de 'Nunca más'. *Somos* 8(408): 6–11.

———. 1985. Apuesta a la conciliación. *Somos* 8(447): 8–14.

Baronetto, L.M. 2010. Juicio al fin. *Página/12*, July 3. http://www.pagina12.com.ar/diario/elpais/subnotas/148778-47774-2010-07-03.html. Accessed 2 August 2016.

Bowlby, J. 1981. *Attachment and Loss, Vol. 3. Loss: Sadness and Depression*. Harmondsworth: Penguin.

Butler, J. 2004. *Precarious Life: The Powers of Mourning and Violence*. London: Verso.

Careaga, A.M. 2009. *Leyes: principales instrumentos legales sobre derechos humanos y memoria*, 2nd edn. Buenos Aires: Instituto Espacio para la Memoria.

Cháves, G.L. 2005. *La masacre de Plaza de Mayo*. La Plata: De la Campana.

Cibeira, F. 2003. Hay que separar la paja del trigo. *Página/12*, July 8. http://www.pagina12.com.ar/diario/elpais/1-22457-2003-07-08.html. Accessed 2 August 2016.

CONADEP. 1986. *Nunca Más: The Report of the Argentine National Commission on the Disappeared*. New York: Farrar Straus Giroux.

Currier, J.M., J.M. Holland, and R.A. Neimeyer. 2006. Sense-Making, Grief, and the Experience of Violent Loss: Toward a Mediational Model. *Death Studies* 30: 403–428.

Díaz Bessone, R.G. ed. 2001. *In Memoriam*, 3 vols. Buenos Aires: Círculo Militar.

Fassin, D., and R. Rechtman. 2009. *The Empire of Trauma: An Inquiry into the Condition of Victimhood*. Princeton, NJ: Princeton University Press.

Feierstein, D. 2006. Political Violence in Argentina and Its Genocidal Characteristics. *Journal of Genocide Research* 8(2): 149–168.

———. 2008. *El genocidio como práctica social: entre el nazismo y la experiencia argentina*. Buenos Aires: Fondo de Cultura Económica.

Freud, S. 1968 [1917]. Mourning and Melancholia. In *The Standard Edition of the Complete Psychological Works of Sigmund Freud*, 7. ed. J. Strachey, 243–258. London: Hogarth Press.

Giussani, P. 1987. *¿Por qué, doctor Alfonsín?* Buenos Aires: Sudamericana/Planeta.

Hinton, D.E., and A.L. Hinton, eds. 2014. *Genocide and Mass Violence: Memory, Symptom, and Recovery*. Durham, NC: Duke University Press.

Holst-Warhaft, G. 2000. *The Cue for Passion: Grief and Its Political Uses*. Cambridge: Harvard University Press.

Kirchner, N. 2003. *Discurso del Señor Presidente de la Nación, Doctor Néstor Kirchner, ante la Honorable Asamblea Legislativa*, May 25, http://nuevamayoria.com/ES/BIBLIOTECA/documentos/discurso_kirchner.pdf. Accessed 15 Jan 2010.

Kirmayer, L.J., R. Lemelson, and M. Barad, eds. 2007. *Understanding Trauma: Integrating Biological, Clinical, and Cultural Perspectives*. Cambridge: Cambridge University Press.

Kleinman, A. 1999. Experience and Its Moral Modes: Culture, Human Conditions, and Disorder. In *The Tanner Lectures on Human Values*, ed. G.B. Peterson, 355–420. Salt Lake City: University of Utah Press.

Kleinman, A., and J. Kleinman. 1991. Suffering and Its Professional Transformations: Toward an Ethnography of Experience. *Culture, Medicine and Psychiatry* 15(3): 275–301.
Kwon, H. 2006. *After the Massacre: Commemoration and Consolation in Ha My and My Lai*. Berkeley: University of California Press.
Lozada, M. 2008. *Sobre el genocidio. El crimen fundamental*. Buenos Aires: Capital Intelectual.
Malamud-Goti, J. 1990. Transitional Governments in the Breach: Why Punish State Criminals? *Human Rights Quarterly* 12: 1–16.
Mántaras, M. 2005. *Genocidio en Argentina*. Buenos Aires: Autores Editores.
Marchesi, A. 2005. Vencedores vencidos: las respuestas militares frente a los informes 'Nunca Más' en el Cono Sur. In *Memorias militares sobre la represión en el Cono Sur: visiones en disputa en dictadura y democracia*, eds. E. Hershberg and F. Agüero, 175–210. Madrid: Siglo Veintiuno de España Editores.
Martín-Baró, I. 1989. Political Violence and War as Causes of Psychosocial Trauma in El Salvador. *International Journal of Mental Health* 18(1): 3–20.
Meierhenrich, J. 2006. A Question of Guilt. *Ratio Juris* 19(3): 314–342.
Neimeyer, R.A. 2001. Meaning Reconstruction and Loss. In *Meaning Reconstruction and the Experience of Loss*, ed. R.A. Neimeyer, 1–9. Washington, DC: American Psychological Association.
Pertot, W. 2006. El juicio fue la suma de la historia. *Página/12*, October 1. http://www.pagina12.com.ar/diario/elpais/1-73818-2006-10-01.html. Accessed 2 August 2016.
Pisani, S. 1990. Instó Menem a una definitiva reconciliación. *La Nación*, June 17.
Potash, R.A. 1980. *The Army and Politics in Argentina, 1945–1962: Perón to Frondizi*. London: The Athlone Press.
Procuraduría de Crímenes contra la Humanidad. 2016. *El estado de las causas por delitos de lesa humanidad en Argentina. Balance y desafíos*. Buenos Aires: Ministerio Público Fiscal.
Ramos Padilla, J.M. 2006. *Chicha. La fundadora de Abuelas de Plaza de Mayo*. Buenos Aires: Editorial Dunken.
Ricoeur, P. 2006. *Memory, History, Forgetting*. Chicago, IL: University of Chicago Press.
Robben, A.C.G.M. 2005a. *Political Violence and Trauma in Argentina*. Philadelphia: University of Pennsylvania Press.
———. 2005b. How Traumatized Societies Remember: The Aftermath of Argentina's Dirty War. *Cultural Critique* 59: 120–164.
———. 2011. Silence, Denial and Confession about State Terror by the Argentine Military. In *Violence Expressed: An Anthropological Approach*, eds. M. Six-Hohenbalken and N. Weiss, 169–186. Farnham: Ashgate.
———. 2012. From Dirty War to Genocide: Argentina's Resistance to National Reconciliation. *Memory Studies* 5(3): 305–315.

———. 2014. Massive Violent Death and Contested National Mourning in Post-Authoritarian Chile and Argentina: A Sociocultural Application of the Dual Process Model. *Death Studies* 38: 335–345.

Robben, A.C.G.M., and M.M. Suárez-Orozco, eds. 2000. *Cultures Under Siege: Collective Violence and Trauma*. Cambridge: Cambridge University Press.

Roht-Arriaza, N. 2005. *The Pinochet Effect: Transnational Justice in the Age of Human Rights*. Philadelphia: University of Pennsylvania Press.

Shear, M.K. 2010. Exploring the Role of Experiential Avoidance from the Perspective of Attachment Theory and the Dual Process Model. *Omegai* 61: 357–369.

Stroebe, M., and H. Schut. 1999. The Dual Process Model of Coping with Bereavement: Rationale and Description. *Death Studies* 23: 197–224.

———. 2001. Meaning Making in the Dual Process Model of Coping with Bereavement. In *Meaning Reconstruction and the Experience of Loss*, ed. R.A. Neimeyer, 55–73. Washington, DC: American Psychological Association.

———. 2010. The Dual Process Model of Coping with Bereavement: A Decade on. *Omega* 61: 273–289.

Torre, J.C., and L. de Riz. 1993. Argentina Since 1946. In *Argentina Since Independence*, ed. L. Bethel, 243–363. Cambridge: Cambridge University Press.

Valentine, C. 2006. Academic Constructions of Bereavement. *Mortality* 11: 57–78.

Verbitsky, H. 1995. *El vuelo*. Buenos Aires: Planeta.

Vezzetti, H. 2003. *Pasado y Presente: Guerra, dictadura y sociedad en la Argentina*. Buenos Aires: Siglo Veintiuno Editores.

Walter, T. 1996. A New Model of Grief: Bereavement and Biography. *Mortality* 1: 7–25.

———. 1999. *On Bereavement: The Culture of Grief*. Buckingham: Open University Press.

Young, J.E. 1993. *The Texture of Memory: Holocaust Memorials and Meaning*. New Haven, CT: Yale University Press.

CHAPTER 5

Organizing Norwegian Psychiatry: Security as a Colonizing Regime

Inger Lise Teig

Introduction

The terrorist attack of 22 July 2011 shocked the Norwegian nation.[1] For most Norwegians the attack was unexpected. What threatened to become a national trauma was quite successfully brought within the language and legal procedures of democratic society. The terrorist event, however, exposed some essential dilemmas of psychiatric treatment regimes that had not formerly been brought into public debate in Norway. The terrorist court case pointed to some limitations of the diagnostic apparatus' approach to the question of the terrorist's rationale and his possible mental disorder. The court case exposed how medical, moral, and political aspects were intertwined in the classification of the terrorist act and the terrorist's mental state.

This chapter focuses on certain critical events preceding the terrorist attack and the subsequent court case in 2012. The chapter does not analyse the Breivik case but focuses on some developments and tensions in psychiatry that were exposed by this case. The purpose of this chapter is to demonstrate how psychiatry—as a social system of practice—is a domain that is becoming more critical in the current risk society. We could even

I.L. Teig (✉)
Department of Global Health and Primary Health Care, University of Bergen, Bergen, Norway

V. Broch-Due, B.E. Bertelsen (eds.), *Violent Reverberations*,
DOI 10.1007/978-3-319-39049-9_5

regard current transformations of psychiatric treatment regimes as diagnostic of crucial social processes linked to securitization, risk, accountability, and managerialism (see also Teig 2015). Trauma—as an unpredicted and uncontrolled violent event—occupies a central defining role, as the unthinkable and impossible risk.

The Breivik case upset the assumed security of daily life and exposed a generalized need to achieve control. The event also exposed controversies within the field of forensic psychiatry, more specifically concerning the risk aspect of mental illness and the treatment regime for the most seriously ill. Within the field of Western contemporary psychiatry, the protection of the public from potentially dangerous patients is a recurrent concern. Forensic psychiatric services face a particular challenge in attaining the right balance between patient rights and safety for other patients, staff, and the public (Urheim et al. 2011:41). The linking of psychiatric illness to security and risk has been analysed as a reshaping of both the management of mental health and of rationalities and strategies of control (Rose 1996, 1998, 2002). Western societies are becoming increasingly preoccupied with risk; thus, there are more attempts to control troubling or unpredictable people, traits usually associated with the mentally disordered. Giddens (1991) describes modernity as a juggernaut inducing anxiety that threatens our 'ontological security'. In this chapter, 'ontological security' is analysed in the light of what Smith refers to as the 'sequestration of experience'. By this, she means the removal from social life those experiences and events that demand our *moral* attention (Smith 2002). The moral and existential questions associated with madness—what it *is*, its continuum with normality, and how to best enable re-integration for 'the mad'—*disturb* the taken-for-granted security of our lives and produce the sequestration of specific experiences associated with madness.

This chapter analyses the 'sequestration of experience' that encourages the establishment of certain abstract systems within the current regimes of psychiatric treatment. Specified and rigid routines, managerial risk modules, and clinical guidelines for professional work are established with the intention of delivering trust and security for the general population, framed within discourses of individual rights and transparency. Media discourses systematically portray the psychiatric patient 'as a danger for the public', and the discourses of security scandals, irregular episodes, danger, and trauma contribute to produce changes in the organization of psychiatric treatment. The case described here shows that the considerations that interfere in the treatment practices of mental patients have increasingly less to do with medical knowledge and more with organizational and social considerations. The notion of 'security' has become central within the legal framework of health care, in mass-media discourses, as well as in a concrete institution of Norway. The chapter draws attention to the correlation between a pronounced and increasing managerialism in psychiatric institutions, society's preoccupation with risk, and the consequent reductive localization of danger in the individual patient.

Sources of Data

The chapter builds on organizational ethnography the author conducted from 2006 to 2008 at a large public psychiatric hospital.[2] This hospital had then recently been merged with several university psychiatric clinics and local district psychiatric centres and organized as an autonomous hospital division given a wider budgetary responsibility. The material is based on ethnographic research gathered through participant observation between spring 2006 and autumn 2007 and 32 semi-structured interviews with clinical workers (mainly psychiatrists), administrators, and managers of the hospital, with follow-up interviews during 2008 and 2009. The interviews followed an interview guide with a list of themes and questions, partly common for all the interviewees, but also individually adjusted to the specific organizational situation for the person in question. The ethnographer participated in senior management meetings, clinical meetings, seminars, courses, and daily events and talked with clinical staff (psychiatrists, nurses, and other health professionals), administrators, and managers throughout 16 months, two to three days a week. Notes were made at all events, meetings, and seminars. Field techniques were semi-structured interviews, observations, and analyses of internal documents. A systematic classification of newspaper articles concerning the hospital was done using the media archive search tool Retriever. The electronic version of two local newspapers with the search query of the name of the hospital for the years 2006 to 2008 was used with the secondary search queries of 'escapes' and 'irregular episodes' in combination with the name of the hospital.

Selection, data collection, and analysis were carried out in accordance with a 'situational analysis' approach that put weight on the event (the situation). This ethnographic method emphasizes that the event or situation is never merely illustrative or a gimmick of a theory but has its own particularity that operates in a social order that integrates macro dynamics into its micro practices (Kapferer 2005). The data generation was performed by studying actors and their roles in a particular incident and then tracing these actors through other incidents and in this way, I could link the varied incidents to one another in order to identify the structural contradictions and the resolving mechanisms in the social order. By scrutinizing particular situations, especially conflicts, as complexes of connected incidents that occur in the field, one can identify the mechanisms underlying the development of the situation ('the event'). The event brings its elements together in a unique way that potentially contains transformative possibilities. In order to achieve any form of anthropological explanation and understanding of an event (Evens and Handelman 2005, 2006; Kapferer 2005), we must attend to the understanding that micro dynamics are integral within larger processes.[3] This analysis of sequences of events over quite a long period where the same actors were involved in a series of different situations enabled me to trace how events chain on to others and how they were linked to one another over time (cf. Mitchell 1983). Van Velsen emphasizes the strengths of the extended-case perspective, arguing '[...] when several or most of the actors in the author's case material appear again and again in different situations, the inclusion of such data should reduce the chance of cases becoming merely apt illustrations' (Van Velsen 1979:140). Likewise, I use the extended case method to investigate how episodes revealed the actual formation of practices that were linked to other situations over time. The empirical descriptions of practices that are extended out of the local situation displayed the very formation of a new regime of management taking place in a society and fuelled by a complex range of processes at different scales.

The Risky Patient and the Organizational Context

In Norway, the processes of de-institutionalization of the psychiatric health services started in the 1970s and the 'total institutions' were gradually reduced to institutions directed more towards shorter stays and to treatment rather than 'storage'. This de-institutionalization was a movement away from 'an institutionally based system of segregative control', as Scull (1977:64)[4] from the UK also has noted. The local district psychiatric centres were established in the early 1980s and were thought of as more localized, accessible, and differentiated mental health services. The establishment of these centres parallels the development of community psychiatry in other Western countries and of the establishment of community mental health centres (Busfield 1986; Rhodes 1991). The number of beds[5] in the hospitals was at its highest in 1973 with 13,000, and it was reduced to 5000 beds in 2005 (Dullum 2007:97). Treatment services that used to be the responsibility of the hospitals, such as long-term care, nursing work, practical training for patients, were now defined as primarily municipal and the responsibility was assigned to local centres or general practitioners. The empowerment of the patient evolved as an important objective and governmental value, and the turning towards individual needs and rights became manifest in mental health politics from the late 1990s (Norvoll 2002:140). A governmental reform programme—the *Mental Health Care Action Plan*[6]—was implemented in 1999 in order to strengthen the de-institutionalization process and to improve the coordination between the hospitals and local psychiatric centres. The transfer of patients to these local centres in the mid-80s was part of a non-hierarchical model for psychiatric health care. The idea was that the patient herself should become an expert. Patients who had committed violent or deadly acts represented a challenge to this model of patient autonomy. This patient group was evidently seen as a threat to the public. The general perception of psychiatric patients in general as a threat has increasingly been publically expressed, as by a local politician in a local newspaper: 'It is unthinkable that psychiatric patients should have a more liberal situation than inmates in prisons'. However, as several psychiatrists reported in in-depth interviews, the patient group in general was fairly comparable with the group of patients from earlier periods, and the character of the patient group had not changed since the 1990s. The patients did not present a greater risk for community than earlier, as Urheim et al. (2011) have reported.[7] It is thus difficult to predict which patients are most prone to violence and almost impossible to identify in advance those capable of extreme violence. Even though the prevailing view among clinicians indicates a clear relation between practicing less punishment and the reduction of risky situations, the need to restrict the autonomy of the mentally ill in general dominated among *non*-clinicians, as illustrated by the politician above.

Whether the psychiatric patient was a danger per se for general society or not was a major factor in the organizing of health care services of the hospital in the present case. Rose refers to the UK and argues that there has been a change in the language, from dangerousness to that of risk when referring to psychiatric patients. He claims that madness has always been associated with danger and unpredictability but that the discursive change from dangerousness to risk in the 1990s points to a transformation in understanding and responding to mental health problems (Rose 2002:211). This material demonstrates that the questions of security and public safety became increasingly important to the hospital's organization and treatment. The increased demand for protection of the general population reoriented the focus to risk and security procedures.

Escapes as Producer of Social Trauma

Throughout its long history, the hospital of the present case regularly experienced episodes of patient escape,[8] but the majority of the escapes were quite innocent, according to reports from hospital workers. Incidents that were categorized as 'escapes' involved patients who had misunderstood the plans for their treatment, disagreed with the treatment plans, missed the bus back, or wished to prolong their leave. These episodes were seen as irregular episodes that were mainly unproblematic but still undesirable for the hospital. The routine was to report every 'escape' (that is unplanned absence) to the local police, regardless of the medical condition of the patient. The police consequently started searching for the missing patient. During my period of observation, a few escapes became deeply problematic as they resulted in traumatic social and personal events. In public debates and media coverage, these episodes were presented as symptoms of serious organizational problems and mismanagement that exposed a hospital in crisis. The incidents were commented upon by involved actors, politicians, and readers, and they sparked a public debate about safety routines of the hospital and about the public risk posed by psychiatric patients in general. Editorials and letters to the newspapers portrayed a 'regime of fear',[9] referring to the internal organizational conditions and the lack of security for the public (the societal consequences of organizational problems). The picture drawn up by this media discourse presented a wide public mistrust of an allegedly mismanaged hospital and of professional workers who lacked the competence to handle dangerous patients. The condensed timeline in Table 5.1 (see also Appendix below) intends to give an impression of the major headlines that figured in the media from the start of the upheavals until 'peace is restored'.

The course of the events was submitted to a public investigation by the Board of Health Supervision in order to find who was to blame, how internal practices could be improved, and how similar occurrences could be avoided in the future. 'This is about our trustworthiness as a psychiatric hospital; we can't handle any more such cases now', one of the senior

Table 5.1 Timeline of the incidents

2006
20 February—Maximum security unit in crisis (news article)
08 April—Patient attacked a health worker and escaped (news report)
22 July—Investigating the hospital (news report)
24 July—Third time he escaped. Accused for murder (34), was categorized as 'not presumed escaping' (news article)
30 July—The ticking bombs (headline for several news articles)
30 July—How dangerous are they really? (news article)
01 September—Chief psychiatrist is called on the carpet (news article)
20 September—Wants to make a stop of the escapes (news report)
22 December—Another escape from the NN [the hospital] yesterday evening (news report)
2007
02 January—The fog of the hospital (chronicle by health worker)
14 January—What will people think? (chronicle by clinician)
16 February—Misplaced patients at the NN [the hospital]. Should have been discharged long ago (news article)
23 May—Thirty-nine captured in the NN [the hospital]-trap (news report)
13 October—Trial on labour legislation is the only way out (reader's letter)
14 November—The NN [the hospital] workers oppose the 'regime of fear' (news article)
2008
16 May—The NN [the hospital] rejects the accusations (news article)
23 May—We did not receive a warning from the health worker (news article)
08 July—Considers to submit an appeal in the whistle blower case (news case)
09 July—Hope to restore peace at the NN [the hospital] (editorial)

managers stated in a meeting partly dedicated to these media cases. 'We must concentrate much more on safety from now on', another manager replied. Internal organizational conditions were revealed to the 'outside world' and the hospital's security policy, security routines, managerial practices, professional judgements, and the very trust of the hospital were questioned in public. The security policy of the psychiatric hospital quickly became a central issue in the local election campaign. A local political party was created and local politicians were mobilized by different actors to advocate for a new mental health policy based upon a more restrictive security regime.

These claims were not unanimous, however; there were large groups of clinical workers who spoke in favour of the specific low-punitive treatment regime of the hospital and worried less about security aspects of the hospital and the alleged risk posed by psychiatric patients. Many refused to characterize the situation as a crisis or as a 'regime of fear' and argued against this in news commentaries and reader's letters. The situation quickly became tense with different groups of actors who deeply disagreed about the situation for the mental health sector in general and for this hospital in particular.

Before analysing how the events challenged the taken-for-granted sense of security of the general population, I present local accounts of what 'really happened' in this period of crisis.

Event 1: A Presumed Medical Misjudgement

One of the episodes that were publicly described involved serious human injuries after an alleged medical misjudgement of a patient's medical condition. Newspapers and non-medical commentators blamed the hospital for not preventing such an episode. The hospital and the individual health worker involved in the treatment of the patient were accused of being unable to predict whether the patient was dangerous and posed a threat to anyone. There was a public call to the hospital to take action in the sense of organizational procedures and professional responsibility. Clinicians described this episode as a tragic event and disagreed on the medical misjudgement argument as the outsiders used. They explained the event as caused by the increased claims for earlier discharges and the lack of available beds. One psychiatrist who once had been accused of medical misjudgement explained how a public exposure might establish its own logic in the understanding of difficult episodes related to the organizing and treating of patients; she said:

> The press is far more negative than before. I know that our hospital has had meetings with journalists trying to inform them about the way we work and what psychiatry is. I think we thought that we could use the press to make visible important angles of our work and the field of psychiatry. But still … This case uncovered [the case of human injuries after an escape] that the press writes whatever it likes. I have heard people here say that it does not matter what we do. Trying to have an influence upon any cases, we just have to answer questions properly without saying 'no comment'—these last words will also make things worse. It was scary how my case appeared in the media. My world was in a way created anew through the press; I started to think in the terms it was presented. I was sure we had done everything right, in medical terms, but when I was confronted with different episodes and so on, I suddenly did not recognize it. I had been told not to say 'no comment' [by the director], because even this might be used in a negative

> way. Thus, I tried to answer as confidently as possible. So I wanted to give the true version, but even then I was accused of breaching professional confidentiality. But everything had been exposed in the press, and I couldn't separate the different versions. And this deeply upsets me. As I said, the newspapers created my reality as well, and I felt helpless, like I was losing control of myself. I tried to hide myself and was afraid of being recognised when I walked outside my home. It is strange; everything that I thought had been right and thoroughly done suddenly changed, and I became doubtful about things that had been so clear for me. I was naïve, I can see it now. But I still think there is a new global trend for scandalising everything. (senior manager, psychiatrist, interview)

This story describes a dramatic change in the psychiatrist's perception of her own medical judgements. She articulates how her understandings of her own previous medical judgements were transformed in line with how the press presented the same facts. She successively perceived and understood her own story in light of an increased personal responsibility or a reinforced discourse of individual responsibility, security, and rights. She became accountable to the public as her alleged failure of expertise posed a threat to public safety. The public enquiry is described as quasi-legal process where she is explicitly made answerable for her professional judgements and practices. Later in the interview she claimed:

> Further on I would be extremely aware of everything, including all the routines that we often take for granted, but also every details of my medical reports and how things are presented. (senior manager, psychiatrist, interview)

In her reflections, we can see that there is a noticeable turn towards an almost legalistic attention to her own clinical and administrative practices. This turning towards a more individual 'responsibilization' process that we observe here has also been described by Rose (1996, 1998, 2002) as occurring in the health sector in the UK. Rose argues that in the British mental health hospital system the psychiatrist must reflect upon his/her medical decision making regarding the discharge of a patient into the community from the perspective of one who may need to defend the decision in some public tribunal in the future. He depicts the reflections that a psychiatrist must go through:

> [...] were all relevant factors taken into account; were there sound reasons for the decision that can be adduced and justified; would any other competent professional in the same position have made a better decision; would other colleagues consider the decision-making process as meeting standards of good practice? (Rose 2002:222)

Thorough awareness of all relevant factors, also non-medical ones, in a medical judgement process seems to be a relevant description of the situation for professionals at the hospital of this study as well, as the psychiatrist expressed above. Her story clearly revealed a professional's (and a senior manager's) anticipation of being held publicly accountable when failure of expertise occurred, or as in this story, when failure of expertise *was claimed to occur*. We may suggest that the psychiatrist's own perspective was altered in the aftermath of the episode because of her placement as a professional within the nexus of management requirements, individualized responsibility, and general expectations of trust and public safety. The enwrapping of professional judgements within this external and non-clinical logic remained unresolved for the psychiatrist, but as a psychiatrist *and* a senior manager, she became the focal point in this nexus and was thus held accountable for the episode.

Event 2: An Escape

When another irregular episode suddenly occurred one late afternoon, the local newspaper dramatically announced that a potentially dangerous patient had managed to escape from the psychiatric hospital during a trip with some nurses:

> No traces of NN. The police is still searching for the convicted NN who escaped from the psychiatric hospital yesterday evening. [...] He is considered dangerous, and people who see him should not approach him directly but call the police [...]. (Excerpt from a news article after the escape of a security patient)

The police moved quickly out looking for him. The escape received huge attention in the local newspapers while the patient was on the run, and the local newspapers continuously reported every details of the event. Police agents quickly found the patient and brought him back to the hospital without further incidence. The episode became a significant component of the critiques (from the press, from supervisory authorities, and from employees) against the hospital's poor safety routines, the lack of secure 'storage' of patients, and the 'unsuccessful management' of the hospital. One of the senior managers (and also a psychiatrist) was held partly responsible for the escape, and he was advised by the press to reconsider his position. The health workers' understanding and description of the episode were, however, far different from the chaotic picture presented by the press. One of the psychiatrists who was most affected by this episode described the situation in an interview some weeks after:

> This was not a very dramatic event. He [the patient] was never a threat to anyone when he was on the run. But it surely was an inconvenient situation. And you know what? he came to me when they had returned him and apologised to me for causing so much fuss. In the aftermath of this event, the newspapers were in contact with me asking how they could write about this incident. I said to them that I thought it would be a wrong decision to write much about this since the focus upon the particular patient would not be good. Patients don't need this kind of attention, both because of what the patient has done, but also because it leads ordinary people to perceive the patient more as a threat. This patient has already experienced situations of mistrust and anxiety during his leaves. But what the people outside the hospital don't seem to understand is that our patients are not dangerous for everyone at all times, always. This is our problem as well; we don't have unequivocal guidelines for every leave; the leaves are granted upon medical judgements, not on standardized regulations. Our judgements are obviously disputed on other grounds than the medical, and this is very difficult. The question of risk is perceived differently by us than by people outside, and this makes things complicated, as this case has demonstrated.
>
> He further claimed that the treatment situation could become difficult if the focus continued to be on the danger and risk of psychiatric patients. 'Maybe the fences will be rebuilt in the bitter end', he reflected, pointing to what he saw as an unfortunate situation for the patients if they would be subjected to a more restricted regime of treatment with less possibilities for leaves. He added that he had been asked by the press to retire from his position. He laughed, saying that this is a question they keep asking a private sector manager. 'But this is not for us in our world', he concluded. He explained this by saying that the considerations of the danger or risk of a patient is part of medical judgement they keep making every day. 'We must be held responsible for our medical judgements, and this is not about having a position or not. The professional gaze is the most important gaze, whatever happens.' (senior manager, psychiatrist, interview)

As we see here, this psychiatrist's version of the escape episode differs naturally from the one described by the press. Health workers in hospitals are bound by the professional secrecy norm and have difficulties providing the official version with precise details of a specific medical case. This duty of confidentiality explains why significant information about the episode was not publically communicated. However, the huge differences between the accounts of the episode are more likely caused by the actors' entanglement in different discourses. In the news discourse, the presentation of the escape of an allegedly dangerous patient demonstrated a hospital in crisis, with failing security routines. This escape story contributes to the portrayal of the hospital as a poorly managed institution. The psychiatrist's description, on the other hand, situates him as a professional insisting that the principles of medical practice have primacy over accountability to outer bodies or actors 'in the public sphere'. In his description of the event, he opposed the attempts to reshape medical judgments within the logic of public security and risk handling. The psychiatrist described the public outcry for more security as a threat to the ideal therapeutic climate of the patients, and he opposed the moral outcry and sensationalism by refusing to resign. He emphasized his medical responsibility but refused to be held individually accountable to non-professionals. The public calls for more rigorous internal routines, and demands for a more trustworthy hospital, were nonetheless claims that the professionals and managers had to adjust to.

Formations of a Crisis

The irregular episodes intensified public attention towards the hospital for a long period. The press kept up pressure by repeating that it was a huge crisis for the hospital and a threat to the public. The director appealed to the professionals to 'stand together upholding the reputation of our hospital'. Given the situation of an institution that regularly had experienced irregular episodes, there were complex reasons why the above outlined episodes were produced as an overall organizational crisis. Ordinary organizational and managerial procedures proved inadequate to prevent the crisis from running as deep as it did. Power argues that by its nature, reputation embeds a potential unmanageability, and reputation has come to be seen as both at risk and at the limits of conventional management control (2007:129). Power further states '[…] reputation has been described as a new management "paradigm" […] Concerns with reputation have existed [...] a long time. [...] it is the rise of concerns with the reputation of organizations which has come to the fore since the mid-1990s' (Power 2007:130). During the observations, the hospital's reputation had attained an increased significance and was reinforced due to the events and the allegedly lack of security precautions of the hospital. While walking in the corridors at the hospital during this period, health workers frequently confided that they were embarrassed to tell anyone that they worked at this particular hospital. At the same time, they expressed anger and irritation about the biased and negative image that had been publicly presented of their workplace. One of the nurses elaborated this point in an interview some weeks after one of the episodes. She said that employees had been requested by the senior management to think thoroughly about how they spoke of the hospital in non-institutional settings. She was deeply sympathetic to this demand, as she felt resentful of the exposure of her workplace. She had worked at the hospital for 20 years and always felt proud of her work, but now, she said, she felt that everyone outside—for instance, on the bus—could tell from looking at her where she was working. She described her feelings as 'almost paranoia'. Being a clinical worker at a short-term department, she was also deeply worried for the patients because they felt stigmatized and compromised by the negative public attention: 'The saddest thing in this is that the patients are spoken of as dangerous, but they are not'.

The media attention became an important reason for changing organizational routines of patient administration and instigating more security regulations, such as locking more doors, reducing the possibilities for exit, and more restrictions in granting permissions. These reorganizational actions were taken primarily on the basis of a fear of decreasing reputational status of the hospital and fostered by the public discourse about danger and risk associated with psychiatric patients. These were not based on clinical reports or medical needs. The significance of reputation for their daily work can be summed up in the word of one of the senior managers and a psychiatrist in an interview:

> As a manager, I have to convince the staff that the management actually takes the needed responsibility. Unfortunately, the opposite is portrayed in the newspapers these days, and I fear that the staff here eventually will take that for a fact. In many ways, the media creates the truth. People will soon think that the hospital does not work or that we are not doing anything good here, even though we actually do a lot of good work.

The psychiatrist's reflection addressed what Power has called the imperative of managing reputation: '[...] internal governance of the enterprise must become explicitly more outward facing and more formal; the new roles, procedures, and strategies [...] constitute an organizational face for public evaluation' (Power 2007:135). It is the concern with the outside that stands out as significant in the psychiatrist's reflections. The management's concern with the hospital's reputation has contributed to reframing institutional practices, which in turn have consequences for the treatment practices.

Rose (1996) describes a case of a recently discharged psychiatric patient who killed a person in UK in late 1992 and the huge publicity this case attracted. Mr. Clunis (the patient) had been considered fit for discharge by the responsible psychiatrists, but the follow-ups after the discharge failed and Mr. Clunis committed the crime. An official inquiry was initiated and the failure of the mental health system was striking; Mr. Clunis appeared as much a victim of the mental health system as the young man he killed. The mental health services and the psychiatry as such appeared to have failed to cure and to take responsibility for both individual care and social protection (Rose 1996:3). The case led to calls of different kinds: More funds for community care, more emergency beds in hospitals, and more effective planning of discharges. Rose argues that the case of Mr. Clunis describes how new responsibilities and political expectations upon the professionals subjugate professional within a risk logic and a '[...] culture of blame, in which almost any unfortunate event becomes a "tragedy" which could have been avoided and for which some authority is to be held culpable' (Rose 1996:4). Risk and security become a value in their own right.

The calls for structural reorganization and new regulations of the mental health services that the Clunis case produced have similarities with what followed the public attention of the irregular episodes at the hospital of my study. The public attention became influential insofar as the professionals' obligations were redirected into prediction and security matters. The professionals were increasingly held responsible for predicting risk in order to protect the general community from dangerous persons. The failure of individual clinicians to cope with risk prediction resulted in the establishment of control procedures and routines that held professionals individually accountable for the trust in the hospital.

Inadequate organizational procedures for handling irregular episodes and the public discourses of crisis, trust, and risk in the aftermath made the situation for the hospital of my study quite difficult, as described here.

What constituted the series of events and the ensuing organizational process as a crisis were not the events 'in themselves' but the framework of (legalized) individualized responsible leadership, the regime of control and sanctions, and discourses of rights, danger, and trust that the actors were entangled in. As we have seen, the crisis event ran deeply into the hospital organization, not because the events of irregular episodes threatened the stability of the organization, but rather because the mental health workers' professional practices were significantly shaped and performed under 'the shadow of the law' (Rose 2002:222). In order to avoid irregular episodes from reoccurring, health workers and managers were reoriented into the administration of risk and reputation. Professionals' pivotal focus in handling patients seemed to be an achievement of a '[...] secure containment of risk' (Rose 2002:218). The management's strategies of handling the crisis events described in this chapter addressed issues of trust rather than medical practices and judgments. The problem of predicting and preventing risk in clinical practices was revealed, and 'madness' as the core of this problem of prediction became '[...] emblematic of the threat to the community' (Rose 2002:232) by an institution which was allegedly in need of stable and reliable management in order to prevent failure from occurring. The management and the individual professional were entangled in public discourses of security and crisis, and this became obvious when they failed to prevent 'threats to the community' from occurring.

Rights Discourses Colonizing Moral Considerations

The Minister of Health holds the overall responsibility for Norwegian hospitals. However, during the upheavals following the irregular episodes at the hospital, the Minister of Justice took the responsibility for the crisis and stated to the press that he found it very important to stop every patient escape from Norwegian psychiatric hospitals. Consequently, the Ministry of Justice initiated a committee to report on the procedures for handling patients convicted of crimes and who are mentally unsuited for imprisonment. The report concluded that patients unsuited for imprisonment should be legally sentenced to two months of compulsory psychiatric treatment at a psychiatric hospital.[10] The conclusion answered the psychiatric legal question clearly but did not propose concrete solutions to the general issue of escapes from psychiatric institutions.

Several professionals reacted negatively to this proposal. They argued that psychiatric patients should be kept outside the penal system and that it would be very unfortunate to criminalize this group of patients. 'These persons are the health care system's responsibility, preferably under compulsion and not by the use of the legal court system', some of them claimed to the press.[11] Power (2007:172) emphasizes that '[...] legalization is becoming a significant mode of reputational risk management' in both private and public organizations. By giving manifest attention to the legal aspects of escapes, the Minister of Justice contributed to the formalistic and legalistic reformation of psychiatric treatment. This legalistic aspect is also emphasized by the fact that it was the Minister of Justice and *not* the Minister of Health who addressed the problem of patient escapes. This governmental act exemplifies what Smith has argued: '[...] ethical codes and law have increasingly come to govern the sites where moral thinking might be expected to hold sway' (Smith 2002:60). Discretion is part of professionals' responsibility of choosing adequate therapeutic means in order to deal with the complexity of the patient's individual health situation. When the committee suggested to strengthen the legal sanctions against a specific group of psychiatric patients, rights discourses contributed to 'colonize' moral professional thinking. Rights and legal codes were thus foregrounded in place of professional discretion and ethical professional codes.

Conclusion

This chapter has described how several irregular episodes during a certain period at a Norwegian psychiatric hospital came to be constituted as critical events, within a discourse of organizational crisis. It was not the episodes in themselves but how they were framed within a nexus of managerialism, discourses of rights, risk, and security that constituted the events as a crisis that was hard to handle for the people involved. It was not a crisis in the sense that organizational operations broke down, that treatment could not be performed, or that professionals were not cooperating. The notion of 'risk' and the 'sequestration of experience' of mental illness has led to the establishment of specified and rigid routines, managerial risk modules, and clinical guidelines for professional work. The episodes were configured or formatted into a larger public discourse of a hospital in crisis, creating a social trauma and threatening public security. The reason why these episodes came to have such consequences for the hospital's internal organization was that they interacted with and reinforced a new regime of individualized responsibility, security, and risk handling. Managerial and abstract systems were established in order to remove or 'sequestrate' the potential moral and social threatening aspects of mental illness.

I have explored how episodes affected the treatment and even the conceptualization of the psychiatric patient through the management of the psychiatric hospital and through the work and perceptions of professional work. I argue that the managerial reactions were largely responses to the outsiders' call for general security and risk management rather than professional medical judgements or requests. When the professional health workers and the hospital as a public institution failed to protect the local community from dangerous psychiatric patients escaping, as we have seen in this case, both the legitimacy of the professionals' judgements and the trust in the hospital came under attack. The professional judgement, based on diagnosis, prognosis, and constantly reviewed treatment plans, became disputed and mistrusted by outsiders. The professionals became answerable to other criteria than medical ones and were subjected to acute and public demands of efficient risk handling, transparency, and safeguarding of public security; the 'outside has been brought in' (cf. Power 2007:139) in a more powerful way. The treatment of patients was recast into an administrative management of risk in the sense of preventing 'madness' from becoming a trauma for the individual himself, the health worker, and the general population. Security became an important part of the treatment regime directly through stricter organizational routines and professional practices. What Rose calls 'the logic of prediction' (Rose 1996:16) has replaced the 'logic of diagnosis' in the sense that principles other than medically defined principles became central in the definition and organization of the treatment services of the hospital. Instead of purely medical considerations, 'folk models' about certain types of mental illness forced themselves upon the therapeutic contexts and lead to changes in the way the hospital was organized and the way it treated patients. Sustaining public trust in the management of the hospital and in the professionals was contingent upon whether and how risky episodes could be avoided.

As pointed out above, demands for more information about internal routines, better coordination between different institutional levels, development of tighter professional standards or codes of conduct, and more meticulous reports and inspections were proposed and instigated by lay people outside the hospital, by clinical workers, and by governmental actors. These demands were not seeking total surveillance of professionals but were imposed upon seemingly free professionals who were nonetheless held accountable for the consequences of 'failed' judgements, 'failed' decisions, and 'failed' organizational arrangements. What was critical in this period was the intriguing part of contemporary (risk) management: '[A] pervasive fear of the possible negative consequences of being responsible and answerable, of being required to produce decidability in the face of the undecidable' (Power 2007:203). Management of health professionals materializes as a critical practice insofar as decisive decisions could still produce unexpected consequences due to the lack of total control over the unforeseen.

The 'objects' of psychiatry will probably never be completely predictable, and this may, within the current dominant logic of risk and security, lead to a stronger use of coercive means in treatment practices. Violent acts are difficult to prevent and predict, also when it comes to psychiatric patients' future acts. The reformulation of psychiatric treatment practices within a security discourse has contributed to essentializing psychiatric patients in general as risky and violent individuals. This reemphasizing of control and security matters gradually risks secluding the psychiatric patient ('the risky individual') away from society, a 'sequestration' of mental illness that disturbs our sense of control quite contrary to the intentions in governmental plans of empowerment and 'decarceration' of this specific patient group. In seeking total control over these patients, we risk trampling over the autonomy and human rights of individuals who are in a deeply vulnerable position.

Appendix: A Chronological Timeline of Headlines of Local Newspapers

2006

Maximum-security unit in crisis—February 20 (news article)
Insurrection at the NN [the hospital]—February 20 (head news title)
Praises the working environment—February 21 (news article)
Health with muzzle—February 21 (editorial)
The truth about the NN [the hospital]—February 25 (editorial)
The NN [the hospital] is rebuked after the suicide of a mother—March 18 (news article)
The hospitals are silent—March 18 (news report)
The responsibility slips away after discharge—March 18 (news report)

Threatening to cut up doctor—March 21 (news report)
Psychiatric health worker ran amok—April 5 (news report)
Inmate attacked a health worker and escaped—April 8 (news report)
Eighteen-year-old will be sentenced for violence against nurse—April 11 (news report)
Was killed by knife while daughter (10) was in the house—July 22 (news article)
Investigating the hospital—July 22 (news report)
Does not separate security patients from other patients—July 23 (news article)
Third time he escaped. Accused for murder (34) was categorised as 'not presumed escaping'—July 24 (news article)
Have to introduce separate psychiatric prisons—July 24 (news article)
Impossible guarantees—July 25 (editorial)
Strange that the hospital didn't ask for guard—July 25 (news article)
This must never happen again—July 25 (news article)
The family of the victim requires an investigation of the routines—July 25 (news report)
For the society's best—July 28 (reader's letter)
The ticking bombs—July 30 (headline including several news articles)
How dangerous are they really?—July 30 (news article)
Do not know what triggered the murder—August 1 (news article)
Patient sentenced for murder threatened LL [health professional]—August 3 (news article)
Armed patient sent alone in taxi—August 10 (news article)
Asked armed patient to take a taxi to the NN [the hospital]—August 10 (news report)
Won five years struggle against the NN [the hospital]—August 16 (news article about a former patient)
Required to take a leave, claim compensation—August 21 (news article)
The police warn against dangerous murderer (33)—August 22 (news article)
I will return—August 22 (news report citing a patient)
The police: Should have been spared for this—August 22 (news article about the affected family)
Family hides from escaped murderer—August 23 (news report)
The convicted murderer jumped over the fences—August 23 (news report)
Crime and punishment—August 23 (editorial)
The Health Supervision investigates the case—August 23 (news report)
Is watched over day and night—August 23 (news report)

What is it with the NN [the hospital]?—August 24 (chronicle)
Mistook inmate for member of staff—August 24 (news report)
We have done too bad work—August 29 (news report)
The police are upset about chief psychiatrist violating the professional secrecy—August 31 (news article)
The NN [the health enterprise] will not answer—August 31 (news report)
The family is shocked—August 31 (news report)
Chief psychiatrist is called on the carpet—September 1 (news article)
About danger within psychiatry—September 4 (chronicle by patient)
The maximum security unit at the NN [the hospital]—September 4 (reader's letter from clinicians)
The NN [the hospital]-workers beaten up by inmate—September 8 (news report)
Wants to make a stop of the escapes—September 20 (news report about the Minister of Law's intentions)
Raped at the NN [the hospital]—September 20 (news article)
The NN [the hospital] gets harsh critique—December 21 (news report)
The NN [the hospital] promises to put things straight—December 21 (news report)
Another escape from the NN [the hospital] yesterday evening—December 22 (news report)
The hospital admits harsh critique—December 22 (news article)

2007

The fog of the hospital—January 2 (chronicle by health worker)
The NN [the hospital]—a destructive hospital—January 3 (reader's letter)
Less fog at the NN [the hospital]—January 3 (chronicle by clinicians)
What will people think?—January 14 (chronicle by clinician)
This was a very unlucky mistake—January 30 (news article)
I am not dangerous to the public—February 3 (news article citing the patient)
Surely people react, but they do not know me—February 3 (news article)
The maximum-security unit—February 3 (News article)
Delicate TT [political party] conflict about the NN [the hospital]—February 13 (news report)
RR [local politician] withdraws from TT [political party]—February 14 (news article about political consequences of the upheavals at the hospital)

Misplaced patients at the NN [the hospital]. Should have been discharged long ago—February 16 (news article)
Foreign experts will investigate the NN [the hospital]—February 28 (news article)
This is how they will heal the NN [the hospital]—March 8 (news article)
Patient convicted for murder (29) escaped from the NN [the hospital]—March 8 (news report)
Psychiatric patients suffer more than enough and should not be wrongly exposed by the media—March 26 (reader's letter from a patient)
Talks about the MM [a specific case]-murder for the first time—April 16 (news article)
Cannot explain why he killed—April 17 (news article)
Still day fines at the NN [the hospital]—April 17 (news article)
He could not deal with intimacy—April 20 (news article)
Happy day for NN [the hospital]—April 24 (news article)
Action plan approved and day fines stopped—April 24 (news article about organizational steps)
The PP's [press agency] psychiatry coverage—April 30 (reader's letter)
Relief after sentence of murder—May 4 (news article)
Prisoners become more dangerous under strict regimes—May 21 (news article)
Thirty-nine captured in the NN [the hospital]-trap—May 23 (news report)
Health workers at the NN [the hospital] were reported [to the police] for breaching the professional secrecy'—July 5 (news report)
The NN [the health enterprise] is taken to court—September 10 (news article)
Whistle blowers lost their job—October 8 (news report)
The NN [the hospital] receives a giant fine because of corridor patients—October 2 (news report)
Trial on labour legislation is the only way out—October 13 (reader's letter)
FF [a minister] interferes in the case of whistle blowing—October 14 (news article)
Ambiguous about whistle blowing—October 15 (news report)
Time to make a diagnosis of the NN [the hospital]—October 19 (reader's letter)
The NN [the hospital]-workers oppose the 'regime of fear'—November 14 (news article)

The press stigmatizes the entire hospital—November 15 (news report)
Muzzle on staff—December 15 (chronicle)
Professional terminology: restructuring. The truth: destroying—December 21 (reader's letter, patient)
Heroes and troublemakers—December 22 (editorial)
New political party born out of the hospital troubles—December 23 (news article)

2008

I'm about to die, I thought—March 16 (news article citing a health worker)
The hospital's fines are cancelled—May 7 (news article)
The NN [the hospital] rejects the accusations—May 16 (news article)
The assumed whistle blowing was vague—May 20 (news article)
Claims that the management threatened with police report—May 22 (news article)
We did not receive a warning from the health worker—May 23 (news article citing the management)
Claimed that it was safe to make a warning—May 27 (news article)
I am deeply disappointed—July 8 (news article citing the whistle blower)
Considers submitting an appeal in the whistle blower case—July 8 (news article)
Hope to restore peace at the NN [the hospital]—July 9 (editorial)

Notes

1. I thank all participants in the workshop 'Reassessing Trauma and Violence: Reframing the Bodily, the Spoken and the Self' for insightful comments and helpful advices. I am also deeply grateful to Kjetil Fosshagen, who has read, discussed, contributed insights to the argument, and offered encouragement for this work.
2. The psychiatric hospital is a separate division in a local health enterprise. The Norwegian specialist hospital services (somatic and psychiatric) were reorganized into five regional health enterprises and numerous local health enterprises in 2002, as a result of a large-scale reform in 2001. The ownership was transferred from counties to the central state.

3. The ethnographic extended-case or situational analysis (both terms refer to the methodology associated with Gluckman) is an ethnographic method developed by the British anthropologist Max Gluckman at the Manchester School of Social Anthropology. Gluckman proposed through this method to trace the relationship between the general and analytical statements through the dynamic particularity of the case. The empirical investigation of particular situations of conflict was one of Gluckman's strong ideas in order to identify mechanisms underlying the conflict. He argued that by taking the actors and their roles in any particular incident and tracing these actors through other incidents, one could link the varied incidents to one another and identify the mechanisms operating in the relevant social order (Evens and Handelman 2006). For Gluckman, it was in the event and the situation the suggestions for analysis were to be found, and the event or situation was never merely illustrative or a gimmick (Kapferer 2005). The idea was to scrutinize particular situations, especially conflicts, as complexes of connected incidents that were occurring in the field, in order to isolate and identify the actual mechanisms that were underlying the development of the situation/the conflict. The concept of the situation as crisis demands an understanding that micro dynamics are always integral within macro forces.
4. In Scull's description of this transition, it is not a move from mental hospital care to community care but from segregation in the asylum to neglect and misery within the community. He argues that the main reason for this new policy in the UK was economic considerations. He introduced the concept of 'decarceration' to denote that 'segregative modes of social control became, in relative terms, far more costly and difficult to justify' (Scull in Busfield 1986:328). This kind of economy-based argument is reflected in the statements from some of the psychiatrists in this study when speaking critically about the de-institutional process of moving patients out of the hospitals.
5. Similar to what Jones and Sidebotham (1998:7) describe, it is also a normal practice in Norwegian psychiatric hospitals to refer to patient numbers in terms of 'beds', even though the fact is that most patients are ambulant.
6. The Mental Health Care Action Plan 1998–2008 [*Opptrappingsplanen for psykiatri*] was proposed in 1997 as the latest plan in the process of de-institutionalization. The Plan was

based upon the white paper no. 25 (prop. no. 25 1996–1997) Openness and entirety: About psychiatric illnesses and health services. In 2006, the Mental Health Care Action Plan was extended two years, until 2008, due to the necessity for more time to implement municipal arrangements, such as housing facilities, etc.

7. The method for measuring risk and potential acts of violence is based on the clinical instrument of HCR-20 among others.
8. Escapes from psychiatric hospitals are normal incidents, as also Strauss et al. (1964/1981) describe from a large American state mental hospital in the 1960s. They describe how escapes happened quite frequently.
9. The title is from an article in the local newspaper that critically debates the situation at the hospital.
10. See the Governmental Report no. 48, 2008; the Mæland Report.
11. http://www.dagensmedisin.no/nyheter/2008/11/28/vil-tvangsinnlegge-plagsomme-personer/ (accessed May 25, 2012). See also the view from The Norwegian Medical Association http://www.legeforeningen.no/id/168011.0 (accessed May 25, 2013).

References

Busfield, J. 1986. *Managing Madness. Changing Ideas and Practice*. London: Hutchinson.

Dullum, J. 2007. Fra oppbevaring til risikohåndtering? Om nedbygging av de psykiatriske institusjonene. [From storage to risk handling. About the de-institutionalization process of the mental health institutions] Ph.D. thesis, University of Oslo.

Evens, T.M.S., and D. Handelman. 2005. The Ethnographic Praxis of the Theory of Practice. *Social Analysis* 49(3): 1–11.

———, eds. 2006. *The Manchester School: Practice and Ethnographic Praxis in Anthropology*. New York: Berghahn Books.

Giddens, A. 1991. *Modernity and Self-Identity*. Cambridge: Polity Press.

Jones, K., and R. Sidebotham. 1998. *Mental Hospitals at Work*. London: Routledge.

Kapferer, B. 2005. Situations, Crisis, and the Anthropology of the Concrete: The Contribution of Max Gluckman. *Social Analysis* 49(3): 85–122.

Mitchell, J. C. 1983. Case and Situational Analysis. *Sociological Review* 31(2): 187–211.

Norvoll, R., ed. 2002. *Samfunn og psykiske lidelser. Samfunnsvitenskapelige perspektiver—en introduksjon [Society and mental illnesses. Perspectives from social sciences—an introduction]*. Oslo: Gyldendal.

Power, M. 2007. *Organized Uncertainty. Designing a World of Risk Management.* Oxford: Oxford University Press.

Rhodes, L.A. 1991. *Emptying Beds. The Work of an Emergency Psychiatric Unit.* Berkeley: University of California Press.

Rose, N. 1996. *Inventing Our Selves.* Cambridge: Cambridge University Press.

———. 1998. Governing Risky Individuals: The Role of Psychiatry in New Regimes of Control. *Psychiatry Psychology and Law* 5(2): 177—195.

———. 2002. At Risk of Madness. In *Embracing Risk. The Changing Culture of Insurance and Responsibility*, eds. T. Baker and J. Simon. Chicago, IL: The University of Chicago Press.

Scull, A.T. 1977. *Decarceration: Community Treatment and the Deviant: A Radical View*. Englewood Cliffs, NJ: Prentice-Hall.

Smith, C. 2002. The Sequestration of Experience: Rights Talk and Moral Thinking in 'Late Modernity'. *Sociology* 36(1): 43–66.

Strauss, A., L. Schatzman, R. Bucher, D. Ehrlich, and M. Sabshin. 1964/1981. *Psychiatric Ideologies and Institutions.* New Brunswick, NJ: Transaction Books.

Teig, I.L. 2015. The Formation of 'Managementhood' in a Psychiatric Hospital. *Dialectical Anthropology* 39(1): 1–25.

Urheim, R., K. Rypdal, T. Palmstierna, and A. Mykletun. 2011. Patient Autonomy Versus Risk Management: A Case Study of Change in a High Security Forensic Psychiatric Ward. *International Journal of Forensic Mental Health* 10: 41–51.

Van Velsen, J. 1979 [1967]. The Extended Case Method. In *The Craft of Social Anthropology*, ed. A. Epstein, 129–152. Oxford: Pergamon.

Other Sources

Governmental Report no. 48, 2008; the Mæland Report.

http://www.dagensmedisin.no/nyheter/vil-tvangsinnlegge-plagsomme-personer/ http://www.legeforeningen.no/id/168011.0

http://www.ba.no/nyheter/article2301555.ece

http://www.regjeringen.no/en/dep/jd/pressesenter/pressemeldinger/2008/nye-tiltak-overfor-visse-utilregnelige-1.html?id=509410

http://www.bt.no/nyheter/lokalt/--Vi-har-gjort-for-daarlig-jobb-1814091.html

http://www.bt.no/nyheter/lokalt/Varslere-i-nytt-parti-1871135.htm

Law of April 28, 1961, no. 2. Lov om psykisk helsevern [law on mental health].

Law of June 19, 1969, no. 57. Lov om sykehus [law on hospital].

Law of July 2, 1999, no. 61. Lov om spesialisthelsetjenesten m.m. [law on specialist health care].

———, 1999a, no. 62. Lov om etablering og gjennomføring av psykisk helsevern [law on establishing and implementation of mental health].

———, 1999b, no. 63. Lov om pasientrettigheter [law on patient rights].

Law of June 15, 2001, no. 93. Lov om helseforetak [law on health enterprises].

Prop. to the Odelsting no. 48 (1997–1998). *Om lov om endringer i sykehusloven og i lov om psykisk helsevern* [*law about changes in the hospital law and in the mental health law*].

Prop. to the Odelsting no. 66 (2000–2001). *Om lov om helseforetak m.m.*[*Law about health enterprises*].

Prop. No. 25 (1996–1997). *Åpenhet og helhet. Om psykiske lidelser og tjenestetilbudene* [*Openness and entirity. About mental illness and the health services*].

Prop. No. 63 (1997–1998). *Om opptrappingsplan for psykisk helse 1999–2006* [*the Action plan for mental health 1999–2006*].

White paper NOU 1996:5—*Hvem skal eie sykehusene?* [*Who should own the hospitals?*]. Oslo, Ministry of Health.

——— 1997:2—*Pasienten først! Organisering og ledelse i sykehus* [*The patient first! Organizing and management of hospitals*] Oslo, Ministry of Health.

CHAPTER 6

Dis-assembling the Social: The Politics of Affective Violence in Memorandum Greece

Rania Astrinaki

Several years have elapsed since Greece entered the realm of the so-called sovereign debt crisis, bailout loan treaties and memoranda of austerity measures.[1] As is evident by now, this 'crisis' served as a political tool (Agamben 2013), as an opportunity for 'accumulation by dispossession' (Harvey 2005), for the violent neoliberal re-engineering of state, economy and society—allegedly necessary for salvation from catastrophe. This tool has been enforced at a paralyzing speed through assemblages of techniques of governance (Ong 2006) implementing 'the shock doctrine' (Klein 2007), and making Greece the first country in the old EU nucleus to be subjected to the IMF 'theory', initially conceived for the South, and to 'evolve toward Africa' (Comaroff and Comaroff 2012).

A 'state of emergency', never officially declared, has been invoked in order to legitimize dismantling the welfare state, labor relations and social rights, selling off public assets and effectively dispossessing low and middle classes. Such a 'state of exception' (Agamben 2005) or, perhaps, a

R. Astrinaki (✉)
Panteion University of Social and Political Sciences, Athens, Greece

V. Broch-Due, B.E. Bertelsen (eds.), *Violent Reverberations*,
DOI 10.1007/978-3-319-39049-9_6

politics of exception (Ong 2006),[2] has come to constitute the normal rule of production and regulation of the juridical, political and social order.[3] Moreover, *the economy* has colonized politics transforming it into a business of economy experts where (neoliberal) economic rationality has subjugated the political and the social (Athanasiou 2012; Brown 2005).

As so-called collateral damages, recession, unemployment and poverty have exploded, beggars and homeless filling the streets and the number of suicides have increased dramatically. With growing numbers of people fed on kitchen-soups and hundreds of thousands stripped of health care, racism against immigrants, even Nazism, seems a solution for many social segments. As wealth is being redistributed upwards, a social and humanistic crisis of immense proportions unfolds, threatening increasing segments of Greek society.

Political liberalism, already evacuated from politics in the past two decades, is now evacuated from liberalism as well (Kioupkiolis 2014), for neoliberal 'restructuring' necessitates an authoritarian shift (Klein 2007). As political authority migrates toward transnational oligarchic politico-economic centers, democracy is severely curtailed; mainstream Greek media merged with the executive; public contest and debate have been largely suspended; political rights restricted. State violence has become routinized in public spectacles of 'law and order', where 'law' is increasingly produced by the police in situ and 'order' consists in managing the chaos generated by the warlike mode of transformation (cf. Rigi 2009). The biopolitical camp is a reality for undocumented immigrants and other vulnerable social groups; Golden Dawn murderous activities fill in the gaps (cf. Dalakoglou 2013a). In memorandum Greece, the violence of everyday life has been inscribed in the cityscape of Athens: closed-down shops, rolled-up bedclothes of the homeless, people rummaging rubbish bins, riot police anchored in central street corners and police motor units patrolling the streets have become part of it. This violence, more than spectacular, is a 'slow', accumulative violence that works insidiously, creating milieus fertile of fear and trauma as Broch-Due and Bertelsen (Chap. 1) point out.

Yet, protests have been strangely thin. Struggles are dispersed, failing to merge into a single wave and to secure support by wider segments of society. An exception was the so-called Squares movement which sparked off big waves of protest between May 2011 and March 2012. Protest, however, has lost momentum: in spite of tectonic changes in the political scenery in favor of the Radical Left in the elections of 2012 and although the coalition government (between Conservatives and Socialists) formed in their wake voted for on an agenda of renegotiating the loan agreements, such a government nonetheless fully enforces further austerity measures and the use of coercive power.[4]

A million and a half unemployed seem hidden in the recesses of public life. The youth, including the students, once the vanguard of Greek politics, are peculiarly politically absent, although 60 percent are unemployed, the rest precarious, and all faced with gloomy life-perspectives. This de(im)mobilization does not necessarily imply consent to the 'reform'. Dissent, discontent and exasperation are widespread yet seem contained, deflected and neutralized—impervious to transformation into substantial resistance, let alone to an alternative political project.

How to explain the apparent tolerance to dispossession from rights, institutions and wealth, to forceful disciplining and subjugation? How to account for this endurance accommodation to own and others' social suffering that ultimately translates into practical compliance and consent? These are the questions I will grapple with in this chapter, drawing on interviews with some of my students, on discussions I had with many more, and on my own experience, in living and 'monitoring' 'crisis'. Rather than capturing the imaginative tropes in which people symbolically subvert/resist 'crisis' (Chap. 10),[5] I will reiterate Gledhill's suggestion that we put the whole of politics back in anthropology (2009:29). And I will elaborate on Gutmann's remark (2013) that political compliance, resignation and passivity remain an uncharted territory in anthropology, through attending to the crisis of political practice and imagination in a society in crisis before this current 'crisis' (cf. Dalakoglou 2013b).

Taking my cues from the shattering of post-dictatorship political imaginaries during the 1990s and from political subjectivities as revealed in recent youth mobilizations, I will explore students' political subjectivities during 'crisis' as evinced in my ethnographic research. I will show that these are dominated by imaginaries of denial, disempowerment, shock, anxiety, numbness, fear and mistrust, as well as by disaffection vis-à-vis politics altogether. I will argue that, rather than being 'natural' effects of the 'crisis-shock' and trauma, they have been actively engineered by politics of affective violence aiming to render hegemonic the idea that the neoliberal 'reform' is ineluctable. These politics strive to dismantle the very idea of the political[6] and the collective through discourses and practices that disintegrate forcefully the political and social fabric. They are politics of social enmity, mistrust, guilt, fear and uncertainty that introduce double binds, dilemmas and confusion in the social body and generate for individuals a mental gap (Sideris 2014) and a sense of social chaos.

Here, I must clarify my subject position. Writing from within the space of 'crisis', being subjected to the violence, destruction and social suffering it entails, I cannot rely on a detached observer position—anthropological accounts convey partial *and* positioned truths (Abu-Lughod 1991). Academic work critical of the neoliberal rationality creates the space from which I approach both the 'Greek crisis' and my interlocutors' views.

Shattered Political Imaginaries

The image of Greek society tolerating with stoicism successive shockwaves of revenue and right cuts, that astonishes even foreign observers, contrasts heavily with its turbulent political history. Democracy was won through intense struggles—most often waged in contexts of harsh repression, especially between the 1920s and mid-1970s—which created a sense of *demos* and diffused political imaginaries (Taylor 2004) of collective agency and power.[7] In these struggles, youth, especially university students, were prominent, as in the movement for Democracy and Free Education (1964–1967) and the Polytechnic School Uprising against the military dictatorship in 1973.[8]

Politicization lost momentum in early 1990s when neoliberalization (Gledhill 2004:340) was initiated through the violent promotion of neoliberal ideas by the private media industry established in late 1980s (Sevastakis 2004), which diffused ideals of consumerism and private benefits, then through the 'restructuring' of state and economy.[9] These developments shattered political imaginaries and eclipsed collective concerns, establishing a consensual post-democracy: political involvement was confined to voting for a mainstream party and was exchanged for real or phantasized affluence obtained through client relationships, corruption and bank loans, while sovereign power slipped into the hands of political and corporate elites (Kioupkiolis 2014).

However, massive, long-lasting youth movements continued to emerge in the 2000s.[10] The 'Defend Article 16 movement', a year-long student mobilization in 2006–7, canceled government projects to amend Constitution article 16 (providing for free higher education in public universities) and allow private universities. In December 2008, the murder of a 15-year-old youth by the police sparked a two-week-long violent, politically leaderless and decentralized youth uprising (with massive participation of high school students), which subsequently transformed into a colorful young 'multitude' performing peacefully in different places for two months. These so-called December events puzzled for their sudden eruption and vanishing, radical forms of political action and non-articulation of a socio-political project. They largely constituted a break with post-dictatorship politics and imaginaries, raising questions about the kind of political subjectivities they entailed and produced.[11]

When 'crisis' erupted in 2009, however, relatively few people below 30 participated in protests, which were thin anyway: its sudden 'irruption' and the force of discourses attributing 'crisis' to corruption and excessive consumption of the whole citizenry produced shock and collective guilt. Only one massive demonstration took place on Greece's submission to the European Financial Stability Facility in May 2010; but the tragic burning to death of three people by petrol bombs thrown inside a bank building during it, an act officially attributed to all protesters, intensified guilt and wrought demobilization.

The 'Squares movement' of *Aganaktismenoi* (Indignant) in May 2011 brought a temporary change. A peaceful 'December', it rested on social media networking (as the 'Arab Spring' and Spanish *Indignados* movements) and on direct democracy processes, along with carnivalesque performances ridiculing mainstream politics and politicians.[12] Leaderless, socio-ideologically heterogeneous and opposed to fixed political agendas, it challenged received ideas of organized movements, attracting young (and older) people never having engaged in politics. The Indignant multitude faded in mid-summer and vanished when Syntagma Square was violently evacuated by riot police. Meanwhile, it helped revitalize the trade-union movement, generating several huge demonstrations between May 2011 and March 2012 (dissipated with warlike violence by riot police and ending in violent clashes between police and groups of protesters). It also inspired legion protests, from takeovers of workplaces and movements of disobedience to verbal or physical assaults on high-ranking politicians, held responsible for the 'crisis'. Social unrest provoked anticipated elections in June 2012 which revealed dramatic political changes: the hitherto marginal Coalition of Radical Left (SYRIZA) rose from 4.60 percent in 2009 to 26.89, the Socialist Movement climbed down from 43.92 to 12.88 percent, and the Neo-Nazi Golden Dawn entered Parliament with 6.92 percent of votes.[13]

The 'Squares' and other movements of that time showed that austerity policies had shattered the post-democratic contract for lower and middle classes. They both revealed and enhanced people's disaffection with dominant political parties and the political system. However, they also revealed disaffection with organized politics altogether. Thus, although the 'Squares movement' left important potentialities for re-inventing democracy and political subjectivity,[14] disquieting questions about the possibilities to build an alternative remained. For despite the emergence of intense social creativity aiming at stimulating collective action (social clinics and pharmacies, barter communities and so on), with many grassroots collectivities springing up in the country,[15] these proved slow in mobilizing people beyond limited circles of activists to form social movements *stricto sensu*.

Paradoxically, massive mobilizations seem to have effected disempowerment, frustration, and weariness, and have peculiarly declined since June 2012, despite SYRIZA's expanding power—or maybe because of it: people seem to be waiting patiently for SYRIZA to win the elections and settle matters once in government, in what has been termed in the Greek political jargon 'conferral politics'.[16] Only islands of struggles have emerged. Meanwhile 'crisis' becomes a regime for country-wide transformation and, along with the material lives of people, it profoundly changes their subjectivities. This may be seen in younger generations' socio-political 'structure of feeling' (Williams 1977) to which I will now turn.

Even as the 'Squares movement' can be credited mainly to young people, its sudden appearance and vanishing (as 'December' before it) also highlighted the puzzling political subjectivities of the generations raised in the last two decades. Moreover, unlike the 'Defend article 16 movement' and 'December', it cannot be attributed to those aged below 25, who were not a remarkable presence. Although 45.5 percent of the age group 18–24 voted for SYRIZA, youth participation in protests is rather low. So is students' even when protests concern education reforms.[17] Participation in Student Union Assemblies is considerably lower than in 2006, while in the elections for Student Councils, the fractions influenced by the right wing and the socialist party (very strong in the past, due to indulging in clientelist politics) obtained much higher records than the parties in the national elections. Participation in conferences on 'crisis' is rather limited and so is engagement in political organizations. The imaginaries of politicized 'dynamic minorities' in universities seem to no longer impinge on their peers. Thus, whereas one might expect (judging from past experience) that universities would foster a space of debate on 'crisis', resistance to deregulation policies and socio-political re-imagination, they largely remained a space of numbness.

Disempowerment as a Structure of Feeling

At the micro-level of my classes at university, students seem scantily informed on 'crisis', describing it with fragments of official discourse: debt, the spendthrift state, excessive consumption or the markets. My comments regarding the effects of 'crisis' on their lives are met with expressionless replies, such as 'we know, we'll be unemployed, or precariat'—uttered as if they were talking about the life of someone else. With few exceptions, students are hardly alert to important events and when they are, they seem to consider them trivial. This lack of awareness also concerns protests: several days after the 'Indignants movement' broke out, few of the 60 students in my class knew what it was about and even fewer went to Syntagma Square for a first-hand experience. Emblematic struggles, waged by local or professional communities, were known to even less. When asked what they consider doing faced with a gloomy future, they reply by shrugging their shoulders, saying 'Nothing we can do' or 'We'll see'—or they say, jokingly, 'We'll emigrate'. Discussions in corridors and cafés turn around course-related activities or entertainment and smart shopping; hardly ever about 'crisis' and politics. In this context, left-wing political activists are discouraged and have disappeared from their emblematic spots in campus.

It seems that students live in some 'state of denial' (Cohen 2001), expecting 'crisis' to end, as the term connotes—a view propagated by official discourses; or that they have resigned, even accommodated, to their gloomy life-perspectives.[18] With post-dictatorship political imaginaries shattered and the subsequent post-democratic contract broken, what socio-political imaginaries drive their lives in the conjuncture?

With these issues in mind I proposed to my students to participate on a voluntary basis in discussions concerning 'crisis'. Nine students volunteered, all originating from the crumbling lower-middle and middle classes, all strongly motivated in their studies, also, as it turned out, in discussing the 'crisis', several espousing left-wing ideas. The picture given by participants was more complicated than that evinced in the classroom.

Moira and Manos related the Greek 'crisis' 'to global domination ... it is part of the crisis of the [capitalist] system and the shift from industrial to finance capital. Greece is the weak link'. So did Sophia, underlining 'the moral punishment character of austerity measures'. Stella 'followed the "crisis" spreading throughout Europe' and feared that the 'EU may break up.' Anna suggested that 'debt and corruption serve as pretext for the measures', pointing to the unconstitutionality of most recent laws.

Ilia was adamant, however, that 'this is a Greek crisis of values: client-relations, corruption, tax evasion … have become a mentality; there is no control, no limit. Surely it is the state's and the politicians' fault, but don't we vote for them? Therefore we are all responsible.' Dimitris and Christos, initially convinced by official allegations that 'measures' would 'save the country' and eliminate state corruption, were prompted to doubt by discussions in classrooms. Dimitris now sees that 'behind politicians' discourses lies something else, this mystery … but I don't have a clear picture and counter-discourses are not illuminating'. Christos admitted to an unreliable knowledge, because 'you never know what they [power-holders] hide and what they let you know, so what you know may be false or half-true'. Irini's image was even hazier. Although she blamed Greek politicians and politics for the 'crisis', she also sensed 'that the power milieu is mysterious and obscure, remote; it could be out of Greece, at a global level; we are governed by people we cannot even see, and we can't understand'.

Resonances with the picture presented in classrooms were visible. Although all students were aware of the 'reform' effects in socio-economic life, including their own, and all (except for Ilia) resented and opposed them, they seemed little informed about the relation of Greek 'crisis' to global governance demands for 'deregulation' and EU quasi-neocolonial restructuring in favor of the economically stronger North. They had to a limited degree sought to scrutinize 'crisis' through examining opposed politico-economic viewpoints—formulated by distinguished (systemic and left-wing) economists, socio-political theorists and institutions—or attended the numerous discussions organized these years. All (including those of far-left convictions) remained within received wisdom, amalgamating it in a *bricolage* with critical viewpoints picked up here and there. Most relied on mainstream media for information—even those mistrusting them; few resorted to the handful of heterodox radios, newspapers and social media that were available.

Thus, in discussions dominated issues ultimately framed by overarching hegemonic, orientalizing and moralizing 'crisis' discourses: exorbitant state expenditure, corruption, clientelism, excessive consumption, immunity, impunity, unaccountability—even as these were questioned. The implicit query 'are we to blame?' was pervasive. Unlike the multiple, multisemic and heteroglossic 'speech genres' analyzed by Bertelsen (Chap. 8), the 'stories', through which my interlocutors attempted to re-order and re-inscribe meaning to their dis-ordered world, were predominantly monologic and 'reconciled' historical fragments, colonized by official discourses. Yet rather than re-ordering, they transpired confusion and puzzlement about 'crisis' effects and perspectives—a mystification by power.

This mystification is associated with students' strong intimidation by the 'economy' media-discourses: all pointed to their unintelligibility and confessed inability 'to make head or tail'. This relates, among other things, to the fragmentary and incomprehensible warlike media 'economy talk', through which official 'crisis' discourses are enforced; to the storming measures' promotion; and to the official silencing or blurring of alternative discourses. It engenders a sense of powerlessness, which discourages from delving into 'crisis things' or leads to 'give up on understanding', as several students declared.

But this might not be the whole story: 'We are more concerned about personal than social affairs', Manos acknowledged self-reflexively. Pointing to the depoliticization *habitus* formed in the 1990s, this statement reveals that the quest for 'good life', dominant since then, has not lost momentum. Yet, it seems that more than being unconcerned about common affairs, students deny knowledge of 'crisis', avoiding information on new measures because 'it is so depressing, you need antidepressants', as Moira said, or because they 'get mad to hear politicians say it [crisis] is their fault', as Dimitris added. In this 'state of denial', retreating to the private realm seems a solution, if only to exorcize extreme poverty that they fear might eventually befall them as well.

If knowledge is power, the power complex, into which political and corporate elites and media industry have fused, strives to control 'crisis' knowledge in order to enforce 'restructuring' as the only alternative. And it does so through an elaborate politics of affect that diffuses fear, insecurity, uncertainty and, ultimately, powerlessness into the social body. By not re-claiming or contesting that knowledge, students are mystified by power; indeed, induced to a 'structure of feeling' (Williams 1977) of disempowerment, widespread in their talk. Moira feels indignity: 'You can't manage, you live on borrowed money … you lose your dignity'. Likewise, Dimitris feels insecurity; his father is unemployed, his mother provides for the family, taking care of an old lady: 'If granny dies … what will it become of us?' he asked, laughing bitterly. Stella grew up comfortably; now she lives 'the fall', feeling 'threat and fear for the future'. And although all were worried about the rise of the neo-Nazi political party Golden Dawn, Ilia, Irini and Christos acknowledged xenophobia, fear of 'immigrant criminality'—explicitly constructed as a threat by official discourses that reiterate Golden Dawn views. Thus, the state of denial works to split wide open students' imaginaries and life-worlds to the affective politics pursued by the ruling power complex.

Yet, a social body haunted by fear, anxiety, insecurity and uncertainty is a dismembered social body. These emotions seem to concern self and family rather than social wholes. Thus, several students acknowledged, self-reflexively, that 'unless misery or police knocks on our door we are not interested in what is happening'. Indeed, the multiple fears of social collapse, of welfare state collapse and of authoritarianism seemed rather peripheral in this topology of fear. Privatizations of public goods, of health, water and electricity, elicited few comments—although they have been heatedly debated in many *fora* as against public interest. By contrast, claims that 'the welfare state should have been strengthened and help people in this time of crisis' evinced the confusion concerning what 'crisis' is about.

Perhaps unsurprisingly, political agency seemed unthinkable and political horizons closed. When asked what they do against this disaster, most students were puzzled, replying: 'there's nothing we can do!' or 'it's not that we don't react, but we don't know what to do, we are desperate!' Irini said and others echoed in a chorus 'Yes! Desperate!' 'Numb!' 'Shocked!' 'Hopeless!'. Elaborating on this, several invoked a gap in collective (re) action. As Anna said 'public discourses are so focused on finances that they blind us as to what is happening at the socio-political level; people are preoccupied and depressed by their financial difficulties, see nothing beyond them and are unaware of what may happen to them'. As she and others remarked bitingly, 'many people say that people will revolt in a while, but nobody includes him/herself in these people; everybody expects others to revolt, so you wonder who is going to revolt since there is nobody to revolt!' 'But that's the point!' Ilia responded, 'that not even those who grumble day and night go out to the streets!' Upon this, Moira intervened: 'but there are many venues of resistance and social remaking. I don't engage in any, but other people do. Yet these are never reported in mainstream media, only through the Internet. This leaves the impression that nobody resists, that you are alone and helpless.'

What is described here as a 'gap in (re)action', then, is to an extent an effect of power, through muting points of resistance, immobilizing those who might consider acting and, simultaneously, providing reasons for inaction. The students reproduced performatively this gap: they admitted to do nothing but 'wait' for others to act. They rarely (some never) participate in demonstrations nor do they engage in any socio-political activity. Anna put the matter squarely:

> There is a widespread perplexity, especially among people born in the 1990s, because they had a really good life. Our grandparents lived the war, our parents lived dictatorship, but we have lived our whole life in prosperity. When you see your 'status quo' crumbling, you don't know how to deal with it. Revolts, good, but our generation has never lived big revolts,[19] and does not know how it is like. It is not simple therefore to say 'go out to the streets'. This cannot happen. Period!

Echoing Anna, Sophia and Irini invoked a lack of *habitus* in collective action: 'I do not have the habit of going to such events and I am never informed on time; but even when I am and do have time, I finally decide to do something for myself.' Moira pointed out, jokingly, 'Facebook-resistance', remarking that many students' action consists in posting ironic comments or pressing the 'Like' button on comments of others on current events.

Positioned self-reflexively, Manos attributes this to self-interested 'individualism', saying: 'we have lost contact with collectivities. We are rarely preoccupied with social matters, only with ourselves, with defending our material goods. We don't react for fear of losing them …' Dimitris followed this up: 'A competitive individualism is emerging, about who will survive, who will get this or that job, since jobs are few'. 'Meanwhile', Christos remarked, 'we are accommodating to increasingly less; less democracy, rights, money; and it is uncertain whether "crisis" will change our views and habits'. Dimitris corroborated: 'We don't ask for a return to affluence … we only ask for survival'.

If politics means concern for the *polis* being the affair of every citizen, and if the political is a space of power, conflict and antagonism, then students seem alienated from this idea and practice, deprived of the sense of possibility of (collective) political agency and entrusting their lives, increasingly 'bared' of rights, to an external agency the nature of which remains unknown. The actions and aspirations of the 'Defend article 16' generation and of the 'Squares movement' seem far removed from their political subjectivities. Born in early 1990s, they are the true offspring of the Greek post-democratic contract. Shocked and despaired to see it broken, they seem to stick to this 'state of shock/despair', without seeing a possibility for change—eerily echoing the 'no alternative' motto of older generations and official discourses. Instead, they seem to hold onto the *habitus* of good life—that same life against which youths of their generation revolted, as adolescents, in 2008, demanding 'give us our lives back'. Fear for the future seems to generate practices of accommodation to its remains, fostering (fantasies of) hope for managing to preserve them. Could this be a sign of social implosion? Are we witnessing the emergence of the neoliberal subject (Dardot and Laval 2010)? Is there more to this enduring 'state of shock' than the loss of good life? How do they explain this numbness?

Imaginaries of Fear and Mistrust: Social Fabric Dismantled?

There are three scripts that 'explain' such a sticking to a *habitus* that keeps students in numbness. The first is 'There is fear to react', as Irini said, or, squarely, 'I am afraid of police violence', as Sophia, and several others confessed. Yet, on further questioning, nobody recounted any traumatic personal experience except for being tear-gassed, mentioned only by Moira and Anna: the rest spoke on vicarious knowledge, mediated by mediatic knowledge. It seems, therefore, that police violence has achieved a capacity of long-distance intimidation and disciplining: by metonymy, through the theatrical performance of the riot police's constant urban presence, random pre-emptive arrests before major protests (only to release those arrested later) and occasional police intrusion into self-governed institutions (e.g. schools and universities) on the pretext of crime prevention; by harsh materiality, through attacks against protests and frequent invasions or violent evacuations of alternative social structures. The doctrine of 'law and order' communicates the government's will to regulate the total social space and to discipline bodies within it to the neoliberal rationality in the name of security: in a highly symbolic move, it is the riot police in full gear that most often undertakes this regulation.

Yet more than such overt violence, a phantasmatic mediatized police violence is implied in this intimidation. As media reports on protests carefully silence political claims and transmit solely the spatially confined clashes between police and small groups of protesters, the media represent the latter as *the* 'reality' of demonstrations, creating a virtual, fictional reality which insinuates that any protester runs the risk of being struck by riot police. A multi-level mediatic violence of representation is implicated in these powerful sense-wise images (cf. Feldman 1994): police is represented as exercising defensive, law-preserving, violence; protesters wholesale as merely people doing violent things ('people throwing stones here and there' as Christos remarked), as potential irrational agents of violence and disorder, who threaten the life of 'defenseless consumers/ citizens' and oppose 'the reforms necessary for the salvation of the country' by promoting their vested interests, against public interest. Protests themselves, along with all sites of resistance and alternative social action, thereby become imaginatively transformed into threatening sites of lawlessness and disorder.

The second script refers to struggles' perceived ineffectiveness: 'They will never change things', Christos affirmed (and several others agreed), 'whenever people happen to gather and block off Syntagma Square, for a day or two—there is no effect! Nothing changes! No matter how much one tries, power allows no alternatives'. While a *doxic* (Bourdieu 1977) omnipotence of the power complex to act at will looms threatening, protests that were in the past conceived as blocking (in metaphor, but often also in reality) the omnipotent flow of power are now, conversely, perceived as undesirable obstacles to the normal flow of urban socio-economic activity, yet also to the flow of that threatening power itself. An ambiguous imaginary of power as an object of desire, mixed at once with fear and critique (cf. Aretxaga 2003), seems to subtend the mystification by power and to inhabit students' political subjectivities, materializing in their social activity. It has superseded and discarded a long-established idea in European and Greek political history: that massive popular mobilization is one of the few means of empowerment, of intervening in political decisions, available to the subaltern. The very ideas of democratic agency and sovereign rights claims now seem negatively valued. How to explain this loss of social memory of what social struggles have achieved, even in the recent past—showing a deep post-political turn?

The third script, illustrated by the oft-repeated phrase 'I don't trust anybody', might be illuminating in this regard. Disregard, discredit and contempt vis-à-vis the hitherto governing parties (Socialist and right-wing) and their politicians were widespread among my interlocutors. They blamed both for self-profiting rule and for building a corrupt, clientelist state and political system that encouraged illegality and spread corruption into the social body. 'They created a country of thieves,' Moira remarked, 'in order to reduce their guilt and to ensure support. There is corruption in other countries too, but it is limited at the highest levels and therefore not so visible. In Greece there is a sort of socialism in corruption, everyone can be corrupt.'

These remarks are true: top-level corrupt rule was largely tolerated due to political elites' clientelist politics and tacit acceptance of corruption at lower levels: this was the cornerstone of the post-democratic contract, being also a source of tacit discredit of the dominant political forces and of political alienation, already before 'crisis'.[20] This 'normalcy' was severely upset in 2009 when the then prime minister Papandreou and his government positioned themselves outside the system that the corporate-political elite and their own party had helped create: exonerating themselves from responsibility, they attributed 'crisis' to systemic, all-embracing corruption, clientelist politics, mismanagement and lack of transparency, and incriminated for them the state *in abstracto* and the Greek people as a whole. This artful move, strongly supported by mainstream media and culminating in the famous dictum by the then vice-president 'We all ate it together' (that is, the money), proved an effective affective political tool in harnessing, initially at least, compliance with or tolerance for the coming 'deregulation'.

Although this move initially enraged the Greek citizenry, it provoked a moment of self-reflexivity among majority party voters for their unconfessed complicity in tolerating corruption practices and produced a strong collective sentiment of guilt. It also generated violent recriminations along different lines (party support, profession—even age), pitting one category against the other in search for the 'culprit' in mutual suspicion. This strategy proved effective in eliciting consensus in the successive scapegoating by the power complex of all protesting groups, accusing each of defending vested private interests against public interest. But in the process of 'deregulation', as successive groups were affected, this strategy started backfiring. Charges were reversed: now *people* blamed the parties for 'crisis', holding *them* responsible for corruption, clientelism and favoritism and for implicating them in these practices. Guilt remained, however, and so did mutual recrimination and suspicion as to who were favored.

Mainstream parties were thus further discredited—and so were trade unions, largely controlled by them and backing their politics. Alienation from them was reinforced as they increasingly raised themselves 'above politics', allegedly overcoming their antagonisms and collaborating in government for the 'salvation of the country', and as they increasingly distanced themselves from their voters by promoting measures that deepened real socio-economic crisis. This generated a problem of political representation. 'We have entrusted them to represent us,' Irini said, 'but they don't represent us anymore.'

However, as these parties monopolized hegemony in the political system for decades, they were identified with it, with the idea of the political party and with politics itself. This was translated into profound alienation of large social segments from the political system as a whole, and into discarding and mistrust vis-à-vis all political parties, including those of the radical left (never implicated in corruption). Such mistrust was particularly pronounced in the 'Squares Movement'. The phrase 'All politicians are the same' (that is, corrupt) became the slogan of the conjuncture, buttressing Golden Dawn claims to anti-systemicity.

Similar sentiments were refracted in many students' views. Irini declares she will not vote for any party: 'I think it is crazy to continue voting for parties after all this disaster, all these suicides!' Intense mistrust and suspicion of pursuing self-interested goals enveloped all parties' projects: 'I am not sure those clamoring against this government do it for the good of this country', Dimitris said; 'all they want is to come in power themselves'. Certainly views differed. Moira, Manos and Anna had voted for SYRIZA and Stella for a Trotskyist party. Yet they did so by default as these parties 'did not represent them'. And although they mentioned that only collective struggle in political organizations and social movements could possibly change things, they then 'deconstructed' both—In a 'left-wing version' of Dimitris' words—and abstained from participating in either.

'Left-wing political forces are fragmented, each promoting its narrow political interests,' Stella said. And although SYRIZA has achieved a unification of some of the left-wing political forces, this was also met with mistrust: 'Will they do what they say? Ideologies have crumbled,' Moira remarked. Disappointment predominates; you cannot believe in something or someone and you feel isolated. There isn't a leader to believe in, to induce you to action. These views resonate with dominant ideas that raise neoliberal politics above politics, identifying others' politics with special interests, not with concern for the common good; that declare the end of ideologies while promoting neoliberal ideology and that discard grass-root political participation in conferring the *locus* of politics to an external agency, a circle of specialists or a leader.

Social movements, on the other hand, are 'too small, partial and fragmented' and forms of solidary social action developed in recent years did not prove more inspiring. Few students were even informed of the initiatives present in their own neighborhoods, and although several stated being motivated by volunteerism in established non-profit organizations (e.g. the Red Cross), no one actually engaged in it for lack of time or of commitment. Thus, even as several remarked that one of the good things this crisis brought is solidarity among people, this seems to work only at the level of personal kinship and friendship networks.

As further discussions revealed, however, political mistrust was part of a more generalized trend of social mistrust. Irini expressed doubts as to whether the money raised by different initiatives actually reached their recipients. Others wondered whether people asking for money rather than being really in distress were not profiting from others' compassion for 'crisis' victims to satisfy consumerist desires (e.g. buying an expensive face cream). Several acknowledged having become anesthetized to spectacles of poverty and homelessness and confessed that secretly they feel poverty is these people's own fault. Most importantly, the homeless and those reduced to beggary were depicted in images of social 'otherness': as 'a social group with which no relationship should have been allowed', as an 'annoying presence', as 'invaders' in the students' social world whom the latter often catch themselves stepping aside in order to avoid touching—ultimately as (subjectively perceived) 'human waste' (Bauman 2004).

As discussions developed, I could not help reflecting whether ten years ago it would have been possible to hear similar discourses from students of their kind. Loss of political imagination, disappearance of political agency and conferral of concern for the polis to professionals, pervasive disempowerment and fear, concern for personal welfare, and social mistrust, with a ring of social Darwinism, all these elements indicate the social and political distance covered since the time it was self-evident that students would be in the vanguard of struggles for freedom, equality and social justice. What happens in and to a society when the young, disempowered and intimidated accept precarity as their fate and accommodate social suffering without raising the question of change? Could this be already a sign of profound transformation—indicative of the traumatizing social engineering taking place—a sign of neoliberal subjectification?

Politics of Affective Violence and the Arts of Domination

Of course, there is no simple answer to these questions. The past dominant party politics, the aporias of the Left after the collapse of extant socialism and the neoliberalization of Greek society had already produced a new social and (post)political *habitus* before crisis. The commoditization of social life and quest for private benefits increasingly shaped forms of social bond, personal investments and identifications, forming subjects' identities as consumers (rather than citizens). The break-out of 'debt crisis' in 2009 and the ensuing socio-economic crisis have generated not only shock and social suffering, but other socio-political processes as well. Socio-cultural creativity and critical thought flourished and politics brought forward a left-wing agenda that, although still unstable and uncertain, seems to reverberate across the European South. Crucially, this included also a neo-Nazi agenda impacting the coalition government to an extreme-right turn and appealing to important segments of the political body. Thus, while new narratives of emancipation may be emergent but yet unformed, a regime of authoritarian post-political biopower is consolidating (Kioupkiolis 2014) together with a polity transition away from democracy to disquieting and as yet unknown directions (Christopoulos 2013).

It is in light of these different temporalities that we must explore students' imaginaries and sentiments of denial, disempowerment, confusion, despair, anxiety, fear and mistrust. On the one hand, they evince, as we saw, that good life *habitus* formed in the pre-'crisis' era of affluence seems disrupted but not eclipsed. This continuity has distancing effects in relation to crisis effects and is perhaps enhanced by continuities in the ethnographically documented Greek families' sacrificial effort to ensure a better life for their offspring.[21] Presumably, the effects of consumer imaginaries on identity formation were more powerful in the generations born and raised in this context, who still stick to the identity of the consumer, although the possibility for consumption has considerably decreased. Maybe because, as Stavrakakis (2007) shows, drawing on Lacan, consumption has become a social fantasy that stimulates desire by promising to substitute objects of consumption to the loss of enjoyment. As such it escapes deconstruction—it can only shift to another object. In this perspective, consumption could be seen as an unconscious attempt to exorcize the malaise of everyday life.

At least partly, these imaginaries evidence the depoliticized subjectivities of a generation that has embodied (in the bourdieusian sense) the dismantling of collective commitments and emancipatory visions, the entrustment of political agency to specialists and the discredit of politics, and their corollary, a utilitarian, consumerist individualism. And it might be precisely largely due to this dismantling of the bond between the self and the social/collective (beyond family and kin) that became possible the prevalence and embedding of these imaginaries and sentiments, which could be plausibly translated in the language, and be perceived as indices, of social trauma (cf. Chap. 2).

On the other hand, while these imaginaries are undoubtedly an effect of the shock engendered by 'crisis' eruption, the humiliating, orientalizing discourses and the intensity of the austerity measures, we should be cautious to consider them a necessary response to these developments, because 'crisis' was not in any sense a natural (disastrous) event. Crisis, Roitman (2011) points out, is not intrinsic to a system but a distinction that produces meaning, an axiological problem that marks a moment of truth. As such, it is a blind spot that regulates narrative constructions, allowing certain questions to be asked, while others are foreclosed. And as Lynteris (2011) suggests, following Foucault, crisis reflects the decision of a sovereign nature, which brings to the surface new techniques capturing and new strategies for securing that truth, and must arrange that crisis come at the right opportunity. This becomes clear in the case of Greece which faced serious fiscal imbalance since the early 1990s but was managing. It was therefore a 'sovereign decision' to declare it in 'crisis' in 2009, in the famous phrase by Euro-Group President Jean-Claude Juncker 'the game is over', and to produce 'the moment of truth' which provoked its activation.

As I suggest in this final section, these imaginaries have been actively engineered by the dominant power complex in order to render hegemonic its 'crisis-and-therapy' discourse, to elicit compliance and to foreclose questions about the stakes of this 'crisis' (the neoliberal restructuring of state, economy and society) and the disastrous socio-political effects of the 'remedy'. Assemblages drawing on all technologies of power and domination brought forward by recent theorists have been articulated into a real art of domination. These were not necessarily products of a unified top-down plan. Although they were largely the outcome of collaboration between transnational institutions launched for the first time, they also operated in a rhizomic and warmachinic fashion that kept moving in the process. Yet they all worked toward the same direction, to complete market dominance in Greece and the European South.

The context of this chapter is not the place to analyze these assemblages. I will only succinctly highlight some of them, in attempting to shed light on the students' discourses, practices and subjectivities with relation to the present. But first, let me comment on their internal strategic logic. This has been a repackaging of the 'shock doctrine' (Klein 2007) to fit the doubly particular circumstances of the enterprise: a functional liberal Western-type democracy and (admittedly) the most violent rhythm of 'restructuring' ever attempted in a country. Briefly, Klein designates with this term the orchestrated deregulation of the public sphere by what she calls 'disaster capitalism' implemented in moments of collective shock or trauma (natural disasters, wars, terrorist attacks, debt crisis etc.). For Klein, the 'shock doctrine' draws on the torture metaphor. Torture techniques are designed to put prisoners into a state of deep disorientation, in order to 'soften up' and force them to make concessions against their will. Likewise, traumatic episodes 'soften up' whole societies which, if the 'shock doctrine' is enacted upon them before they slip back into the normal, accept neoliberal policies, giving up things they would otherwise fiercely protect (Klein 2007:16).

Greek society, however, was not under the impact of shock, no matter how defined. Therefore the shock had to be created; and it was. Not only by the irruption of 'debt crisis' per se, but even more so by its processing, staged by three shock strategies, which channeled violence to the social body, by targeting violently the mind and the soul of society first (if I am allowed to use this Ancient Greek triptych for analytic purposes). These strategies had a double effect: they targeted the mind, insofar as they created the 'blind spot' that imposed the official 'crisis and therapy' discourse as the only relevant one, by blurring or even blocking alternative ways of thinking 'crisis' and thus by obstructing oppositional discourses from acquiring cogency; at the same time, they targeted the soul, in so far as they engendered what Ahmed (2004) calls an 'affective economy' of anxiety, confusion, uncertainty and fear that created an agitated state of awareness, which 'softened up' Greek society and paved the ground for (initially) accepting the shock therapy as the only solution, on the promise of salvation.

The first affective strategy, promoted by phantasmagoric mediatic (re) presentations in a monophonic orchestration of information, consisted in creating the affective truth of 'crisis' during the first months after its eruption. Conveyed as an imminent attack by an invisible enemy from without, 'the markets', through an unintelligible financial-economic jargon, it transposed war-time strategies to a civil context, spreading thrill about imminent bankruptcy, euro-exit and the resulting deprivations. As government's discourses were incoherent, and international meetings surrounded by secrecy or contradictory information leaking, all sorts of rumors replaced official information, spreading confusion. The master metaphor 'Titanic sinking' came as a sensory objectification of 'crisis' and recourse to the European Financial Stability Facility as a salvation. Shock and the sensory-affective state of emergency were generated together.

The second strategy consisted in explaining the origins of debt 'crisis' by local deficiencies (corruption, clientelism etc.), silencing external factors. In appropriating saturated pre-crisis public discourses on these matters (Astrinaki 2015), the dominant power complex drew on a common meaningful framework to create a hegemonic discourse, which it then instrumentalized in order to shatter the post-democratic contract, present 'crisis' as a 'Greek moral crisis' and hold the subaltern responsible for moral failure. This strategy diffused guilt among the latter and insinuated the 'remedy' as a therapy of modernizing 'reform' and disciplining. The hegemonic script structured the field of thought and action around the idea of 'no alternative'—premised on the hegemonic ideas of Greece's EU and Eurozone belonging.

These two violences of representation, pointing to an external and an internal 'enemy', respectively, were complemented by a third strategy. Redoubling the cleavage between the ruling class and the subaltern, a state-sponsored politics of social enmity and disguised social violence was launched. In the 'deregulation' of particular professional regimes, salaries, labor and social rights, categories of people defined by profession, age, gender, years of work and labor regime were pitted against each other, in a sort of governmentality (Foucault 2007) 'of enmity', which divided the social body on a 'search-for-the-culprit', punitive basis (Astrinaki 2014). Employees in the private sector were pitted against employees in the public sector, who, one category after the other were morally slaughtered; then employees in the private sector were pitted against selected categories of their kind and this continued *ad infinitum*. As the restructuring deploys and real socio-economic crisis settles, new professions and social categories are demonized and incriminated.

This orchestrated politics of social enmity came to constitute a 'regime of truth', convincing large segments of society of its allegations and constructing multiple replicas of 'the internal enemy' that refracted in different social and professional categories and fragmented the social body. It has spread suspicion and mistrust about the motives of the fellow human, preventing people from defending united basic labor and social rights and displacing liability from the dominant classes horizontally, to the subaltern next door. Moreover, under the shock of the (imminent or real) impoverishment, it has installed a sort of your-death-my-life antagonism: large social segments turned against the targeted groups and vividly agreed with their salary cuts and rights abolition. Conversely, once salaries and rights of one group were curtailed, it found it normal (even wished) that those of other groups be curtailed as well. Each professional or otherwise defined group focused on its own rights and survival, ignoring that those of the others might impact on them. Once this divisive logic was embedded as an 'automatism of common sense' (Bourdieu 1993), it could be multiplied and reproduced in other directions, opposing unemployed to employed, precarious to those securely employed and so on, and diffused in a more capillary fashion. This fragmented social body has lost its sense of community. For important social segments, it re-becomes an imaginary community on a nationalist ground against immigrants, who are blamed for the excessive growth of unemployment that the crisis provoked.

As socio-economic crisis settled, whatever consensus was initially achieved was largely shattered: the large protest movement of 2011–2012, the tectonic changes in the political landscape and diffuse discontent attest to this. But the idea of 'no alternative' to the present political project structures, to this day, the field of thought and action, maintaining a negative hegemony: it has produced a 'common sense' (Gramsci 1971) that sets the terms for thinking and debating, engulfs all counter-discourses and prevents alternative frames of thought and projects from developing. With the social body fragmented, when the strategy of guilt seemed faltering, two other strategies, mobilized all along, were artfully mastered, gaining preeminence in the struggle for compliance: the ones of hope and open fear/threat/repression.

The first takes on a messianic logic: against all socio-economic indices, semi-announced further poverty-generating 'reforms' and lived experiences of increasing suffering and dispossession, fantasies of hope are projected in a communicative storming by the dominant power complex. Constituting a parallel, virtual reality, wrapped up in the so-called success story, they contend that soon suffering will be over; juxtaposing and reconciling the two images becomes a source of further confusion. The second consists in the forcefully promoted idea that whoever protests or insists on exposing the disaster that is taking place is an internal enemy, harming the successful image of the 'country', working against national economy and putting the country at risk of euro-exit. Dilemmas, threat and blackmail are turned into a mode of governance. Meanwhile, warlike regulative action of the executive has produced a sort of 'chaotic mode of domination' (Rigi 2009) and a mode of domination through chaos: the coercive power of the state operates along with complex networks of governmental institutions, private businesses, multinationals and NGOs; power becomes increasingly opaque, state apparatus is increasingly intertwined to informal networks; deregulation produces disorder and lack of meaning in everyday life; and those living in Greek territory are increasingly uncertain about the laws and regulations governing their lives.

It is with these thoughts in mind that I want to come back to the students' numbness and fear. Numbness seems to be an epiphenomenon of this agitated state of awareness and fragmentation of the social fabric; it is produced by this 'affective economy' working out both a psycho-intellectual and a political deregulation that renders possible the acceptance of the socio-economic 'reform'. It is the outcome of multiple double binds (Bateson 1972; Sideris 2014), where thought is jammed by contradictory and mutually conflicting messages, without being capable to work the paradox produced. At one level, you have the official monophonic communicative hurricane of allegations: it is your fault; this 'reform' demands sacrifices from you but saves and modernizes the 'country'; if you resist, you place your interests above it, working for its bankruptcy, Grexit and disaster. At another level, the crude reality: unemployment, misery, despair; if you submit, you are accomplice to them. And at a third level, you are told that there is no alternative and indeed you do not see any, because the contradictory messages generate mistrust and because you do not know: where 'decisions' come from, how this magic thing called economy works, and so on.

Fear is the other side of the coin. In a 'phantomatic mode of production' (Aretxaga 2002) the powerful images of police- and mediatic violence merge with official threats and mythologies of hope to produce a diffuse, inchoate, smoldering, indefinable affective/embodied 'structure of feeling' of fear. Fear is sliding from one 'object' to the other, from police violence to the alleged violence of social agents, to disorder, to the crumbling economy, to loss of good life. This mobility of fear works to stick 'objects' together as signs of threat or danger in an 'affective economy of fear' (Ahmed 2004): fear of a 'spectralized' state violence is refracted and projected, replicated and translated into fear of power, of economic catastrophe, of unemployment and poverty, of the future, of the radical change of society taking place in still unknown directions. And perhaps most importantly: into fear of the other(s)' motives and of changing received ways of seeing and doing. Fear, then, gradually impregnates social imaginaries in ways that contrast with a democratic regime and invoke societies exposed to political violence and authoritarian rule or to post-conflict situations (cf. Chap. 9; see also Green 1999; Robben 2005).

Shock-producing technologies have thus been productive in generating more than the 'softening up' necessary for implementing the socio-economic 'reforms'. They have been traumatropic political technologies for fashioning an (un)political aesthesis, to paraphrase Feldman (2010), that disorient and immobilize subjects, entraps them in the web of 'no alternative' accommodation and in the melancholia of good life, depriving them of the sense of possibility and subjectifying them in this deprivation. By dis-assembling the social body and imbuing it with the misrecognized affective violence of confusion, fear and mistrust, these technologies have proved a masterful art of domination. For they obstruct contesting and undoing the conditions of their production. Undoing these conditions, subverting the traumatropes to the direction of re-claiming agency, re-building the collective and re-locating the self in it, in short, re-inventing the political, these are the challenges young people are faced with if they are to move beyond disempowerment and to reclaim a future beyond trauma, misery and precarity. Will they take them up?

Afterword

The ethnographic present to which this paper refers is 2013 to early 2014. Dramatic changes have occurred since, whose incorporation would add considerable length to this chapter. Widespread discontent provoked anticipated elections in January 2015 and drove 36.34 percent of votes to SYRIZA, not through struggle and conversion to radical left ideas but due to an 'immobile' conferral politics movement in search for hope. Given SYRIZA's promise to renegotiate agreements and debt, promote a mild social-democratic program, relieve those in distress and restrain the 'restructuring' process, its coming to government in coalition with the right-wing party of Independent Greeks initially spurred euphoria.

However, it soon became clear that Greece's European and IMF 'partners' were determined to enforce existing agreements despite their rejection by Greek citizens. Exemplifying Foucault's thesis that 'politics is the continuation of war by other means' (Foucault 2003:48), they orchestrated a war in order to extort the new government's submission to their regime of truth presented as destiny. This political war illustrated the departure of European governance from the founding principle of Europe, democracy, and was waged in tandem with local political and corporate elites and mainstream media. A wide, once more shock-producing arsenal was used, ranging from fear campaign to financial 'asphyxia' and capital controls, to, finally, outright threats of 'Grexit' from the Eurozone (after the July referendum, in which 61.32 percent voted against the agreement proposed by European governance). The new government was finally bent to 'capitulation': breaking its promises, it signed one more 'memorandum' with more austerity measures and neoliberal 'reforms'. Promising, this time, a biased implementation in favor of the weak, Alexis Tsipras won the elections of September 2015 with 35.46 percent of votes.

The interstitial political effervescence of January pre-election weeks and then again of the last pre-referendum days gave way to shock and immobility. All citizens, even SYRIZA voters, remained anxious spectators of the political thriller that would determine their lives. This turbulent process created new traumatropes that thickened the web of 'no alternative' accommodation, enriching the melancholia of good life with the one of hope, and it finally left people 'comfortably numb'. It now seems even more difficult not only for the young but also for the older people, to move beyond disempowerment and to reclaim political agency. More challenging too.

Notes

1. I thank the organizers of the workshop 'Reassessing Trauma and Violence: Reframing the Bodily, the Spoken and the Self' in the University of Bergen, for their lavish hospitality and rich food for thought. I am deeply indebted to all participants in the workshop for their insightful comments, and especially to Nicolas Argenti and Carol Kidron as well as to Bjørn Enge Bertelsen, Vigdis Broch-Due, Tony Robbens and Margit Ystanes. Special thanks are due to Allen Feldman, Dimitra Gefou-Madianou, Takis Geros, Andreas

Notaras and Leonidas Economou for generously offering their critical remarks, and last, but not least, to the students who shared their thoughts with me.

2. This politics consists in excluding groups of subjects from protection (cf. Agamben 2005), yet also in excepting privileged groups from measures implemented, in constructing vulnerable groups as exceptions, spaces of 'graduated' sovereignty and so forth.
3. Constitution article 48 about the 'state of emergency' has never been activated. Yet the state of emergency is constantly foregrounded by the executive in order to promote radical 'structural reforms' through an exceptional legislative practice, that extends executive power into the legislative sphere encroaching also the judicial, in an almost paradigmatic example of Agamben's analysis.
4. The ethnographic present of this chapter is 2013 to early 2014; see Afterword.
5. Cf. Kalantzis 2012; Knight 2015.
6. On the distinction between politics and the political, see Mouffe 2008.
7. Taylor's definition of social imaginaries, as 'the same common understandings that make possible common practices and a widely shared sense of legitimacy' (Taylor 2004:23), refers to imaginaries shared by society as a whole. Here I extend it to fit in conditions of political antagonism, where antagonistic social forces may foster different, even opposed, partially or wholly, social imaginaries.
8. For an analysis, see Kornetis 2013.
9. This 'restructuring' was launched well before recent 'crisis', by the Socialist Party then in government: in 1996–2008, extensive privatizations of public assets were implemented (ranking Greece second after Portugal in EU), state functions were transferred to the private sphere and the state adopted private-sector functioning principles (Stathakis 2014).
10. For an analysis of youth movements since the 1990s, see Giovanopoulos and Dalakoglou 2011.
11. See Astrinaki 2009; Vradis and Dalakoglou 2011.
12. For more information, see Gourgouris 2011; Panourgia 2011.
13. The right-wing New Democracy obtained 29.66 (from 33.47). Golden Dawn retains its power since, despite its criminal practice and the prosecution in criminal court of many of its leading members.

14. For discussions, see Stavrides 2012; Douzinas 2013; Kioupkiolis and Katsambekis 2014; cf. Giovanopoulos and Mitropoulos 2011.
15. See, for instance, Rakopoulos 2014.
16. Cf. Allegralab 2015.
17. Reaction against the higher education 'reform' promoted in 2011 (which dismantled universities' democratic, public and academic character), was rather mild, while dramatic higher education budget cuts (by almost 70 percent) passed unnoticed.
18. It is worth noting that Marie Emily Sørensen, who conducted field research for her MA thesis among young people in a neighborhood of Pireaus, develops similar remarks (Sørensen 2015).
19. This is only partly true. Her generation lived *the revolt* in Greek political culture: December 2008.
20. In the neoliberalizing process of the 1990s, the pattern was complicated by profound transformations in state sovereign power. The latter intertwined to nexuses and networks of corporate power to form a 'corporate state' (Kapferer and Bertelsen 2009), in which corruption became a mode of governance.
21. See, for instance, Friedl 1962; Vlahoutsikou 2015.

References

Abu-Lughod, L. 1991. Writing Against Culture. In *Recapturing Anthropology: Working in the Present*, ed. Robyn Fox, 137–162. Sante Fe: School of American Research Press.

Agamben, G. 2005. *State of Exception.* Chicago, IL: The University of Chicago Press.

———. 2013. Interview to *Frankfurter Allgemeine Zeitung*, Republished by *Epohi*, September 8.

Ahmed, S. 2004. Affective Economies. *Social Text* 22(2): 117–139.

Allegralab. 2015. Exception, Solidarity and Conferral Politics: Crossroads of the 'Greek' Crisis. http://allegralaboratory.net/exception-solidarity-and-conferral-politics-crossroads-of-the-greek-crisis/.

Aretxaga, B. 2002. Terror as Thrill: First Thoughts on the War on Terrorism. *Anthropological Quarterly* 75(1): 138–150.

———. 2003. Maddening States. *Annual Review of Anthropology* 32: 393–410.

Astrinaki, R. 2009. '(Un)hooding' a Rebellion: The December 2008 Events in Athens. *Social Text* 101: 97–107.

———. 2014. Governmantality of Hate in the Greek 'Crisis'. Paper Presented at the Conference *Crisis-Scapes, Athens and Beyond*, Athens, 9–10 May 2014.

———. 2015. Corruption Discourses and Practices as an Instrument for Dismantling the (Social) State in Contemporary Greece. Paper Presented at *Max Planck Institute for Social Anthropology*, Halle Germany.

Athanasiou, A. 2012. *Crisis as "State of Emergency": Critiques and Resistance.* Athens, GA: Savvalas (in Greek).

Bateson, G. 1972. *Steps to an Ecology of Mind.* San Francisco, CA: Chandler Publication.

Bauman, Z. 2004. *Wasted Lives: Modernity and Its Outcasts.* Cambridge: Polity Press.

Bourdieu, P. 1977. *Outline of a Theory of Practice.* Cambridge: Cambridge University Press.

———. 1993. *Sociology in Question.* London: Sage.

Brown, W. 2005. *Edgework: Critical Essays on Knowledge and Politics.* Princeton, NJ: Princeton University Press.

Christopoulos, D. 2013. *In the Risk of Crisis.* Athens, GA: Alexandria (in Greek).

Cohen, S. 2001. *States of Denial: Knowing About Atrocities and Suffering.* Cambridge: Polity.

Comaroff, J., and J. Comaroff. 2012. *Theory from the South or How Euro-America is Evolving Toward Africa.* Boulder, CO: Paradigm Publishers.

Dalakoglou, D. 2013a. 'From the Bottom of the Aegean Sea' to Golden Dawn: Security, Xenophobia, and the Politics of Hate in Greece. *Studies in Ethnicity and Nationalism* 13(3): 514–522.

———. 2013b. The Crisis Before 'the crisis': Violence and Urban Neoliberalization in Athens. *Social Justice* 39(1): 24–42.

Dardot, P., and C. Laval. 2010. *La nouvelle raison du monde.* Paris: La Découverte.

Douzinas, C. 2013. *Philosophy and Resistance in the Crisis: Greece and the Future of Europe.* Cambridge: Polity Press.

Feldman, A. 1994. On Cultural Anaesthesia: From Desert Storm to Rodney King. *American Ethnologist* 21(2): 404–418.

———. 2010. Traumatizing the Truth Commission: Amnesty, Performativity, Intentionalist Teleology and the Event. *e-misférica* 7(2). Digitally available at http://hemisphericinstitute.org/hemi/en/e-misferica-72/feldman, accessed 5 August 2016.

Foucault, M. 2003. *Society Must Be Defended: Lectures at the Collège de France 1975–1976.* New York: Picador.

———. 2007. *Security, Territory, Population: Lectures at the Collège de France 1977–1978.* New York: Palgrave Macmillan.

Friedl, E. 1962. *Vassilika: A Village in Modern Greece.* New York: Holt, Rinehart & Winston.

Giovanopoulos, C., and D. Dalakoglou. 2011. From Ruptures to Eruption: A Genealogy of Post-Dictatorial Revolts in Greece. In *Revolt and Crisis in Greece:*

Between a Present Yet to Pass and a Future Still to Come, eds. Antonis Vradis and Dimitris Dalakoglou, 91–114. London: AK Press & Occupied London.

Giovanopoulos, C., and D. Mitropoulos, eds. 2011. *From the Streets to the Squares: Democracy Under Construction*. Athens, GA: A/Syneheia (in Greek).

Gledhill, J. 2004. Neoliberalism. In *A Companion to the Anthropology of Politics*, eds. David Nugent and Joan Vincent, 332–348. Malden, MA: Blackwell Publishing.

———. 2009. Power in Political Anthropology. *Journal of Power* 2(1): 9–34.

Gourgouris, S. 2011. Democratic Dreams Rage in Athens. http://www.aljazeera.com/indepth/opinion/2011/07/201171985335665864.html.

Gramsci, A. 1971. *Selections from the Prison Notebooks*. New York: International Publishers.

Green, L. 1999. *Fear as a Way of Life*. New York: Columbia University Press.

Gutmann, M. 2013. Beyond Resistance: Raising Utopias from the Dead in Mexico City and Oaxaca. In *New Approaches to Resistance in Brazil and Mexico*, eds. John Gledhill and Patience Schell, 304–324. Durham, NC: Duke University Press.

Harvey, D. 2005. *A Brief History of Neoliberalism*. Oxford: Oxford University Press.

Kalantzis, K. 2012. Crete as Warriorhood: Visual Explorations of Social Imaginaries in Crisis. *Anthropology Today* 28(3): 7–11.

Kapferer, B., and B.E. Bertelsen. 2009. The Crisis of Power and Reformations of the State in Globalising Realities. In *Crisis and the State: War and Social Upheaval*, eds. Bruce Kapferer and Bjørn Enge Bertelsen, 1–26. New York: Berghahn Books.

Kioupkiolis, A. 2014. Towards a Regime of Post-Political Biopower? Dispatches from Greece, 2010–2012. *Theory, Culture and Society* 31(1): 143–158.

Kioupkiolis, A., and G. Katsambekis, eds. 2014. *Radical Democracy and Collective Movements Today: The Biopolitics of the Multitude Versus the Hegemony of the People*. Farnham, UK: Ashgate.

Klein, N. 2007. *The Shock Doctrine: The Rise of Disastrous Capitalism*. New York: Metropolitan Books.

Knight, D.M. 2015. Wit and Greece's Economic Crisis: Ironic Slogans, Food and Antiausterity Sentiments. *American Ethnologist* 42(2): 230–246.

Kornetis, K. 2013. *Children of the Dictatorship: Student Resistance, Cultural Politics and the 'Long 1960s' in Greece*. New York: Berghahn Books.

Lynteris, C. 2011. The Greek Economic Crisis as Evental Substitution. In *Revolt and Crisis in Greece: Between a Present Yet to Pass and a Future Still to Come*, eds. Antonis Vradis and Dimitris Dalakoglou, 207–213. London: AK Press & Occupied London.

Mouffe, C. 2008. *On the Political*. London: Verso.

Ong, A. 2006. *Neoliberalism as Exception: Mutations in Citizenship and Sovereignty*. Durham, NC: Duke University Press.

Panourgia, N. 2011. The Squared Constitution of Dissent. In *Beyond the Greek Crisis*, Hot Spots Forum, Cultural Anthropology. P. Papailia, ed. http://www.culanth.org/fieldsights/252-the-squared-constitution-of-dissent.

Rakopoulos, T. 2014. The Crisis Seen from Below, Within and Against: From Solidarity Economy to Food Distribution Cooperatives in Greece. *Dialectical Anthropology* 38: 189–207.

Rigi, J. 2009. Post-Soviet Formation of the Russian State and the War in Chechnya: Exploring the Chaotic form of Sovereignty. In *Crisis of the State: War and Social Upheaval*, eds. Bruce Kapferer and Bjørn E. Bertelsen, 53–82. New York: Berghahn Books.

Robben, A. 2005. *Political Violence and Trauma in Argentina*. Philadelphia: University of Pennsylvania Press.

Roitman, J. 2011. Crisis. In *Political Concepts: A Critical Lexicon*, online journal, The New School for Social Research, http://www.politicalconcepts.org/2011/crisis.

Sevastakis, N. 2004. *Common Place Country*. Athens, GA: Savvalas (in Greek).

Sideris, N. 2014. *Devil's Gospel: Political Psychology of Crisis*. Athens, GA: Metechmio (in Greek).

Sørensen, M.E. 2015. Living with the Crisis as If It Was Not There: An Anthropological Inquiry into Young People's Engagement with the Greek Economic Crisis. Unpublished Master Thesis, Department of Anthropology, University of Copenhagen.

Stathakis, G. 2014. *The Veer*. http://www.protagon.gr/?i=protagon.el.post&id=30624.

Stavrakakis, Y. 2007. *The Lacanian Left: Psychoanalysis, Theory, Politics*. Edinburgh: Edinburgh University Press.

Stavrides, S. 2012. Squares in Movement. *South Atlantic Quarterly* 111(3): 585–596.

Taylor, C. 2004. *Modern Imaginaries*. Durham, NC: Duke University Press.

Vlahoutsikou, Christina. 2015. *For the Children's Good*. Athens, GA: Nisos (in Greek).

Vradis, A., and D. Dalakoglou, eds. 2011. *Revolt and Crisis in Greece: Between a Present Yet to Pass and a Future Still to Come*. London: AK Press & Occupied London.

Williams, R. 1977. *Marxism and Literature*. Oxford: Oxford University Press.

CHAPTER 7

Re-Assessing the Silent Treatment: Emotional Expression, Preventive Health, and the Care of Others and the Self

Maria Tapias

'Trauma' provides an important and paradigmatic framework among Western societies that helps link an individual's exposure to extreme circumstances of past violence, natural catastrophes or other deleterious injury to present day suffering and manifestations of distress (Fassin and Rechtman 2009). Violent events such as war, political violence, rape and natural and man-made disasters can undoubtedly have traumatic effects but the framework of 'trauma' has been less adept at helping explain the effects of ongoing *chronic* stresses related to poverty, precariousness, hunger, depression, domestic violence and other social ills (Dickson-Gómez 2002). Violence and poverty create systemic vulnerabilities in the social fabric and deeply reconfigure sociality and trust reshaping ways of being and ways of interacting with others (Broch-Due 2005, see also Chap. 9). Across cultures, physical and psychological manifestations of distress and violence often emerge in 'folk illnesses' and other health concerns (Dickson-Gómez 2002; Desjarlais and Kleinman 1997; Jenkins 1991; Tapias 2006a, b)

M. Tapias (✉)
Professor, Department of Anthropology, Grinnell College, Grinnell, IA, USA

V. Broch-Due, B.E. Bertelsen (eds.), *Violent Reverberations*,
DOI 10.1007/978-3-319-39049-9_7

and hence, medical anthropologists have called for a wider conceptualization of trauma and closer examination to how everyday violence insidiously affects health and well-being (Farmer 1996; Kleinman et al. 1997; Scheper-Hughes 1992).

In this chapter I examine how everyday violence as experienced through economic precariousness, the effects of immigration policies and other social and structural barriers related to immigration (such as fear of deportation and failing social relations) destabilize sociality, intimacy and trust among Bolivian migrants and their family members back home and among Bolivian migrants in Spain and how this reconfiguration, in turn, is embodied into numerous preventive health practices and wellness concerns. Of particular note, I am interested in exploring how concerns about the wellness and susceptibility of loved ones and concern about one's very own tranquility and vulnerability are managed through practices of silence, obfuscation and non-disclosure. Silence provides a subtle cultural mechanism through which relations of power and intimacy are contested, subverted and/or negotiated. When narrativity is self-censored and strategically silenced, what are the reasons for doing so? What are the risks of talk for Bolivian migrants? I posit that the silence and non-disclosure surrounding the personal, social and economic struggles migrants face in their host country can be instrumental in helping sustain sociality and intimacy and indeed enable resilience in the face of such hardship. As a meaningful speech act, silence reveals as much as it conceals.

One important therapeutic approach Western psychiatry relies upon to treat multiple forms of trauma and violence is individual and group talk therapy. The globalization of talk therapy (which may occur through individual *testimonios*, debriefing sessions, group therapy, the retelling of trauma stories and other forms of remembering) in response to personal experiences of trauma and violence often rests on an assumption that a gradual or cathartic release of emotions can have deep healing properties individually and collectively at appropriately managed times (see Chap. 1). Increasingly, however, psychologists are attuned to how the social and cultural backgrounds of those in need of assistance shape the effectiveness of such approaches. Indeed, there has been considerable debate on the benefits of psychological debriefing post-trauma and a greater recognition of the fact that privileging active coping through 'talk' fails to recognize that in some contexts it can be harmful and that resilience and healing can take many different shapes across cultures (Bonanno 2004, see also Chap. 8). For example, some healing systems may focus more on ritualistic or spiritual dimensions of healing. In this chapter I ask for closer attention to the relationship between talk and local conceptualizations of the body, emotions, risk and vulnerability. Drawing upon ethnographic research conducted in Bolivia and among Bolivian migrants in Spain, I argue for a more in-depth understanding of the cultural value and motivations surrounding silence and/or non-disclosure in different contexts. Among the Andean Bolivians I have worked with, the enactment of silence is seen as a form of 'preventive' health (Escandell and Tapias 2010). That is, to remain silent in the face of hardship can protect the self from the ill wishes of others or can prevent distress and possible illness in those one loves. These practices complicate assumptions underlying the 'universal' therapeutic value of talk in non-Western contexts. Ethnographic inquiry into the multiple meanings of silence in different cultures offers a more context-sensitive understanding of the therapeutic strategies searched for and comfort levels associated with personal disclosure. It also helps reveal the multiple ways intimacy and trust are wounded by migration.

Methodology

This chapter draws upon qualitative research conducted in both Bolivia and Spain in the summers of 2006, 2007, 2008 and 2010 and from over two years of extended ethnographic fieldwork carried out in the late 1990s in the Cochabamba region of Bolivia. Participant observation and in-depth and conversational interviews were conducted among members of nearly 30 transnational families in both Bolivia and Spain. Initial interlocutors interviewed in Bolivia enabled the expansion of the research sample, as many relatives and friends migrated and provided vital contacts in Spain. Interviews in Bolivia focused on the multiple factors that influenced people's decisions to migrate as well as the broad impacts migration had on family and social relations, emotions, health and wellness concerns. The interviewees resided in the region of the Valle Alto and the city of Cochabamba as well as in Barcelona, Madrid and Bilbao. Migrants in Spain were a heterogeneous population that reflected the linguistic, ethnic and social distinctions prevalent in Bolivia, although the groups interviewed for this chapter were of Quechua ancestry.

Migration, Sociality and Emotions

As a cultural anthropologist, my work has examined the intricately interwoven aspects of emotions, health and globalization in the lives of Andean Bolivians. In Bolivia's hesitant relationship with globalization, I have asserted that the turmoil around economic instability and political volatility is not only manifested in public spheres (such as participation in popular protests) but also, more intimately, in the visceral and emotional suffering experienced by men and women (Tapias 2006a, b, 2015). By examining women's emotion narratives and paying attention to the physical, psychological and social effects of the 'violence of everyday life' (Scheper-Hughes 1992) I have approached health and the embodied manifestations of distress as a distinct arena that sheds light on the subtle links between the political restructuring of states and the private anxieties women experience under enduring political and economic precariousness. My long-term fieldwork with Quechua- and Spanish-speaking market women in Bolivia has enabled me to explore the ways women link emotions stemming from poverty, domestic violence, and social conflict to numerous 'traditional' ailments as well as illnesses regularly treated by biomedical practitioners. Furthermore, underlying implicit 'rules' of sociality and everyday interactions are concerns that the 'accumulation' of emotions such as rage, sorrow, longing, desire, jealousy, envy and disillusionment (all emotions common to the migratory experience) can lead to numerous ailments among adults and can be inter-generationally transmitted to children through women's/mother's bodies (Tapias 2006a, b).

Throughout the 1990s and 2000s, one vital mechanism through which many Bolivians have coped with the state's failure to address rampant un- and underemployment has been through out-migration. Migration, however, has also posed numerous challenges that have strained sociality and consequently impacted beliefs about health and illness. Spain was one of several destinations for Bolivian migrants seeking better employment opportunities. According to the Spanish national statistical office (INE 2007) there were 140,740 Bolivians residing in Spain in 2006. The Spanish embassy in Bolivia, however, estimated that at the peak of the migratory wave, closer to 300,000 Bolivians were residing in Spain and of these, approximately only 20 % of them held legal residency and work permits (Bárbulo 2007). The rest endured the expected stresses of being undocumented and often exploited.

In the late 1990s this inter-continental migratory flow was driven by a combination of factors such as Spain's demands for cheap labor and economic growth, and a stagnant and uncertain economy in Bolivia (Izquierdo 1996; Solé and Parella 2003). Fluency in Spanish further facilitated migrants' entry into Spain's informal economy, generally in the agricultural and construction sectors for men, and in domestic and care work for women. When employed, women migrants were often better paid and had greater job security than men. These gendered economic opportunities were catalyzed by the feminization of the Spanish labor market (Solé and Parella 2003). As Spanish women became increasingly integrated into the labor market, numerous gender role transformations and needs emerged within households, creating the demands for domestic help and care work for children and the elderly.

In 2008, with the onset of the global economic crisis, migrants experienced significant intensification of stress as wages decreased while competition for jobs and the need to retain a job increased. In Catalonia alone unemployment rates climbed to 11.8 % in the last quarter of 2008, compared to 6.6 per cent a year earlier. The migrant population was even more deeply affected with unemployment rates reaching 20.2 % among foreign workers. Among the migrant population, unemployment has been particularly high for males (22.2 %) compared to females (17.4 %). These losses have been most felt in the construction and agricultural sectors (Pajares 2009). By 2013 official unemployment rates in Spain continued to soar at 27 % unfolding not only a process of 'return migration' but also the 're-emigration' of Spaniards to other areas of the European Union.

The intent of most men and women interviewed in Spain was to return to Bolivia after earning enough income to open businesses, buy land and/or build a home. Indeed, prior to the economic recession of 2008, many migrants were able to make a living in Spain and send remittances home but the decision to migrate nonetheless had deep social and intimate repercussions. In the early 2000s migration to Spain was described as a 'craze' (*una locura*), a 'wave' that many people wanted to join and benefit from. People spoke of the ample job opportunities available: in construction, agriculture and in child and elderly care. This optimistic view of migration as 'an opportunity too good to pass up', and 'a pathway to economic prosperity' belies and obfuscates the often contentious and tempestuous processes through which decisions to migrate are made. In many cases, parents and spouses were skeptical and weary of the numerous risks of migration. For example, prior to 2007 Bolivians were not required to secure visas before travel to Spain. While at first sight this would seem to encourage migrants to migrate (in that one could travel freely as a tourist), in actuality this meant that the risk of deportation was randomly determined at the border: after migrants had already incurred significant debt (and if border control agents were skeptical that 'tourists' were indeed 'tourists'). Many young adults migrated without their parents or spouses' approval or 'blessing' and this significantly stressed familial ties. It also prevented migrants from fully disclosing difficulties and discrimination they faced during their migratory trajectory to loved ones back home out of fear of being reminded that they had been 'told so'.

The ensuing fragmentation of households also placed a significant emotional toll on transnational families. In addition to the expected sadness, sorrow and pining often associated with being separated from loved ones—children or elderly parents left behind often felt abandoned, even when remittances were forthcoming. Intimate relations were stressed not only by physical separation but also by changing gender roles, particularly when wives provided a household's main source of income and supported men back home. Suffering also ensued when remittances were not sent home, making the emotional costs of migration too high to bear.

Many of the men and women interviewed were unprepared for the difficulties and challenges they encountered upon their arrival to Spain. Anticipating a relatively easy integration into the labor economy many, in fact, found it very difficult to initially find employment. In addition, the hardship of the first few months was exacerbated by the fact that social networks were found to be non-existent or fragile, at best. Ironically, most interviewees had been persuaded to emigrate by family members and friends already abroad. During phone conversations, relatives and friends in Spain regularly spoke of the abundance of work opportunities and the ease with which one could find work. They spoke of monthly salaries earned in Euros which were ten times the amount that could be earned in Bolivia. Upon arrival in Spain, however, newer migrants found it much more difficult to establish themselves than they had been lead to believe and found that they could not count on much financial help or emotional support from relatives and friends. Thus, the reality of their experiences did not match the promises of economic prosperity and opportunity portrayed by relatives and friends. Some experienced severe exploitation, both by Spaniards and their fellow Bolivians; others experienced illnesses, others feelings of abandonment and loss of hope. While some found work immediately, others often spent months in search of steady employment and fell further into debt. Those lucky to find work quickly were nonetheless frustrated by the small remittances they could send home. Migrants spent several months and sometimes years, repaying debts accrued in order to travel to Spain.

The profound strains on sociality in Spain engendered mistrust and competition and social tensions emerged amongst migrants as people compared their relative successes and failures to the experiences of others. As people navigated these new economic terrains emotional stress was a regular part of their experiences abroad. Insofar as rules of sociality were reshaped by migration, so too were 'traditional' beliefs about emotions, the body and health. As emotions 'traveled' across borders, the ways they were expressed in Spain and communicated to loved ones back home were also reshaped. Emotional expression, constructs and embodiment were reconfigured, reinforced and contested by the challenges posed by migration.

In this chapter I explore how undocumented migrants cope with the anxieties of finding themselves in an unfamiliar physical and social context (often lacking reliable social networks) and in competition with other migrants for sources of employment. What new ways of feeling and interacting with others emerge in the process of migration and how does this influence the care of self and of others? I seek insight into these questions by focusing on particular communication strategies deployed in the context of migration: practices of silence, secrecy and obfuscation. An understanding of these practices requires being attuned to enduring as well as emergent views of the body, emotions, risk and vulnerability. Prior to an exploration of these views, however, I consider how cultural and linguistic anthropologists have explored the phenomenon of silence.

The Anthropology of Silence

Over 40 years ago, anthropologist Keith Basso called for increased attention to practices of silence and why it may be deemed a culturally appropriate response in particular contexts among the Western Apache. Following Hymes (1964), Basso argues that in examining modes of communication, attention should not only be focused on the codes, channels and expressions people enact but also to the instances in which people decide to refrain from verbal behavior (Basso 1970: 215). Basso ultimately argues that keeping silent among the Western Apache is prevalent when interlocutors believe their relationship to others is ambiguous and/or unpredictable. Similarly, I examine practices of silence and non-disclosure to reveal how migration strains social relations and as a way to provide insights into the ways beliefs about emotions persist in new contexts.

Other anthropologists have since examined the multiple meanings and functions of silence (see Chap. 3). While silence is often seen as analogous to invisibility, many scholars stress that an absence of articulation does not necessarily always mean an absence of voice (Leap 1999), power (Lakoff 1995) or the denial of an occurrence or risk (Chapman 2006; Wood and Lambert 2008). Robin Lakoff, reflecting on the meanings of silence in gender relations, also notes that 'it is easier to perceive what is there as meaningful, as opposed to discerning the meaning in the absence of a phenomenon' (1995: 25). Furthermore, many medical anthropologists have examined how people often communicate through the body and the numerous illnesses and symptoms that affect it, particularly when voicing distress is not possible or even dangerous (see Dickson-Gómez 2002; Rebhun 1993; Scheper-Hughes 1992; Tapias 2006b for discussions of *nervios* and other manifestations of the embodiment of distress). Feminist anthropologists have also examined silence, but more particularly, the phenomenon of silencing within gender and other power relations. They have focused on the myriad ways women and other minoritized groups have been silenced through interruptions, the control of discourse topic, non-response and interpretive control (Bucholtz and Hall 1995; Lakoff 1995). While these studies examine how people are silenced, attention also needs to be focused on silence as an agentive communication strategy that people may deploy in particular contexts.

I consider the occurrences of silence and 'not telling' among Bolivian migrants from two perspectives. The first unfolds transnationally as migrants conceal the suffering they fear might worry family members back home (and vice versa). The second occurrence is viewed within the context of Spain where migrants may hide information from one another. The practice of not telling and camouflaging experiences of suffering or relative success seeks to prevent the onset of future health problems. In the transnational context, protecting loved ones from hardship stories are motivated by the desire to prevent them from getting sick from sorrow or preoccupation. When carried out in Spain, practices of non-disclosure and secrecy are active efforts to protect one's own health from the envy and bad wishes of others. An understanding of these practices requires appreciation of how emotions are embodied in Bolivia and (re)constructed in

Spain. What migrants and family members intimately tell one another and, more importantly, what they hide, demonstrates the extent to which 'traditional' health beliefs about the body, illness and affect remain vibrant.

The Embodied Physicality and Sociality of Emotions at Home and Abroad

The conceptualization of emotions among my interlocutors had both physical and social dimensions and makes salient the ways the body's boundaries are perceived to be porous and permeable. During my extended fieldwork in Bolivia, people spoke of emotions such as rage and sorrow (two of the emotions most commonly linked to ill health), as if they were 'fluids' or substances that accumulated in the body or were transformed into other harmful substances. Rebhun, working in Brazil, has examined how emotions were viewed as 'energy' which acted according to the 'same physical properties as water' (Rebhun 1994: 366, 1999). Similarly, in Bolivia, both the etiological explanations for how emotions made people sick and the treatments used attested to this physicality. For instance, emotions were said to accumulate in the body when not expressed and this posed noxious effects on the body. If people did not find a means to express their emotions, these could also be transformed into other substances which then had to be eliminated to avoid illness. These views of emotions as 'fluids' are part of a larger hydraulic view of the body where equilibrium not only of hot and cold qualities (present in the body and ingested through foods and medicines) but of the flow of substances and fluids are central to the maintenance of good health (Bastien 1987; Classen 1993; Hammer 1997; Tapias 2006a, b).

The physicality of emotions is also inextricably tied to sociality. While accumulated emotions could cause illness in the actual person experiencing them, the emotions one's behaviors engendered in others could also cause ill effects. Additionally, emotions did not just affect those who 'felt' things such as sorrow, anger or envy. Rather, emotions could also be 'passed' on to others. Specifically, a mother could transmit her sorrow or rage (against injustice, violence, poverty or other forms of distress) to her child through her breast milk or through the placenta. Or finally, the envy that one individual feels towards another could have physical effects on others through the deployment of sorcery. This transmission of emotions fits within a larger belief system concerning the body, corporeality and sociality among Andeans and also shapes ideas of what constitutes 'health risks'.

The burgeoning scholarship on emotions in the last two decades has only recently begun to examine how emotions and embodiment are closely interlinked with migratory processes (Escandell and Tapias 2010; Ewing 2005; Velayutham and Wise 2005). Wise and Chapman (2005) note a lack of attention to how affect intersects with the new experiences migrants have as they encounter cultural difference. In the case of Bolivian migrants, attention must be directed to the 'traditional' beliefs about emotions and the body in Bolivia where emotions are perceived to have a direct effect on bodily wellness and where bodily injuries, in turn, can cause emotional distress.

Immigration processes pose numerous interesting challenges to how emotions are conceptualized. For example, social scientists have long examined the culturally constructed aspects of emotions and affect. They argue that emotions, rather than being 'pre-cultural', are very much shaped by the cultural 'matrix' in which emotions manifest themselves, which makes it difficult to describe the experience of people who straddle multiple cultures (Ewing 2005: 226). Certainly, the contexts that define emotions and the power dynamics inherent in social relations that shape their expression change with the migratory experience. Nonetheless, upon arrival to their host countries, migrants do not simply embrace or reject the discursive elements that shape expression in the host country, nor do they 'forget' or solely privilege the local discourses from their own home countries. The socio-cultural matrices that shape emotions are broader and more intricately woven. The 'cultural context' relevant to Bolivia-Spain migrants is very much a transnational one that borrow elements from multiple sites. As such, emotions in this transnational arena not only have 'local' meanings, manifestations and effects specific to each country but also a recombined 'local' meaning which makes sense only when embedded within the transnational cultural trajectory of the migrant life. Thus, how a migrant conceptualizes emotion is shaped not only by the emotional constructs he/she travels with but also by the new moral systems, social rules, opportunities and constraints encountered through migration.

Silence and the Care of Others

Because of the availability of new technologies, migrants were able to regularly communicate with loved ones back home (Vertovec 2004a). In spite of this frequent, sometime daily, communication migrants often remained silent or simply did not disclose stories that reflected the hardships they faced or the depths of their own suffering. In general, they selectively disclosed information to key people in the household, usually siblings or cousins close to their age, but rarely disclosed to others the multiple stresses that could accompany their migratory journey: unemployment, diminishing savings, ethnic and gender discrimination or health problems among others. While conversations with family members could occur frequently, via cheap phone calls or the Internet, these interactions were closely self-monitored and self-censored. Similar behaviors were deployed by relatives who remained behind. The silence and self-censoring make sense when considering the important role that emotions are seen to play in a person's overall health.

Joaquín, a shopkeeper interviewed in Bolivia, for example, reflects the mutual censoring he and his wife enacted as they were separated. He recounted the story of how he and his wife decided she should emigrate to Spain. In 2000, Joaquín and Isabela were doing well financially. Together, they owned four taxis, which were subcontracted to other drivers, and a small restaurant/grocery store. Joaquin and Isabela had two children and that year, when their youngest child turned a year old, as is custom, they decided to have a birthday celebration inviting many members of the community, relatives and *compadres*. They hired a band and splurged on food and drink. He recounts:

> At the time, I had the taxis, I had lots of work. When my daughter turned one we threw a big party and a little while after the party, I noticed that things started to go wrong. I started to lose money, I had to sell my taxis and everything was going badly. There was lots of envy. So my wife and I decided that she should go work in Spain to earn money so we could start over. She had a cousin there who told her there was lots of work. So she left for the Canary Islands … She's suffering …. she misses our children. It's been so long—almost two years. She tells me 'Sometimes I get sick, but I don't want to tell you, because I know you will also start to worry and get sick yourself'. I also don't want to tell her anything that is going on here—if we get sick, the kids or I—because you can start to feel very bad there as well. I just about conceal everything so that she doesn't worry, so that she doesn't suffer, so that she doesn't feel so afflicted.

Joaquin's decisions not to disclose suffering to his wife were fueled by his desire to prevent her from feeling worse and worrying about him and their children. Indeed, while interviewing migrants and their family members, conversations were often interrupted by ardent requests such as: 'Please don't mention these things to my family', Don't tell my mother', 'Don't say anything to my sister'. Such remarks do not necessarily signal a lack of trust in relatives but rather a careful selection of those with whom they would share details of their adversities. A consideration of the ramifications of expression at home and abroad (Vertovec 2004b), coupled with awareness of how emotions are embodied, help contextualize these requests for non-disclosure. Migrants were mindful of the ill effects that sorrow, preoccupation and pining could have on family members (elderly parents and grandparents, people debilitated by illnesses or loved ones in general) and were likely to censor what they told certain family members about their own health and suffering. Experiences of gender and ethnic discrimination, sexual harassment, unemployment and conflicts with siblings, roommates and others were concealed in efforts to spare those far away from suffering and illness. Lucia, a young woman who had interrupted her college education in Bolivia to try her luck in Spain, faced weeks of unemployment and hunger and once employed, experienced sexual harassment. Yet despite being very close to her sisters, she did not speak of these conflicts with her family, particularly since her father had warned her of the risks she would be taking and did not approve of her departure. Her sister Anna sensed the difficulties Lucia was facing during their regular phone conversations and asked me to relay the following message to her: 'Tell her to come home. The sacrifices she is making are not worth it; the emotional costs of emigrating are too great to compensate for the little bit of money you can make.'

Non-disclosure and silence regarding personal suffering in conjunction with efforts not to worry family members were a regular feature of many narratives collected in Spain and Bolivia. Most migrants' social networks were fragile and they lacked the social capital that could have eased their stay abroad. Nonetheless, they remained silent on the topic of their suffering or the multiple challenges they face. Such efforts were an act of love and were active efforts to preserve and protect, from afar, the intimate ties they had with their relatives The same effort to protect loved ones from negative information by 'not telling' was also visible in Bolivia. While most people suspected their loved ones in Spain withheld information, they engaged in similar practices. The distress of numerous interviewees in Bolivia was readily apparent as they actively sought to hide problems or health issues from relatives abroad.

Silence, Envy and the Care of the Self

Concern for the health of others is not the only factor motivating practices of silence and non-disclosure. The management of silence is also enacted in the care of the self. In a context of stiff competition for employment and resources, mistreatment by employers, isolation and loneliness, Bolivian migrants regularly complained about the lack of solidarity between compatriots. While clearly not all relationships were always guarded, there was a prevalent view that relations could be very strained and this shaped the types and depth of friendships and intimate relations one could forge. When migrants maintained their distance from others or suppressed information from others, the motivations behind such practices were different from active efforts to conceal information from relatives back home. Central to the apprehension about disclosing too much information to fellow Bolivians were concerns about the proliferation of envy and the possibility that the envious may resort to sorcery and affect a migrant's economic success, or in more extreme cases, physically affect their health. Silence and concealment thus remained a form of 'preventive health', but these practices were intended to protect the self, rather than the health of loved ones. In the context of migration, concerns about envy and active efforts not to be the *source* of envy provide a rich arena to observe the effects of global inequalities and how these inequalities are intimately experienced among community members. Furthermore, talk of envy, and the silence that seeks to guard its inception from occurring, grants insight on the precariousness of newly forged social networks and how ideas of reciprocity and collaboration are challenged by migration.

In Spain, the unequal accessibility of economic opportunities and social success between different migrants ensured a vibrant ground for the proliferation of envy. The discourses of envy and competition that circulated among Bolivians in Spain (who are often members of the same family or community back in Bolivia) were fueled by the constraints and opportunities posed by the receiving labor market (Hondagneu-Sotelo 1994; Fernandez-Kelley 1983; Menjivar 2003; Sassen-Koob 1984). Furthermore, the narratives of envy and competition, while shaped by adverse labor conditions, were also an intricate part of 'traditional' discourses and folk constructions of illness and misfortune and a reflection of rules of sociality in Bolivia (Crandon 1983, Crandon-Malamud 1991; Hammer 1997; Hawkins and Price 2001; Tapias 2006a, b; Van Vleet 2003). As migrants traversed borders, they forged new social ties and developed new networks. These fragile ties and networks, however, were strained by the hardships of migration and were not always very dependable. Indeed, throughout interviews envy was regularly evoked as people tried to explain conflicts with others and as they navigated between the pull they felt between meeting the expectations of the community of migrants and their own desires and aspirations to get ahead and find ways to prosper.

The unpredictability and uncertainty surrounding whether people would prioritize their own self-interests or meet moral obligations to the collective community engendered widespread mistrust and a profound lack of confidence in one's networks. In both Bolivia and Spain, migrants and their family members and friends lamented 'there is no fraternity among Bolivians'; 'there is no trust (*confianza*).' This disillusionment usually expressed through stories of mistreatment from their *propios paisanos*, their very own countrymen or even family members or *compadres*. The realities of migration stressed these relationships, often to the point of disbanding them (Menjívar 1995; Napolitano Quayson 2005).

Throughout interviews migrants spoke of how disheartening and disappointing it was to come to the realization that relatives and friends would not share contacts, charged them exorbitant rents, spread lies to disrepute them or took advantage of their vulnerability. In Bolivia, these relations between relatives and friends were likely to be on a more equal footing, but in Spain, the newly arrived were very dependent on and often disappointed by their relatives. Because of the lack of trust in the available networks, migrants often feared that if they succeeded economically, they would be the target of envy and this would dampen their success or negatively affect their health.

In light of this lack of trust and concerns about their own vulnerability and well-being, migrants were careful with the information they disclosed to others. This was particularly the case if things were going relatively well for them, that is, if they were gainfully employed and in some instances able to send home remittances. People did not freely share information about their economic situations, their earnings, savings, or the amount of remittances they were able to send to Bolivia. In 2008, at the cusp of the economic crisis in Spain, Teresa, a cleaning lady who held numerous jobs, pleaded for me not to share information about her with her three roommates. Many workers were beginning to feel the effect of the economic decline as Spaniards were no longer able to afford the domestic services these women provided. While earlier that day, we had all shared a meal and they all seemed very fond and supportive of one another, Teresa was keenly aware and self-conscious about her good fortune regarding employment and was concerned her roommates would be envious. In many ways, the decision to migrate, although not easy, had gone well for Teresa. Upon arrival to Spain, she had 'inherited' numerous jobs from a cousin who had returned to Bolivia and who recommended Teresa to her employers. Somewhat embarrassed she told me: 'I arrived in Barcelona at 5:00 p.m. on a Wednesday and was working at 7:00 a.m. on Thursday morning.' Teresa actively cleaned seven households and the public areas of an apartment building each week. With good reason, she felt closely watched by her roommates who wondered how many sources of income she actually had since she was never home. Teresa recounts:

> It's just that there is a lot of *miramiento* (vigilance). People are envious. I tell them I only clean 4 houses and that on the other days I go to an agency to look for work. If they knew how many jobs I had they would say I was selfish and would envy me. I just want to make enough money to go back home to my three daughters. I cannot afford to lose any of my jobs.

Teresa was acutely aware that her own good fortune could fuel the envy of others. As such she felt the need to conceal as many details about her work life as possible, less she make herself vulnerable to other people's ill wishes. While her entire plan to migrate extolled a significant emotional cost (by being away from her daughters), she was determined to succeed. She worried that others would view her as ambitious and 'selfish' because of the number of jobs that she held (thus preventing others from prospering as well). She was convinced that if others knew of her good fortune, she might be envied, they might resort to sorcery to harm her and she might be at risk of losing one of her jobs. All of Teresa's interactions with her roommates were guarded and secretive. When the topic of work came up, she often tried to direct the conversation elsewhere. Like Teresa, many other migrants guarded information from others, evading questions in social settings or providing vague answers to people's questions.

Among Bolivian families the stresses and hardship produced by migration are believed to be the triggers of illnesses among migrants themselves and/or their relatives back home. The link between emotions and health influences how migrants administer and share personal difficulties with relatives and with fellow migrants. Practices of non-disclosure and secrecy tangibly demonstrate the relationship between bodily and emotional health, and are a concrete and ongoing linkage between people at opposite ends of the migratory chain or within the same community of migrants. Controlling emotional expression, that is, carefully selecting what information to share with others, and what to keep concealed, is a tangible way of *managing* the ill effects that emotions can cause others or oneself.

Conclusions

In this chapter I have called for greater attention to practices of silence in different contexts and its relationship to conceptualizations of the body, emotions, risk and vulnerability. Beginning in the 1990s and throughout the first decade of the new millennium, emigration to Spain was one of the principal economic strategies that many Bolivians relied upon to earn a better living and provide a better life for their loved ones. The emotional costs of migration, however, are often very high. Families can be fragmented for years at a time and they are forced to forge new forms of intimacy with one another. As shown in this chapter, the withholding of information from relatives in Bolivia and vice versa is an act of concern for a loved one's health. The withholding of information from fellow migrants in Spain is an act of self-care. When examining the case of Bolivians in Spain, we can see that beliefs and concerns about emotions such as sorrow, preoccupation and envy continue to underpin the interactions migrants have with their family members and with fellow Bolivians in Spain. As one considers how migrants in Spain and relatives in Bolivia communicate and interact with one another and how migrants in Spain communicate among themselves, it becomes apparent that the regularity and speed with which information is shared and the instability of newly forged social networks unravel new self-monitoring practices regarding their emotional lives. Migrants rely on silence, white lies and non-disclosure not only to protect others and to give themselves a sense of security but also to provide a way to sustain sociality and intimacy. This self-monitoring reflects 'traditional' beliefs that physical pains unleash emotional harms and, vice versa, that emotional harms can manifest themselves as physical pains. In transnational communication, contact through cheap phone calls and the Internet stimulates increased censorship in the routine conversations migrants have with family members. Thus, they tell one another about their lives and distress but also mutually consider how their own suffering affects the emotional states of those from whom they are separated. Among migrants in Spain similar communication strategies emerge but for different reasons.

The migrants interviewed often feared the proliferation of envy and the potential dangers it posed to one's employment and well-being. In Spain migrants never boasted about their success and emphasized the emotional and physical sacrifices they had to make to be where they were. Through appreciation of how emotions operate and are conceptualized in Bolivia, we can better understand migrants' self-monitoring practices in both arenas and the concerns migrants have about disclosing information about themselves to others. The silence and obfuscating strategies that migrants and family members deploy are instrumental in helping sustain intimacy and indeed enable resilience in the face of social and economic hardship.

References

Bárbulo, T. 2007. Último vuelo sin visa para los bolivianos. *El País*, April 1.

Basso, K.H. 1970. 'To give up on words': Silence in Western Apache Culture. *Southwestern Journal of Anthropology* 26(3): 213–230.

Bastien, J. 1987. *Healers of the Andes.* Salt Lake City: University of Utah Press.

Bonanno, G.A. 2004. Loss, Trauma, and Human Resilience: Have We Underestimated the Human Capacity to Thrive After Extremely Aversive Events? *American Psychologist* 59(1): 20–28.

Broch-Due, V. 2005. Violence and Belonging: Analytical Reflections. In *Violence and Belonging: The Quest for Identity in Post-colonial Africa*, ed. Vigdis Broch-Due, 1–40. London: Routledge Press.

Bucholtz, M., and K. Hall. 1995. Introduction: Twenty Years After Language and Women's Place. In *Gender Articulated: Language and the Socially Constructed Self*, eds. Kira Hall and Mary Bucholtz, 1–22. New York: Routledge.

Chapman, R. 2006. Chikotsa-Secrets, Silence and Hiding: Social Risk and Reproductive Vulnerability in Central Mozambique. *Medical Anthropology Quarterly* 20(4): 487–515.

Classen, C. 1993. *Inca Cosmology and the Human Body.* Salt Lake City: University of Utah Press.

Crandon, L. 1983. Why Susto? *Ethnology* 22(2): 153–168.

Crandon-Malamud, L. 1991. *From the Fat of Our Souls.* Berkeley: University of California Press.

Desjarlais, R., and A. Kleinman. 1997. Violence and Well-Being. *Social Science and Medicine* 45(8): 1143–1145.

Dickson-Gómez, J. 2002. The Sound of Barking Dogs: Violence and Terror Among Salvadoran Families in the Postwar. *Medical Anthropology Quarterly* 16(4): 415–438.

Escandell, X., and M. Tapias. 2010. Transnational Lives, Travelling Emotions and Idioms of Distress Among Bolivian Migrants in Spain. *Journal of Ethnic and Migration Studies* 36(3): 407–423.

Ewing, K.P. 2005. Immigrant Identities and Emotion. In *A Companion to Psychological Anthropology*, eds. C. Casey and R. Edgerton, 225–240. Oxford: Blackwell.

Farmer, P. 1996. On Suffering and Structural Violence. *Daedalus* 125(1): 261–283.

Fernandez-Kelly, P. 1983. *For We Are Sold, I and My Peope: Women and Industry in Mexico's Frontier*. Albany: State University of New York Press.

Fassin, D., and R. Rechtman. 2009. *The Empire of Trauma: An Inquiry into the Condition of Victimhood*. Princeton, NJ: Princeton University Press.

Hammer, P. 1997. 'To be a woman is to suffer': The interplay of Illness, Emotions, and the Body in Quechua Women's Experiences. Ph.D. thesis, University of Illinois.

Hawkins, K., and N. Price. 2001. From International Policy to Local Reality: Women's Reproductive Health Strategies in el alto, bolivia. In *Managing Reproductive Life: Cross-Cultural Themes in Fertility and Sexuality*, ed. S. Tremayne, 52–70. New York: Berghahn.

Hondagneu-Sotelo, P. 1994. *Gendered Transitions: Mexican Experiences of Immigration*. Berkeley: University of California Press.

Hymes, D. 1964. Introduction: Towards Ethnographies of Communication. In *The Ethnography of Communication*, eds. J.J. Gumperz and D. Hymes, 1–34. American Anthropologist, Special Publication, 66(6) part 2.

INE. 2007. *Demografía y población*. Instituto Nacional de Estadística. Online at: http://www.ine.es/inebmenu/mnu_cifraspob/htm

Izquierdo, A. 1996. *La inmigración inesperada: La población extranjera en españa (1991–1995)*. Madrid: Trotta.

Jenkins, J. 1991. The State Construction of Affect: Political Ethos and Mental Health among Salvadorean Refugees. *Culture, Medicine and Psychiatry* 15: 139–165.

Kleinman, A., V. Das, and M. Lock, eds. 1997. *Social Suffering*. Berkeley: University of California Press.

Lakoff, R.T. 1995. Cries and Whispers: The Shattering of the Silence. In *Gender Articulated: Language and the Socially Constructed Self*, eds. Kira Hall and Mary Bucholtz, 25–50. London: Routledge.

Leap, W. 1999. Language, Socialization, and Silence in Gay Adolescence. In *Reinventing Identities: The Gendered Self in Discourse*, eds. Mary Bucholtz, A.C. Liang, and Laurel A. Sutton, 259–272. New York: Oxford University Press.

Menjívar, C. 1995. Kinship Networks Among Immigrants: Lessons from a Qualitative Comparative Approach. *International Journal of Comparative Sociology* 36(1–2): 219–233.

———. 2003. *Through the Eyes of Women: Gender, Social Networks, Family and Structural Change in Latin America and the Caribbean*, International Studies in Social Science. Ontario: de Sitter.

Napolitano, Q.V. 2005. Social Suffering and Embodied States of Male Transnational Migrancy in San Francisco, California. *Identities* 12(2): 335–362.

Pajares, M. 2009. La Inserció Laboral de la Població Immigrada: L'estat de la Immigració a Catalunya, 1–27. Barcelona: Fundavio Jaume Bonfil. http://www.fbofill.cat/publicacions/la-insercion-laboral-de-la-poblacion-inmigrada

Rebhun, L. 1993. Nerves and Emotional Play in Northeast Brazil. *Medical Anthropology Quarterly* 7(2): 131–151.

———. 1994. Swallowing Frogs: Anger and Illness in Northeast Brazil. *Medical Anthropology Quarterly* 8(4): 360–382.

———. 1999. *The Heart is Unknown Country: Love in the Changing Economy of Northeast Brazil.* Stanford, CA: Stanford University Press.

Sassen-Koob, S. 1984. Notes on the Incorporation of Third World Women into Wage Labour Through Offshore Production. *International Migration Review* 18(4): 1144–1167.

Scheper-Hughes, N. 1992. *Death Without Weeping.* Berkeley: University of California Press.

Solé, C., and S. Parella. 2003. The Labour Market and Racial Discrimination in Spain. *Journal of Ethnic and Migration Studies* 29(1): 121–140.

Tapias, M. 2006a. Always Ready and Always Clean? Competing Discourses of Breast-Feeding, Infant Illness and the Politics of Mother-Blame in Bolivia. *Body and Society* 12(2): 83–108.

———. 2006b. Emotions and the Intergenerational Embodiment of Social Suffering in Rural Bolivia. *Medical Anthropology Quarterly* 20(3): 399–415.

———. 2015. *Embodied Protests: Emotions and Women's Health in Bolivia.* Urbana: University of Illinois press.

Van Vleet, K. 2003. Partial Theories: On Gossip, Envy and Ethnography in the Andes. *Enthnography* 4(4): 491–519.

Velayutham, S., and A. Wise. 2005. Moral Economies of a Translocal Village: Obligation and Shame Among South Indian Transnational Migrants. *Global Networks* 5(1): 27–47.

Vertovec, S. 2004a. Cheap Calls: The Social Glue of Migrant Transnationalism. *International Migration Review* 4(2): 219–242.

———. 2004b. Migrant Transnationalism and Modes of Transformation. *International Migration Review* 38(3): 970–1001.

Wise, A., and A. Chapman. 2005. Introduction: Migration, Affect and the Senses. *Journal of Intercultural Studies* 26(1): 1–3.

Wood, K., and H. Lambert. 2008. Coded Talk, Scripted Omissions: The Micropolitics of AIDS Talk in an Affected Community in South Africa. *Medical Anthropology Quarterly* 22(3): 213–233.

CHAPTER 8

Multisemic Speech Genres as Vehicles for Re-inscribing Meaning in Post-conflict Societies: A Mozambican Case

Bjørn Enge Bertelsen

Beyond material destruction and human suffering, civil wars entail the violent transformation and erasure of existential, social, relational, cosmological and ontological meaning (Maček 2014; Whitehead 2011; Hoffman 2011; Robben 2010).[1] In fact, it has been argued that modern wars are destructive *in extremis* precisely due to their comprehensive, mediated nature and with a dynamic encompassing and engulfing the realm of everyday life (Whitehead and Finnström 2013). Further, and as Butler (2009) has argued, ongoing mass mediation not only ceaselessly distributes war across living rooms globally but also establishes certain frames of war wherein human life and its loss are cast as grievable or ungrievable—thus inculcating and normalising both the continuing of warfare generally as well as the wars continually waged at Euro-American peripheries (see also Joxe 2002). It might also be argued that the myriad forms of the war machine of the twentieth and twenty-first centuries reflect a double dynamic of increased securiticisation and violence that characterize societ-

B.E. Bertelsen (✉)
Department of Social Anthropology, University of Bergen,
Bergen, Norway

V. Broch-Due, B.E. Bertelsen (eds.), *Violent Reverberations*,
DOI 10.1007/978-3-319-39049-9_8

ies nominally at peace—such as the global North (see, e.g., Fassin 2013 [2011]; Bertelsen and Zagato 2015).

Away from flickering TV screens displaying precision warfare inherent to necessary wars against 'terrorists', war on the ground is concrete: the large-scale violence that ravaged predominantly rural Mozambique from 1976/77 to 1992 razed hundreds of thousands of homesteads, maimed bodies and broke vital and life-sustaining agricultural cycles. It also, however, produced effects that transcend the temporal confinements into singular violent events or periods of warfare (Nordstrom 1997). Since the formal peace agreement was signed in 1992 at the national level between both the Frelimo government and Renamo insurgents, the two warring and later political parties predominantly communicate that the civil war era has ended. Simultaneously, however, bellicose moral and political dimensions of the civil war are still regularly evoked and invoked by both parties in heated political debates, election rallies, and so on, making the civil war still loom large in popular and political discourse alike. The waxing and waning of civil war rhetoric—often following electoral campaigns or other significant political temporalities—commonly result in violence mimicking on a lesser scale that of the civil war, especially as armed confrontations between alleged Renamo groups and various forces of the government security apparatus started again in 2012 (Reuters 2013). One example of this was in mid-May 2014 when confrontations between alleged Renamo groups and Special Forces units of the government (the so-called FIR—*Força da Intervenção Rapida*) left numbers of policemen as well as Renamo-affiliated dead (Mozambique News Reports 2014). Further, the situation of low-intensity warfare and threats of large-scale war continue with Renamo groups forming their own armed police force as well as army bases in mid-June 2015 (see also Igreja 2015). In early 2016 the situation is even graver with around 6000 Mozambican refugees in Malawi having fled fighting between government troops and Renamo close to the Malawi-Mozambique border (UNHCR 2016). Further, attacks on civilians, especially on road transport, have also been resumed, together with an emergent outlawing of Renamo from regular Mozambican politics (Lusa 2016).

The resurgence of violence and fighting from 2012 onwards is reminiscent of how particular modalities of warfare—including Renamo's civil war-style ambushing of policemen—continues to produce a Mozambican political crisis which is the object of major discussion at the national level. In strong and significant ways, the re-emergence of violence from 2012 brings back to life the ghosts of the past—and once again present violence mirroring violence past dominates major national discourses and informs positions.

However, such a presence of the past is significantly also found at the *local level*, identifiable in what one may term post-conflict 're-constructive practices' where, in addition to ritual cleansing and the re-engagement of agrarian cycles of production, the civil war violence remains central to the domain of everyday conversation and storytelling. This chapter will empirically explore such post-war oral practice from a non-national domain. This focus is chosen also as these domains are key loci for countering what Allen Feldman (2004:164–165) terms powerful state-dominated processes of '[p]oliticized anamnesis [which] constantly requires the re-auditing of "residual" marginal, repressed, denied and unreconciled historical fragments that can call the present into question, and to political accountability'. Employing the theoretical apparatus of particularly Bakhtin (1981, 1986), I will argue that oral thematisation in the form of stories is crucial in this respect. Or as Nefissa Naguib (2009:141) states in her work on Palestinian women, '... stories are memories of the past merging with current life'. In addressing 'current life' and past sufferings present, stories are circulated, enacted, contested and appropriated to form, I argue, wholly new and constantly changing *speech genres*. Their social force and importance in post-conflict societies reside in their capacity to transcend the particularities of individual narrators and the dyadic construction of speaker/listener—or therapist/traumatised, for that matter. Thus, in their social settings, multiple and multisemic speech genres effectively address civil war violence by re-inscribing *post hoc* meaning to an emerging, fragile and ambiguous post-conflict social order. Constituting in Feldman's sense 'unreconciled historical fragments' that deny, are ambiguous towards or critique national level discourses, these stories also have critical potential that transcend their localities of production, circulation and appropriation.

What of the Spoken? Reassessing the Critique

The idea, concept and therapeutic practices associated with 'trauma'—routinely premised on the individual as locus for suffering—is the subject of both global distribution and local re-interpretation, as has also been ascertained in this volume's Chapter 1. Increasingly, these approaches to trauma have been challenged especially for their universalist, oral and individual (and, some would say, individuating) characteristics and bias (see, e.g., Breslau 2004) or the tendencies of trauma discourse to emphasise victimhood over resilience (see, e.g., Scheper-Hughes 2008). Particularly, this critique has been launched against a universal application of the notion of post-traumatic stress disorder (PTSD) to contexts of suffering, war and violence (see also Chap. 1).[2]

Englund's early critique (1998) is typical in this regard: In an analysis of Mozambican civil war refugees in Malawi, he argues that the notion of PTSD problematically revolves around discursive therapies, universalised symptoms and the individual. Instead, Englund writes, it is important to acknowledge non-verbal dimensions, such as the roles of bodily practices in the form of mortuary rites and spirit exorcism rituals, which obviate group-individual distinctions. Likewise, scholars such as Werbner (1991, 1995) with Zimbabwean and Lambek (1996) with Madagascan cases have, directly or indirectly, challenged notions of the spoken in terms of individuated, presumably cathartic oral therapeutic practices by proposing, alternatively, to view memory as encompassing bodily, spiritual and other domains of highly contested pasts. Further, and drawing on *longue durée* research on the painful weight of the past among Vietnamese refugees, Knudsen (2005:164) argues succinctly that '... much of the therapeutic community [is] trapped (perhaps unconsciously?) in the nemesis of the neo-Freudian dogma of the healing powers to talk.' A similar critique is launched by Young who, in relation to PTSD's origins in the context of the treatment of US Vietnam Veterans, claims that a predominant logic is 'that every patient conceals a narrative, his pathogenic secret' (Young, quoted in McKinney 2007:266). Further, Fassin and Rechtman (2009 [2007]) have, of course, also made a genealogical critical account of the rise of the political economy of the term 'trauma' as well the universalization of notions such as PTSD. Finally, from a psychiatric and anthropological point of view, Nicolas et al. (2015) question the cross-cultural relevance of the political economy of PTSD and its de facto importance for therapists (see also Moghimi 2012 for an overview of anthropological approaches to PTSD).

These critiques are important correctives to the shortcomings of especially the wholesale application of the notion of PTSD as a global template. However, they have also, perhaps inadvertently, served to sideline the crucial dimension of *the spoken* in contexts of violence in their eagerness to underline non-verbal aspects. Recognising and endorsing this critique, this text will nonetheless re-emphasise this oral domain but stress that it works in tandem with non-oral practices and wider socio-cultural traits of any post-conflict social order. As such, this oral domain should neither be seen as an element of potential therapeutic practices nor be understood prescriptively. Put differently, seeing oral practice in terms of distinct 'speech genres' (Bakhtin 1986), I seek *neither* to privilege the spoken simply in a celebration of a multitude of voices—as in some post-modern literature—*nor* support a recourse to particular formalised and universalist PTSD discourses wherein the empirical diversity is contained—and constrained. Rather, by underlining the dynamic, complex and powerful elements of the spoken, Bakhtinian speech genres are argued to be apt for grasping the fluidity characteristic of *post hoc* addressing of the violent erasure and inscription of meaning characteristic of civil war.

Post-War Fieldwork. A Note on Context, Method and Stories

The Mozambican civil war was the outcome of a range of complex internal and external processes including heavily unpopular state policies implemented in Mozambique after its 1975 independence by the liberation movement Frelimo (Geffray 1990), Southern Rhodesia's and later Apartheid South Africa's policies of destabilisation through the guerrilla movement Renamo (Vines 1996), and the diverging Cold War interests of USA and the Soviet Union (Hall and Young 1997). Evident in its immense human and material destruction, its loss of 1 million lives and its 5 million refugees, the civil war was characterised by violence that may be understood as a force that both erases and inscribes meaning (see also Bertelsen 2004b).

Numerous rural localities were destroyed during the war and it was into such a context I entered to do long-term anthropological fieldwork in the autumn of 1999. In the main site of fieldwork, a rural context that I choose to call 'Honde' outside the city of Chimoio, central Mozambique, people had at the time of the first fieldwork just recently or were still in the process of returning to their war-torn home area. Through participant observation as well as carrying out ethnographic interviews during the initial ten-month period of fieldwork I was able to follow closely practical post-war processes at the local level relating to the allocation of land, the reconstruction of houses, the re-opening of plots, communal and individual rituals of post-war cleansing and so on. Returning at irregular intervals and having until 2016 undertaken a total of 23 months of fieldwork (during the periods 1998, 1999–2000, 2004, 2005, 2007, 2008, 2012,

2013, 2016), the long-term engagement with the community of Honde has provided my ethnographic material with considerable time-depth. In addition to studying Honde, I have carried out repeated fieldworks in a limited number of other urban and peri-urban localities for comparative purposes during the same fieldwork periods.[3]

These multiple and recurring fieldworks span around 17 years and have produced qualitative data on the formation of post-war communities in general, as well as specific knowledge on the social processes related to the war and its violence. One such important social practice in Honde was the stories constantly told and retold in most social settings, when moving through the war-torn landscape or when attending practical chores (see also Nora 1989). I will here analyse the different categories and contexts of stories recounted as these emerged mainly within the fieldwork period of 1999 and 2000, as well as use supplementary material from numerous fieldworks between 2004 and 2016.

Theme One: War as Complex

The theme of war as a complex matter from which meaning is difficult to expound was recurrent and persistently communicated in Honde. Especially, the intricacies of national and international politics influenced perceptions. One variety of such a vision of complexity was conveyed to me by an informant while a group of men sat in the shade of a mango tree at the household of one, drinking a few cups of *nipa* (homemade liquor). Conversations revolved around current politics and the upcoming elections in early December 1999. One man, Eduardo, in his late thirties and a former soldier of FAM (Frelimo's post-independence government's army), recounted the background for the current Mozambican state of affairs: 'Here we had war. *Eh pah*! There was a lot in this zone. First we had the colonial war, and then "the war of Renamo"'. Smiling, an elderly local resident turned towards me as well as addressing the first and said: 'And then you should not forget "the war of Smiti" [Ian Smith]. That was a hard war.'

The war of Smiti refers to the Zimbabwean liberation war fought until independence in 1980. Especially following Mozambican independence in 1975, Zimbabwean guerrillas operated from Mozambican soil and were persecuted there by Southern Rhodesian troops (Bhebe and Ranger 1996). This uneasy relation to Southern Rhodesia/Zimbabwe and its influence on the war in Mozambique were also expressed in another setting in

November 1999 after it had rained furiously for days on end. Working predominantly as peasants, many spend such days of hard rain inside the cooking huts around the fireplace, sleeping, eating and sleeping again—rain suspending the cycle of work and blurring distinctions between night and day. When the rain had finally halted, this did not mean the streams and ditches encircling and criss-crossing the low-lying agricultural plots [*matoros*] had subsided: The news on the radio of floods in the south preoccupied Honde's rainmaker [*tchirenge*], and he voiced his concern for the state of the vegetables he was currently growing.[4] When I accompanied him to inspect these, he contemplated aloud about Zimbabwe's and Honde's interwoven pasts:

> Many of us worked in Zimbabwe before. It was good work, and the pay was good. Zimbabwe was much better than here. But then there were problems. Eh! Great problems. The war came, and we are in the centre of the things. We are between Zimbabwe and Mozambique, and that is bad.

One dimension evident here is that of Honde being caught between the violent dynamics of Mozambique and Zimbabwe/Southern Rhodesia. A related experience of being unprotected holds significance as the civil war was waged against Renamo 'bandits' in the view of FAM and Frelimo, and against a repressive government in Renamo's view. This frequently expressed sentiment is here also voiced by the *tchirenge*:

> The war destroyed a lot. When Frelimo came, they came as enemies. When Renamo came, they came as enemies

Other aspects pointing to wider international connections were also, however, regularly addressed. At another occasion I sat again drinking and talking with several middle-aged to elderly Honde residents. The former FAM solider, Eduardo, deliberated on the pros and cons of different weaponry before pointing out international involvement:

> But the war is bad. All the wars are political, only. They are all bad. The problem was Samora [Machel, Mozambican president 1975–1986], but also America. This war came from America. [...] Shit! It is like Bulgaria in Angola. They sold a lot of arms there, these guys. It is like America here that sold arms and did politicking.

Coming from a man who had fought Renamo 'bandits' seven years in the FAM, the view that the war was 'bad' starkly contrasts the Frelimo-held image of a nation threatened by Southern Rhodesian and South African aggression and Renamo's alleged blood thirst. Eduardo's own story of terming the war as 'bad' thus forms an oppositional point to *both* Renamo's and Frelimo's adversely posed narratives by pointing out its suffering and meaninglessness in terms of being 'only political'. In this, Eduardo is informed by his own particular war in which he was captured numerous times and tortured and starved in a Renamo camp before succeeding to escape. But frequently additional elements are also communicated, especially in terms of how the war entailed debasing, anti-human and confusing effects. While aiding Eduardo in weeding his maize plot, he also spoke to me of his time in the FAM and how hard it was to distinguish friend from foe:

> Here in Manica [province] Frelimo were very undisciplined. Frelimo robbed people, beat them, killed them, and said it was Renamo that did it! Will you believe that? You cannot do that!

Donning the garbs of the enemy was widely practiced during the war (see also Nordstrom 1997), effectively making opaque distinctions between groups of armed men. Such experience of the civil war as chaotic and opaque also complements that of the impossibility of a 'just war'. Many former combatants and non-combatants alike stressed that the civil war was 'dirty' or 'unjust', often explicitly in comparison to the preceding liberation war (1964–1974) fought by Frelimo against the Portuguese colonial rule.[5] What is conveyed by such stories is the civil war's complexity understood in terms of 'bad', 'dirty' or 'unjust' in keeping with memory also always being a moral discourse (Werbner 1995). However, the civil war was also spoken of in more unequivocal terms.

Theme Two: War as Liberating or Destructive

The many stories that also cast the civil war as either simply 'liberating' or 'destructive' seemingly mimic the national meta-narratives of Renamo and Frelimo where the latter portray the former as destructive bandits and the former, conversely, claimed the war as one of liberation against Frelimo tyranny. Contrasting the absoluteness and rhetorical purity of such national antagonistic narratives, the stories circulating in Honde are made more opaque by setting, position and political affiliations. Crucially, the fluidity of these expressed perceptions is dictated by the social context of oral practice and does *not* necessarily reflect individual positions or experiences. An example of this dynamic emerged in the following case where António, a prominent Honde Frelimo supporter, told me and several visitors from Chimoio about the alleged lack of local support for Renamo:

> No-one here supported Renamo. Renamo only controlled them with arms. Local people were recruited with machetes. White [shiny] weapons were used. They do not make any noise at all. You just cut. My five brothers were taken by Renamo. Now it is only me left.

He added that prior to Renamo's arrival, in Honde there was no *aldeia comunal*—a communal village system introduced by Frelimo post-independence and integral to attempts at modernisation of the rural sector (Bertelsen 2016; see also Coelho 1993). However, after Renamo came, António said, people were in 1982 brought to *aldeias comunais* by FAM for protection.

At one level, such a story may be understood as reflecting political conflict: Renamo rhetorically defined the *aldeias comunais* variously as inimical to peasantry and 'tradition' or as Communist repression. Beyond its protective purpose, Frelimo defined *aldeias comunais* in terms of communal agrarian production and as a means for rationalising peasant production. Also, such national narratives are continuously appropriated locally, and António's claim that there was no *aldeia comunal* in Honde may be perceived as such an adaptation. Interestingly in doing so, he invoked the *negative* image of *aldeias comunais* as being repressive enclosures partly reflecting Renamo rhetoric. Conversely, Renamo sympathisers posit the existence of *aldeias comunais* as the *raison d'être* for what it saw as Renamo's war of liberation wherein its war machine destroyed statal, anti-traditional institutions (Bertelsen 2009a, 2016).

Thus, these different stories seemingly express multiple dimensions, relating both to war's *ontology* (i.e. whether or not there existed an *aldeia comunal* in Honde) and *causality*. However, treating violence and trauma as identical to individual experience and that which is verbalised is a dangerous analytical impasse as, for instance, Knudsen (2005) and Das (1997, 2015) have also argued: António, in this case, explained to me in a different setting how he benefited from Frelimo's communal agricultural aspirations and became comparatively well off with a goat, a bicycle and other material goods, only to be impoverished by the war that followed. Further, although acknowledging prevalent anti-Frelimo sentiments in Honde, he countered pro-Renamo arguments by underlining Renamo destruction: As there was no *aldeia comunal* before 1982, there was no rationale for Renamo's violence.

This highly ambivalent relation between experience and what is verbalised is also illustrated by another setting where several elderly men, António, the *tchirenge* and I conversed under yet another mango tree. As usual, the conversation oscillated between crops, soil and politics. Speaking of the latter, *tchirenge* said:

> The war against the Portuguese [1964–1974] changed a lot. When we had Frelimo afterwards they did away with all the tradition, all the *régulos* [chiefs]. We had nothing, only party secretaries. That was bad. Then came the war of Dhlakama [civil war] and it changed again. He wanted us to do rituals, to have a *régulo*.

As the *tchirenge* sat and recounted his version in this setting, António nodded, seemingly in agreement, despite having frequently provided me and others with a different version. This 'stifling' of António by the *tchirenge*'s story is interesting as an indicator of authority and influence in terms of which stories carry the greatest contextual currency—what Feldman (2004:167) calls the 'social being of narrative truth'. It also illustrates the complex relations between stories, politics and context, bearing in mind that at another occasion, in the quote above, the *tchirenge* gave complementary views on the war and its actors, saying both Renamo and Frelimo came as enemies. This corresponds more closely to his personal experience of harassment, destruction and flight. However, there is also a sense that an *order* has been regained by 'the war of Dhlakama' in the rituals of old re-acknowledged, the *régulo* [chief] returned and, in that respect, societal structures (and also his status as rainmaker) partly re-instituted. Conversely, for António the destructive war entailed an un-ordering of the local community and practices.

War, the Extraction of the Spoken and 'Life History'

Stories told and their setting, contents and nature are entry points into Mozambican perceptions of violence and war—an important feature being that stories are often recounted with several present. During fieldwork, I recorded a host of formally near identical stories revolving around the same events, themes and locations, sometimes elaborating in great detail and at other times narrated matter-of-fact-like. Frequently expressed in oral practice, but by no means unproblematic, these stories arguably constitute a powerful and dynamic social form of generalised post-conflict experience and knowledge. In keeping with this argument people often therefore *do* draw on and vocalise strands of these experiences in telling stories as (if) they are crucial features of Honde's past and present.

My material thus contradicts Dolan and Schafer's (1997:18) findings that in post-war Mozambique there was a general lack of a 'willingness to talk'. In interviewing and asking people direct questions, vocalising direct experience cannot, perhaps, be expected and may account for such unwillingness to speak. Rather, by long-term fieldwork and taking part in social life, the 'talk' is a social and not necessarily individual phenomenon integral to everyday life—not matter to be extracted from it to be re-inserted into formulaic contexts of therapy or mined through questionnaires. A related problematic has also perhaps shaped Carolyn Nordstrom's (1997) otherwise highly valuable work. The stories collected through Nordstrom's 'runway-strip anthropology' privileging '... *topic* and a *process* rather than a *place*' (1997:10, italics in original) was to a large extent based on multiple short fieldworks during the civil war. Neither being in for the long haul through a lengthy one-place fieldwork, nor focusing on the specific 'social life of stories', Nordstrom is thereby prevented from assessing and accessing generalised stories that circulate and are enacted, and also to effectively differentiate these from those seen as personal and idiosyncratic, yet important and listened to.

An example of the latter category is Jorge's story, a man persecuted by Renamo for his Frelimo involvement. António and I had gone to visit him, and we sat under a courtyard tree, shaded from the midday sun, together with some of Jorge's neighbours. We had just finished a meal of *sadza* (maize-meal porridge) and fried eggs when Jorge apologised profusely for being unable to 'follow the tradition' and serve chicken. This lack of meat, he explained, was the fault of the Renamo soldiers, spurring him on to narrate his war experience:

> I lived here in Honde before the war, working on the fields like everyone else. One day Renamo came, and I was taken away. They brought me and some others to [...]. There I was undressed completely and beaten

> under the threat of guns. I was questioned: 'Where do you work?' I did not answer, but I think they knew I had been working a bit with Frelimo. Others were set free. To me they shouted 'I will kill you', and they beat me. Then they shot me in my right foot, and in my right shoulder. They also stuck a bayonet in my back when I had fallen to the ground. They left me and sat around smoking marihuana, not paying attention. Me and one of the others ran away naked. The other had lost a lot of blood. I had to leave him by a river to go and get help. He died there. I came naked to my house. My whole family had run away. I ran, ran, ran. I came to the main road. A car stopped for me, and drove me to Chimoio. I survived.

Stories and pasts have their own dynamics and settings—some being silenced altogether (Kidron 2009). Knudsen has argued that '[g]iven its situationally constructed nature, a life history is not a story of a life but rather a conscious, or even unconscious, strategy for self-presentation, a legitimization of moves and countermoves and of projections for the future' (1995:29; see also 2005:161–171). Knudsen's position complements Bakhtin's notion of the *speaker* also always being a respondent: 'He is not, after all, the first speaker, the one who disturbs the eternal silence of the universe. And he presupposes not only the existence of the language system he is using, but also the existence of preceding utterances ...' (1986:69). Endorsing these views, examining how stories, as Jorge's, are received, transformed, contested and appropriated is crucial to appreciate the local unfolding of post-conflict processes.[6] The story of Jorge is a personal tale of violence and the madness of the war. It is, crucially, also a story listened to. Yet, it is not a story that has entered circulation to be the subject of continuous re-inscription with meaning through such appropriation. Not all stories can.

Manuel lived near me in Honde and frequently interrupted the storytelling and general conversation of others. He himself, however, was never interrupted. This was due both to his status and stories. In the 1970s and early 1980s, Manuel was part of the national Frelimo party elite and travelled internationally with Mozambican president Samora Machel, as well as serving in the FAM. This background provided him with authority. He was also generally regarded as having 'become mad by war' and all attempts by both *n'angas* (traditional healers) and hospitals to treat him were unsuccessful.[7] Nevertheless, when he talked of war, shouting, waving hands and screaming the message into the face of others (also the anthropologist), Manuel was listened to:

> I was with Samora [Machel] in 1971! In 1971, I tell you! I've been to the army, and I know what it is like! Understanding what goes on is simple. Killing! That is what goes on in war. Do you hear? It is all very simple: The one that dies, dies. The one that lives, lives. That is all.

Manuel's stories were told again and again, but by him only. In one way, he was a living enactment of war, his clothes in rags, his bloodshot eyes testifying to a hard life. Still, he is accorded a voice in Honde's social settings, and his tales are attentively listened to: Despite (or due to) being perceived as mad, for many in Honde he holds a key to the true destructive nature of violence and war. Thus, Manuel is able to verbalise and embody some experiences of war others may not. In local terms, such crucial and profound insight is often expressed by saying 'he/she knows something'—an expression also reserved for allusions to the penetrative gaze and knowledge associated with wielding sorcerous powers.

This, however, is not true for all those perceived mad: In Chimoio's streets and markets there was in 2000 a stark naked man, living on the spoils of the gutters. When he walked the streets, with a supreme disregard for cars and traffic, no one looked at him. Quite the opposite: People were reluctant to acknowledge his existence and averted their gaze. And only hesitantly was his insane condition explained to me—unanimously pointing to the madness of war as having contaminated him.

There is a difference in acknowledgement and setting between the madness of Manuel and the naked man: Manuel has a social frame for storytelling, being part of kin relations and enjoys a status in Honde as part of the autochthonous group (*aridzi wo nhika*, 'owners of the land'). Equally important, there is a relation between his personal story and that of the local community. As Connerton (1996:21) points out: 'The narrative of one life is part of an interconnecting set of narratives; it is embedded in the story of those groups from which individuals derive their identity'. Building on Halbwachs, Connerton asserts that groups '... provide individuals with frameworks within which their memories are localised and memories are localised by a kind of mapping. We situate what we recollect within the mental space provided by the group' (1996:37). Connerton's assumptions highlight some crucial differences between the two men: Manuel is accorded a voice and socially acknowledged within the context of Honde where he originates from and has returned to. The other is naked but *invisibly visible*, devoid of group, kin, status, voice and social context—doubly a relic *of* war and destroyed *by* war.

Although Connerton's assertions are incisive, they do problematically posit a coherent local community ('the group') as providing a 'mental space'. As many other post-conflict localities, Honde cannot meaningfully be analysed as such an integrated 'community'. As we saw above, processes of generating contested and conflicting versions of the past and present—or differentiated 'mental spaces', if you will—exist instead. The case of Honde finds more resonance in the approach suggested by Schmidt (1999:212) building on material from Zimbabwean areas bordering Mozambique, asserting that '... beyond the single meta-narrative of war, a multitude of entangled voices can be heard which are often contradictory and which change over time (...). Hence it is important to look at the processual character of this "text" how it is being made and thus how sense is being made of violence ...'. More than Connerton, Schmidt's perspective sees appropriation and circulation of stories as part of a creative allocation of meaning to a violent past.

The importance of Schmidt's vision of and approach to the presence of the past to analyses of post-conflict addressing of violence can be illustrated by a striking story told by Younas, a young man in Honde in December 1999:

> During the war, a lot of bad things happened here, a lot of bad things indeed. If you walked down the road you would see all sorts of things. Often, you saw people who had had their heads cut off. Or people impaled with the sticks coming out of their mouths or their sides. Often they had bananas stuck in their mouths, just like animals. But no one, not even their families, dared to bury them. The corpses were left to rot. There is still a lot of problems from this. *Eh pah*! A lot of problems, my friend.

When Younas recounted atrocities committed during the mid-1980s to me and a group of elder men in Honde, all nodded in agreement and no one reacted afterwards as Younas' story was immediately followed by another. To me this was surprising as Younas here remembering violence was merely a very young child when the violence 'took place' or 'happened'. The 'whys and wherefores' as to how he could tell the story as (if) he experienced it, why, if and how he saw it and so on, fundamentally questions the perception of a clear-cut linear temporality of violence (see also Nordstrom 1997). However, it also underlines the importance in post-war situations of re-inscribing violence with meaning. This is a process in which '... the self of a memory may be imagined as player in the larger narratives of a community' (Lambek and Antze 1996:xx). It is evident that in Honde, an important dimension of oral practice following the civil war was providing a social space for not only individual recall but also processes that appropriate, re-mould and re-deploy stories of pasts painfully present.

Telling Stories and Creating Speech Genres

> A song is just a song … a narrative is just a narrative.[8]
>
> Maurice Bloch

> [A]n utterance is defined not only by its relation to the object and to the speaking subject-author (and its relation to the language as a system of potential possibilities, givens) but—for us most important of all—by its direct relation to other utterances within the limits of a given sphere of communication.[9]
>
> Mikhail Bakhtin

A central conceit of this chapter has been that confronted with the presence and persistence of a violent past, the circulation of verbalised stories, memories and experiences represents crucial social attempts at re-ordering a world that has been dis-ordered—to re-inscribe social meaning. Such a process—what Das (2000:213) calls 'the social emplotment of stories'—is characterised by communal, collective narratives becoming personal, and some (but not all) individual stories being de-originated, appropriated and retold by many. This process of appropriation and personification of a circulating story was clearly evident in the story told and remembered by Younas above. This voicing of a communal story of atrocities is also subscribing to practices related to meaning, inserting oneself into a shared sociality, re-presenting the community—not to be mistaken for 'life stories' (see also Bourdieu 1987). Moreover, stories in themselves also contribute to constructing a new post-conflict sociality by reshaping meaning in the face of violence's dual capacities for erasure and inscription.

In such a process seemingly idiosyncratic stories are also privileged, as Jorge's and Manuel's, but not necessarily appropriated: They are in some sense 'bearing witness' to, and representing, incomprehensible parts of destruction and erasure of meaning, parts that cannot (yet?) be incorporated into a more comprehensive narrative. Exemplifying this, the FAM soldier Eduardo's story of war's confusion privileges a view often verbalised of the sometimes near impossibility of discerning good from bad. As an effect, the post-war national level Frelimo and Renamo narratives of good and evil do not resonate well with experience and these, therefore, do not circulate widely (see also Sumich 2008).

Bloch's comparison of narratives and songs in the above quote illustrates his questioning of whether narratives are at all helpful in analyses of knowledge of the past. Disagreeing with Bloch, the Honde material demonstrates ways in which experience and knowledge are, indeed, circulated and constructed socially and verbally in different settings. Thus, certain types of knowledge and narratives of the past talking to the present may be seen to reflect each other. Further, what has here been deliberately inaccurately dubbed 'story' may also, and perhaps better, be seen as an 'utterance' in a Bakhtinian sense. In his vision, the utterance (or the story) is an excerpt from a continuum: '[t]here can be no such thing as an isolated utterance. It always presupposes utterances that precede and follow it' (1986:136). It is this complexity where stories/utterances interface and are informed by others that Bakhtin (1986:60, italics retained) terms a 'speech genre' where '[e]ach separate utterance is individual, of course, but each sphere in which language is used develops its own *relatively stable types* of these utterances'.

Firstly, through Bakhtin's well-known concept of 'dialogue', meaning is created and re-negotiated, the dialogue being the fundamental locus of the condensation of meaning. Having taken here the *social* rather than the *individual* and the *dynamic* rather than the *static* as entry points into the *post hoc* verbal addressing of the Mozambican civil war, the concept of speech genres is analytically helpful. Within the Bakhtinian view of speech genres and the interrelation of utterances, the different oral practices dealing with the presence of the past indicate profoundly social processes of construction of non-individual memories in particular post-conflict societies.

Secondly, another dimension of this social process pertains to the heteroglossia of stories: When stories were told, others followed, generating ceaselessly situational rather than static understandings of not merely what constituted the past but also comprising dynamic ways in which to '*languagify*'. A precedence was constructed relating to the continuum of instances and settings wherein individuals may express, contest, support, mirror and frame stories and their lived relational experiences. Such a position is in concert with Das' and Kleinman's (2000:13) assertion that '[t]he question of memory and representation is not only a question of the authenticity of memories [...] but the struggle to author one's stories in relation to representations that seek to impose a different kind of truth on them.'

Thirdly, and again following Bakhtin, how meaning and telling are perceived is also to a great part related to credibility and skill. A case in point in this respect might, again, be how Younas recounted past roadside impalements in Honde how (or as if) he experienced them. By inserting himself into the story, the story becomes true and good. This oral practice makes sense out of continued experience, a perpetual and dynamic reshaping and inscription of novel meaning. In Michael Lambek's words, the narratives should rather be seen as '... vehicles of memory but recognising that they can become more or less objectified, more or less detached from the process of remembering' (1996:243). Generating, appropriating and/or telling a story, personified or de-personified, that circulates therefore becomes a constructive effort in the face of civil war. As such, this oral practice is informed also by local perceptions of knowing and relationality: *Masoko*, meaning 'news' is always asked for, given in and dominates all social settings. *Masoko* is therefore paramount for understanding relations, developments and processes, as well as crucial for navigating the social. Thus, the telling of stories from the war, as if they were news, is also a locally informed way of making sense not merely of current events and gossip but of past events and actions currently and painfully present.

The Inconclusiveness of the Verbalised

The relationship between violence and memory has been stressed strongly in this analysis drawing on some aspects of oral practice in post-war Mozambique. What is evident is that at the level of politics, the extreme violence of the war obviates simplistic distinctions between bellicose parties. At the personal and social level, the erasure and inscription of violence and the destructive dynamic of the war create a festering presence of the past in Honde and other locations which do not resonate with national histories. This ambivalence towards historical representation and violence itself is evident in the stories that circulate in Honde. There, these may be analysed as being re-constructive practices—speech genres within which the fluidity of meaning is socially addressed and contained.

Such an argument resembles Krohn-Hansen's (1994:376) position that in contexts of extreme violence, epistemological and ontological '[q]uestions about what distinguishes human from animal, truth from lies, or civilizing development from savage underdevelopment become habitual'. Following Krohn-Hansen, singular violent acts and the civil war may be approached as a continuum. Such an un-endedness is socially circumscribed and addressed by circulating stories, by creating Bakhtinian speech genres and by listening to stories of atrocities from mad, men, women and youths.

As both Perera (2001) and Malkki (1995) have argued for Sri Lankan villagers and Hutu refugees respectively, post-conflict narratives are habitually concerned with a socio-moral order. Likewise, what I have argued to be the process of establishing speech genres in Honde represents an oral practice which freezes, moulds and generates meaning from a polysemic, fluid and violent presence. These speech genres and their enactment evade, however, simple categorisation by being heteroglossic and in flux rather than being 'monologic' and stable. In a sense, we can follow Bakhtin in claiming '[n]othing is absolutely dead' (1986:xxi). But the circulating stories and the speech genres they are cast in imply or, rather, command the sharing of experiences with neighbouring households, family and wider community: 'Telling' becomes, thus, an exercise neither personal, exhaustive or therapeutic as in PTSD discourse but social and relational. Further and as Mollica (2006:116) argues, '[s]torytelling is a powerful process because of the listener's ability to form pictures of what the teller is saying.' Informed by memory, the mulitple and multisemic stories encapsulate, shape and voice experiences and, in doing so, perhaps relieves some of the burdens harking from the past: Meaning is then re-inscribed into memories of violence in its transformation from *unsocial* and *chaotic* to distinctly *social speech genres.*

The circulation of stories is, however, not insular to a 'community': Shaped by party politics and the national narratives, different, competing versions circulate and are re-negotiated. This is a process that is perpetual and ongoing and the sedimentation of speech genres does not mean these become stable through fixating or locating the meanings of violence to the point of sanitising these. Let me provide two brief examples: Firstly, with the recent resurgence of political violence in Mozambique—mentioned in the beginning of this chapter—notions of war-time identities of Renamo and Frelimo were again actualised, as were war-time practices such as ambushes on buses by alleged Renamo soldiers or indiscriminate attacks on civilian populations in search for 'terrorists' by government forces. In such circumstances and in both 2013 and 2014, my interlocutors drew on formerly established speech genres—some resembling or assuming the shape of official discourses also—to question hegemonic nationally disseminated discourses about Mozambique being at peace. Secondly, in the last few years Mozambican cities have been rocked by urban popular uprisings (sometimes called 'riots' by commentators) primarily directed at the Frelimo-dominated government, as well as rising prices. Crucial to the mobilisation of a vast spectre of people—men and women, young and old—to participate in these *greves* (literally 'strikes'), as they were called, was to re-invent and re-deploy the memory of popular power (*poder popular*): Recalling the hardships as well as the promises of shared wealth under former President Samora Machel (1975–1986), participants appropriated and destabilised discourses of past struggles, including the civil war, to inform chants and slogans that drove participants (see also Bertelsen 2014). In both cases, a violent past is re-actualised and re-deployed in ways that transcend the stability of speech genres or the confines of officialese discourses. Put differently, the process of oral re-inscription of meaning is perpetual, reflect the dynamics of current politics and is crucially informing political action.

A word of caution. An analysis solely privileging the verbalised would effectively mute the unspoken, the everyday practices, the languages of the soil and ancestors and so on. Englund (2005:68) therefore advises us to include social forces and particular realities, underlining that '[b]oth the said and the unsaid must belong to the purview of ethnographic analysis'. Further, Bloch (1998:100) also highlights how we need to explore the 'multiplicity of the representations of the past' where '... what is said can never be equated with memory'. Despite agreeing with both Bloch's and Englund's arguments, nevertheless what 'is said' has been prioritised here.

Conclusion

A two-pronged conclusion may be drawn from this Mozambican case. In addressing the dynamics of post-conflict societies, the spoken needs to occupy an important analytical position. Such analysis needs to be informed by particular socio-political contexts and to be steeped in the crucial historical trajectories of violent erasure and inscription so central to violent conflict. In this respect, speech genres are points of entry that in their plasticity and open-endedness capture ongoing processes of contestation, formation and conflict that shape the trajectory and scope of the oral practices in which these stories are enacted. Secondly, however, the particular oral practices of re-constructing meaning are *not* congruent with the therapeutic and more limited setting of somatising notions such as PTSD. The narrative structuring of PTSD and similar, increasingly global technologies of witnessing and therapy on the one hand and the state-dominated narratives of the past on the other both threaten to (and frequently do) eclipse or erase alternative marginal oral accounts of past political violence neither integral to these state machineries nor to globalised therapeutic knowledge.

This text has been an attempt to counter such processes of eclipsing and erasure of the 'residual' by presenting stories that address, redress and re-inscribe meaning onto that violent canvas that is the Mozambican past—and present (see also Bertelsen 2009b). As such, the text recognises the need that Allen Feldman (2004:167) has identified for scrutinising 'the social being of narrative truth'. Here, this has been done through seeing oral practices as particular Bakhtinian speech genres and highlighting how these are generated out of an ongoing re-formulation of sociality that is non-individual, rooted in oral culture and aimed at continuously addressing the violent past and its places in the present.

Notes

1. This chapter builds on long-term and repeated fieldworks in urban, peri-urban and rural areas in and close to the city of Chimoio, Mozambique, stretching from 1998 until January 2016. I would like to express my sincere gratitude for the profound generosity and hospitality with which I have been met during these stays—without which this chapter and my research in general would not have been possible. *Maitabassa maningue*! Further, my great thanks are also extended to my co-editor of this volume, Vigdis Broch-Due, for involving me in her ongoing research, as well as to all the other authors in this volume for making important and critical comments on early drafts of this chapter, in particular Maria Tapias and Tony Robben. Thanks!
2. See Hanna Kienzler (2008) for an analysis of the long-standing debate between relativist and universalist positions within the PTSD literature of which also the exchange between Joshua Breslau (2004, 2005) and Joop T. V. M. de Jong (2005) may serve as examples.
3. All fieldworks have been carried out in compliance with guidelines developed by the Norwegian national committee for research ethics within the social sciences and humanities (NESH). Permits for field-

works have also been applied for and given by relevant Mozambican authorities.

4. The Mozambican floods of early 2000 were frequently understood to be caused by the leader of Renamo opposition to wreak havoc in Frelimo strongholds in vengeance for alleged election fraud in late 1999 (see Bertelsen 2004a).
5. This resonates with a 1997 survey where 50 % of former FAM fighters in Manica province answered 'don't know' as to the objectives of the civil war (Dolan and Schafer 1997:140; see also Schafer 2007).
6. However, as Knudsen (1995:29) cautions, one should tread carefully because as researchers we are '... gatekeepers to landscapes of emotions'.
7. See also Honwana (1999) and Igreja et al. (2009) for comprehensive and non-conventional analyses of social practices addressing violence in post-war Mozambique.
8. Bloch (1998:111).
9. Bakhtin (1986:122).

References

Bakhtin, Mikhail M. 1981. *The Dialogic Imagination*. Austin: University of Texas Press.

———. 1986. *Speech Genres and Other Essays*. Austin: University of Texas Press.

Bertelsen, Bjørn Enge. 2004a. 'It will rain until we are in power!' Floods, Elections and Memory in Mozambique. In *Rights and the Politics of Recognition in Africa*, eds. Harri Englund and Francis Nyamnjoh, 169–191. London: Zed Books.

———. 2004b. 'The traditional lion is dead'. The Ambivalent Presence of Tradition and the Relation Between Politics and Violence in Mozambique. In *Lusotopie 2003: Violences et contrôle de la violence au Brésil, en Afrique et à Goa*, ed. Camille Goirand, 263–281. Paris: Éditions Karthala and Centre d'Étude d'Afrique Noire (CEAN).

———. 2009a. Sorcery and Death Squads. Transformations of State, Sovereignty, and Violence in Postcolonial Mozambique. In *Crisis of the State: War and Social Upheaval*, eds. Bruce Kapferer and Bjørn Enge Bertelsen, 210–240. New York: Berghahn Books.

———. 2009b. Multiple Sovereignties and Summary Justice in Mozambique. A Critique of Some Legal Anthropological Terms. *Social Analysis* 53(3): 123–147.

———. 2014. Effervescence and Ephemerality: Popular Urban Uprisings in Mozambique. *Ethnos: Journal of Anthropology*. doi:10.1080/00141844.2014.929596.
———. 2016. *Violent Becomings: State Formation, Sociality, and Power in Mozambique*. New York: Berghahn Books.
Bertelsen, Bjørn Enge and Alessandro Zagato. 2015. Introduction: The Event of Charlie Hebdo—Imaginaries of Freedom and Control. In *The Event of* Charlie Hebdo*—Imaginaries of Freedom and Control*, ed. Alessandro Zagato, 1—11. New York: Berghahn Books.
Bhebe, Ngwabi and Terence Ranger. 1996. *Society in Zimbabwe's Liberation War*. Harare: University of Zimbabwe.
Bloch, Maurice. 1998. *How We Think They Think: Anthropological Approaches to Cognition, Memory, and Literacy*. Boulder, CO: Westview Press.
Bourdieu, Pierre. 1987. *The Biographical Illusion*. Chicago, IL: Center for Psychosocial Studies.
Breslau, Joshua. 2004. Cultures of Trauma. Anthropological Views of Posttraumatic Stress Disorder in International Health. *Culture, Medicine and Psychiatry* 28: 113–126.
———. 2005. Response to 'Commentary. Deconstructing critiques on the internationalization of PTSD'. *Culture, Medicine and Psychiatry* 29: 371–376.
Butler, Judith. 2009. *Frames of War: When is Life Grievable?* New York: Verso.
Coelho, João Paulo Borges. 1993. Protected Villages and Communal Villages in the Mozambican Province of Tete (1968–1982). A History of State Resettlement Policies, Development and war. Unpublished Ph.D. thesis, University of Bradford.
Connerton, Paul. 1996. *How Societies Remember*. Cambridge: Cambridge University Press.
Das, Veena. 1997. Language and Body: Transactions in the Construction of Pain. In *Social Suffering*, eds. Veena Das, Margaret Lock, and Arthur Kleinman, 67–91. Berkeley: University of California Press.
Das, Veena, and Arthur Kleinman. 2000. Introduction. In *Violence and Subjectivity*, eds. Veena Das, Arthur Kleinman, Mamphela Ramphele, and Pamela Reynolds, 1–18. Berkeley: University of California Press.
———. 2015. Beyond Trauma, Beyond Humanitarianism, Beyond Empathy: A Commentary. *Medicine Anthropology Theory* 2(3): 105–112.
Dolan, Chris, and Jessica Schafer. 1997. *The Reintegration of Ex-Combatants in Mozambique. Manica and Zambezia Provinces*. Oxford: University of Oxford.
Englund, Harri. 1998. Death, Trauma and Ritual: Mozambican Refugees in Malawi. *Social Science and Medicine* 46(9): 1165–1174.
———. 2005. Conflicts in Contexts. Political Violence and Anthropological Puzzles. In *Violence and Belonging: The Quest for Identity in Post-Colonial Africa*, ed. Vigdis Broch-Due, 60–74. London: Routledge.

Fassin, Didier. 2013 [2011]. *Enforcing Order: An Ethnography of Urban Policing*. Cambridge: Polity Press.

Fassin, Didier, and Richard Rechtman. 2009 [2007]. *The Empire of Trauma: An Inquiry into the Condition of Victimhood*. Princeton, NJ: Princeton University Press.

Feldman, Allen F. 2004. Memory Theaters, Virtual Witnessing, and the Trauma-Aesthetic. *Biography* 27(1): 163–202.

Geffray, Christian. 1990. *La cause des armes au Mozambique. Anthropologie d'une guerre civile*. Karthala: Paris.

Hall, Margaret, and Thomas Young. 1997. *Confronting Leviathan: Mozambique since Independence*. London: Hurst.

Hoffman, Danny. 2011. *The War Machines: Young Men and Violence in Sierra Leone*. Durham, NC: Duke University Press.

Honwana, Alcinda. 1999. Appeasing the Spirits: Healing Strategies in Postwar Southern Mozambique. In *Religion, Health and Suffering*, eds. J.R. Hinnels and R. Porter, 237–255. London: Kegan Paul.

Igreja, Victor. 2015. Amnesty Law, Political Struggles for Legitimacy and Violence in Mozambique. *International Journal of Transitional Justice*. doi:10.1093/ijtj/ijv004.

Igreja, Victor, Wim Kleijn, Beatrice Dias-Lambranca, Douglas A. Hershey, Clara Calero, and Annemiek Richters. 2009. Agricultural Cycle and the Prevalence of Posttraumatic Stress Disorder: A Longitudinal Community Study in Postwar Mozambique. *Journal of Traumatic Stress* 22(3): 172–179.

Jong, J.T.V.M.d. 2005. Commentary. Deconstructing Critiques on the Internationalization of PTSD. *Culture, Medicine and Psychiatry* 29: 361–370.

Joxe, Alain. 2002. *Empire of Disorder*. Los Angeles, CA/New York: Semiotext(e)/MIT Press.

Kidron, Carol A. 2009. Toward an Ethnography of Silence: The Lived Presence of the Past in the Everyday Life of Holocaust Trauma Survivors and Their Descendants in Israel. *Current Anthropology* 50(1): 5–27.

Kienzler, Hanna. 2008. Debating War-Trauma and Post-Traumatic Stress Disorder (PTSD) in an Interdisciplinary Arena. *Social Science & Medicine* 67: 218–227.

Knudsen, John Christian. 1995. When Trust is on Trial: Negotiating Refugee Narratives. In *Mistrusting Refugees*, eds. John Christian Knudsen and E. Valentine Daniel, 13–55. Berkeley: University of California Press.

———. 2005. *Capricious Worlds: Vietnamese Life Journeys*. Berlin: LIT Verlag.

Krohn-Hansen, Christian. 1994. The Anthropology of Violent Interaction. *Journal of Anthropological Research* 50(4): 367–381.

Lambek, Michael. 1996. The Past Imperfect. Remembering as Moral Practice. In *Tense Past: Cultural Essays in Trauma and Memory*, eds. Paul Antze and Michael Lambek, 235–254. New York: Routledge.

Lambek, Michael, and Paul Antze. 1996. Introduction: Forecasting Memory. In *Tense Past: Cultural Essays in Trauma and Memory*, eds. Paul Antze and Michael Lambek, xi–xxxviii. New York: Routledge.

Lusa. 2016. Mozambique Reinstates Mandatory Military Escorts on National Roads. News article published online. http://clubofmozambique.com/news/mozambique-reinstates-mandatory-military-escorts-on-national-roads/. Accessed 20 Feb 2016.

Maček, Ivana. 2014. *Engaging Violence: Trauma, Memory and Representation*. New York: Routledge.

Malkki, Liisa. 1995. *Purity and Exile: Violence, Memory, and National Cosmology Among Hutu Refugees in Tanzania*. Chicago, IL: University of Chicago Press.

McKinney, Kelly. 2007. 'Breaking the conspiracy of silence': Testimony, Traumatic Memory, and Psychotherapy with Survivors of Political Violence. *Ethos* 35(3): 265–299.

Moghimi, Yavar. 2012. Anthropological Discourses on the Globalization of Posttraumatic Stress Disorder (PTSD) in Post-Conflict Societies. *Journal of Psychiatric Practice* 18(1): 29–37.

Mollica, Richard. 2006. *Healing Invisible Wounds: Paths to Hope and Recovery in a Violent World*. Orlando, FL: Harcourt.

Mozambique News Reports. 2014. Cease Fire After 6 Renamo Attacks in 6 days on N1. *Mozambique News Reports* 253: 1–2.

Naguib, Nefissa. 2009. *Women, Water and Memory: Recasting Lives in Palestine*. Leiden: Brill.

Nicolas, Guerda, Anna Wheatley, and Casta Guillaume. 2015. Does One Trauma Fit All? Exploring the Relevance of PTSD Across Cultures. *International Journal of Culture and Mental Health* 8(1): 34–45.

Nora, Pierre. 1989. Between Memory and History: Les lieux de mémoire. *Representations* 26: 7–24.

Nordstrom, Carolyn. 1997. *A Different Kind of War Story*. Philadelphia: University of Pennsylvania Press.

Perera, Sasanka. 2001. Spirit Possessions and Avenging Ghosts: Stories of Supernatural Activity as Narratives of Terror and Mechanisms of Coping and Remembering. In *Remaking a World: Violence, Social Suffering, and Recovery*, eds. Veena Das et al., 157–200. Berkeley: University of California Press.

Reuters. 2013. Police Killings, Ambushes Put Mozambique Peace on Edge. Reuters news item, reproduced on Voice of America website 10 April 2013, retrieved 15 June 2013 from http://www.voanews.com/content/police-killings-ambushes-mozambique-peace-violence/1638821.html

Robben, Antonius C.G.M. 2010. Chaos, Mimesis and Dehumanisation in Iraq. American Counterinsurgency in the Global War on Terror. *Social Anthropology* 18(2): 138–154.

Schafer, Jessica. 2007. *Soldiers at Peace: Veterans and Society After the Civil War in Mozambique*. New York: Palgrave.

Scheper-Hughes, Nancy. 2008. A Talent for Life: Reflections on Human Vulnerability and Resilience. *Ethnos* 73(1): 25–56.

Schmidt, Heike. 1999. Neither War Nor Peace: Making Sense of Violence. In *Dynamics of Violence: Processes of Escalation and De-escalation in Violent Group Conflicts*, eds. G. Elwert, S. Feuchtwang, and D. Neubert, 211–225. Berlin: Duncker & Humblot.

Sumich, Jason. 2008. Politics After the Time of Hunger in Mozambique: A Critique of Neo-Patrimonial Interpretation of African Elites. *Journal of Southern African Studies* 34(1): 111–125.

UNHCR. 2016. UNHCR Stresses Asylum Right of Mozambicans Fleeing to Malawi. Article published online 18 February 2016. http://www.unhcr.org/56c5daaa9.html. Accessed 20 Feb 2016.

Vines, Alex. 1996. *Renamo: From Terrorism to Democracy in Mozambique?* London: James Currey.

Werbner, Richard P. 1991. *Tears of the Dead: The Social Biography of an African Family*. Edinburgh: Edinburgh University Press.

———. 1995. Human Rights and Moral Knowledge: Arguments of Accountability in Zimbabwe. In *Shifting Contexts: Transformations of Anthropological Knowledge*, ed. Marilyn Strathern, 99–116. London: Routledge.

Whitehead, Neil L. 2011. The Cannibal War Machine. *Counterpunch*, Weekend edition, July 2011, pp. 1–3.

Whitehead, Neil L., and Sverker Finnström. 2013. Introduction: Virtual War and Magical Death. In *Virtual War and Magical Death: Technologies and Imaginaries for Terror and Killing*, eds. N.L. Whitehead and S. Finnström, 1–25. Durham, NC: Duke University Press.

CHAPTER 9

Violence, Fear, and Impunity in Post-War Guatemala

Margit Ystanes

'*Guatemala, the land of eternal status quo*',[1] a friend of mine sometimes comments when the news reports yet another setback for the advancement of justice, democracy or human rights in his country. This is a pun on 'Guatemala, the land of eternal spring',[2] which the small Central American country is often termed because of its favorable climate. Spring, of course, symbolizes rebirth, life, growth, vitality, renewal—all indicating a hopeful, forward-looking, sturdy social body and an ever-regenerating natural environment. While this image of Guatemala is widely used in the marketing of the country as a tourism destination, it makes a stark contrast to how the people I have worked with conceptualize their society. Instead of vitality and optimism, the sense that society as well as social interaction contain some degree of danger forms their daily choices and experiences in both subtle and pronounced ways. This conceptualization emanates from a complex interweaving of past and present experiences; the civil war, new kinds of violence that affect postbellum Guatemala and their compound effects on social relationships. As such, it exemplifies how certain modalities of trauma may 'continue to move through [the] tissue, blood, bones and minds of those affected' (Chap. 1).

M. Ystanes (✉)
Department of Social Anthropology, University of Bergen, Bergen, Norway

V. Broch-Due, B.E. Bertelsen (eds.), *Violent Reverberations*,
DOI 10.1007/978-3-319-39049-9_9

The Agreement on a Firm and Lasting Peace[3] formally ended Guatemalan civil war in 1996. The 36 years long war was fought between the Guatemalan state—headed by a succession of right wing military dictators during this period—and various leftist guerrilla groups. The Guatemalan population was exposed to unimaginable violence during the civil war (see e.g. CDH 1999; Manz 1995; Zur 1994; Nelson 2009; Hale 2006; ODHAG 1998). Activists, students and intellectuals were murdered and disappeared, and in the countryside, whole villages suspected of sympathizing with the guerrillas were massacred. The violence was particularly intense during the early 1980s, when the majority of massacres took place. It is estimated that about 200,000 people were killed or disappeared during the civil war, and that the Guatemalan army and paramilitary forces are responsible for 93 % of the atrocities (CDH 1999).

Today, although the civil war officially ended 20 years ago, Guatemala remains an extremely violent society. The capital is considered one of the most dangerous cities on the planet, and many feel life is more unsafe now than during the war (see also Thomas et al. 2011:2). Indeed, an evaluation report from NORAD (Norwegian Agency for Development Cooperation) states that a full implementation of the peace accords has not been possible and that the increase in violent crime has led to murder rates being higher in recent years than they were during the internal conflict (NORAD 2011:38). People's experience of fear is related to the very real risk of violent crime any Guatemalan faces as he or she leaves her house, to the continued presence of political violence, to environmental destructions and the risk of illness and to conceptions of social relationships (Ystanes 2011). In agreement with the critique of an individualizing and universalizing approach to trauma (see Chap. 1), I argue that the collective trauma experienced by Guatemalans cannot be reduced to residing in individual psyches. Neither is it likely to be 'the same' as traumas endured by people who find themselves in other circumstances and other historical moments. In the Guatemalan context, harrowing experiences did not end with the signing of the 1996 Peace Accords but continue to emanate from and work upon the very social fabric in which people exist. The foremost symptom of this ongoing process is endemic political fear, which in turn has profound societal consequences. This fear contributes to reproducing impunity and inequality, and as such, facilitates the cumulative and slow violence (see Chap. 1) that continues to mark Guatemalan society.

Political Fear and the Legacy of Civil War

Fear affects the human experience in fundamental ways. Corey Robin argues that there is considerable ambiguity in the way fear has been approached by Euro-American political leaders and philosophers. While many have paraphrased Michel de Montaigne's famous declaration that 'The thing I fear most is fear', fear is also widely considered to arouse a heightened state of experience:

> It quickens our perceptions as no other emotion can, forcing us to see and to act in the world in new and more interesting ways, with greater moral discrimination and a more acute consciousness of our surrounding and ourselves. (Robin 2004:4)

However, Robin discards such conventional understandings of fear and argues for the need to see fear for what it is; 'a symptom of pervasive conflict and political unhappiness' (2004:3) and 'a basic mode of social and political control' (2004:19). I take this as a starting point for my exploration of contemporary fears of violence in Guatemala. I follow Robin's distinction between political and private fear, focusing here on the former; 'fears that emanate from society or have consequences for society' (2004:2). Political fears, then, are different from the personal fears that arise within persons, such as the fear of spiders, and more or less affect that person alone. In contrast, a woman's fear of her abusive husband or a worker's fear of an unkind employer are political fears as they both arise from and help sustain pervasive social inequalities.

I have worked with people who were not targeted by the counterinsurgency campaigns of the 1980s. Almost all of them are *ladinos*, that is, people of mixed origin who tend to emphasize their European ancestry and downplay their indigenous heritage. They are often associated with 'national culture', although traditionally they have been excluded from the Euro-Guatemalan elite and oppressing of the indigenous Mayan population (see e.g. Hale 2006; Nelson 1999; Smith 1995, 1990). These persons' perspective on the fear and danger they experience tends to be focused on the current situation. Every day they are exposed to stories about violent assaults and even death; they read about it in the papers, watch it on television and learn about them from family, friends and colleagues. They remind each other to be careful when leaving the house and coming back. They worry about using public transportation, taking a taxi or going to new places. They are anxious about whether there will be dangerous people there, and if they will get home safely.

The understanding of this situation as an 'eternal status quo' resonates with the potential of war to profoundly reconfigure the social and cultural universe in which it takes place. The violence of war is not its own context; rather, it is embedded in already existing cultures and cosmologies. Nevertheless, it may produce thoroughgoing change in the identities and bonds of family, marriage and gender by penetrating into the most intimate spheres (Broch-Due 2005:15–17). During the Latin American dirty wars, the very aim of state terror was indeed to reconfigure society and political thought. This effort involved attacking people even in their most intimate domains; their selves (see e.g. Feitlowitz 1998; Klein 2007). Trust on all levels—social, personal, even self-trust—was shattered in the process (Manz 1995). Contemporary fears, whether related to physical violence or the social, must be read against this backdrop.

The recent attempts to convict former President General Efraín Ríos Montt for war crimes exemplify the enduring effects of the civil war and the terrorization of the Guatemalan people. Ríos Montt, who presided over the most violent counterinsurgency campaigns of the early 1980s, was charged with genocide and crimes against humanity after his immunity as a congressional representative was lifted in January 2012. During the trial, both prosecutors and judges received threats, and one of the most powerful institutions in Guatemala, the Coordinating Committee of Agricultural, Commercial, Industrial and Financial Associations (CACIF),[4] publically opposed the trial. Their director of communication was removed from the courtroom for photographing witnesses, human rights activists and journalists attending the proceedings. In light of the above-mentioned threats and the far-reaching circulation of material that resembled hit lists, the CACIF representative's behavior was perceived as threatening (Allison 2013).

Throughout the trial, the Attorney General fought continuous attempts to close the process down. It has been suggested that the President at the time, retired General Otto Pérez Molina, was instrumental in this endeavor, motivated by fear that his own role in the genocide will be exposed. Although Ríos Montt was found guilty and sentenced to 80 years in prison on 10 May 2013, the sentence was annulled due to allegations of procedural errors forwarded by his defense lawyers (Grant 2013). After numerous other obstruction and delaying tactics, such as claiming Rios Montt was in too poor health to stand trial and challenging the neutrality of the judge, Irma Jeannette Valdez, the case was suspended indefinitely in January 2015 (MacLean and Beaudoin 2015).

These events bring into sharp focus the ambiguities involved in attempting to achieve justice, democratization and reconciliation, while power is mainly gathered on the same hands as during the counterinsurgency campaigns, and impunity is the norm (see also Feitlowitz 1998 for an analysis of the Argentine case). It is clear that there are also new actors on the scene. As in Latin America in general, the state no longer controls the means and the direction of violence. Instead, violence increasingly appears to be an option for a multitude of actors pursuing all kinds of goals (Rodgers 2002:268; Thomas et al. 2011:2). These activities have lead to a widespread sense of *ingobernabilidad* (ungovernability) that the authorities are unable or unwilling to stop the tide of violence and implement the law.

As people interpret the situation and the increasing fear they experience, they draw on these two narratives about the current situation—one emphasizing the continuity with past state terror and the other foregrounding an essentially new situation of hidden powers. These narratives also sometimes meet, as in the following characterization of the Petén region. Here, the *ingobernabilidad* that so troubles the population is clearly understood as a benefit to the more powerful sectors of society:

> Today, even with laws, institutions and formal politics in force, the sectors with more economic and political power continue to impose their own particular interests on those of the nation and of the majority sectors. The prosperity of their businesses in cattle ranching, agriculture, timber, and some illicit ones such as drug trafficking, is founded on the destruction and degradation of the department's natural environment, in the immutable poverty of the majority of the population, as well as the predominance of ungovernability, corruption and general anomie. (Hurtado Paz y Paz 2007:24)[5]

Hence, the Guatemalan society continues to be marked by far-reaching impunity. In February 2014 Human Rights Watch declared that although impunity rates were reduced from 93 % to 70 % in the last six years, it continues to be a 'cancer that consumes Guatemala' (AFP 2014). In April that year, the International Commission of Jurists (ICJ) stated that there exists an 'impunity pact' in Guatemala that includes systematic attacks on the agents of justice lead by de facto powers (EFE—Guatemala 2014).[6] In the following sections, I will address how this situation affects peoples' day-to-day life and experience. How does it shape their way of being in the world? As we shall see, the ethnography to be presented here speaks to Robin's assertion that political fear severely complicates people's possibilities for acting upon the world, and in this way, helps perpetuate impunity and inequalities.

Before moving on to this, however, I will outline some of the effects of the Latin American 'dirty wars' on selves and social bodies.

The Effects of Terror on Selves and the Social Body

It is clear that the terrorization of Latin American people during the authoritarian regimes of the 1970s and 1980s produced widespread political fear. Studies of these events and their aftermath also show that for many of the survivors, it has been challenging to settle back into an experience of the world not dominated by political fear (see e.g. Green 1999; Feitlowitz 1998; Nelson 2009). The terrorization, however, extends beyond those who were personally targeted and victimized. For example, in Argentina, all of society's institutions—political, military, legal, religious, social and domestic—were mobilized or appropriated for the purposes of clandestine torture and public complicity (Feitlowitz 1998:61). Indeed, the penetration of jargon from government concentration camps into Argentine Spanish illustrates that in some sense the terror of the camps did not just happen to those who were imprisoned there—'in some sense it happened to everyone' (1998:62). Similarly, Whitehead suggests that torture 'invades the subjectivities of both those who suffer it and those who anticipate suffering it', and rebounds on the torturers (Whitehead 2004:13).

In Guatemala, not only institutions but also local communities were appropriated for the purposes of repression, thus deepening the effects of terror on the social body. In large parts of the country, and particularly in indigenous communities, all men from the ages of 14 to 60 were forcibly incorporated into civil patrols (PAC)[7] (Nelson 2009:14). Thus, the state 'directly [involved] every family in every village in the terrorizing of their own community; everyone was implicated in the new order' (Zur 1994:13).[8] The traumas produced by these occurrences are profoundly collective and cannot be argued to reside merely in the psyche of individual victims. Instead, they deeply affect the very social fabric in which people' lives are situated, working upon intimate as well as societal relationships (see e.g. Hale 2006).

While the internal conflict in Guatemala clearly had 'racial' overtones as the most severe repression took place in Mayan communities, it must also be read against the broader canvas of the Cold War and US support for right-wing dictatorships across Latin America. Klein (2007) shows how torture and terror during the 'dirty wars' of the Southern Cone in the 1970s and 1980s were explicitly intended to crush opposition to the implementation of neoliberal economic policies. It is now well known that the CIA manual on 'counterintelligence interrogation' (KUBARK 1963) was employed in the repression of resistance throughout Latin America. It describes various methods for inflicting confusion or pain upon detainees and was based on research into brainwashing techniques undertaken at McGill University in the 1950s.

The methods recommended for breaking down resistance in detainees ranged from staging arrests in the middle of the night, to sensory deprivation and unsettling of normal routines for eating and sleeping, the use of electric shocks, and so on. The aim argues Klein, was to produce 'a blank slate', a *tabula rasa* that could be worked upon and reconfigured into accepting the economic shock therapy and destruction of democracy inflicted upon the populations by the juntas. The McGill researchers eventually concluded that it is not possible to turn a human mind into a blank slate (Klein 2007), yet the methods they developed worked very well to produce and perpetuate political fear. The situation that followed is often referred to as a 'culture of terror' (Taussig 2004), marked by silence and negation of the truth, as well as an abundance of rumors. Fear, of oneself as well as of others, thus permeated selves and the social body:

> In the culture of terror the goal is to turn not only against neighbor and family but, more significantly, inward, directing one's fear against oneself: the enemy is oneself because the individual's motives and actions are subjected to constant scrutiny. Individuals must always prove their loyalty and lack of subversive intent. The eternal question of the government is, when will you reveal your crime? Everyone is perceived as guilty. The object is to prove and constantly re-prove one's innocence. (Manz 1995:157–158)

This undermining of trust even in one's self has devastating effects on the possibility for intimacy and close relationships of any kind. People are mentally isolated from one another, each constantly scrutinizing themselves for dangerous thoughts. Furthermore, official denials of acts of terror, coupled with the very public messages communicated by such incidents as the appearance of mutilated corpses along roadsides, or the witnessing of torture, murders and 'disappearances' make it very difficult to separate the real from the imaginary. As Taussig points out, this is an aspect of the power of terror:

> the epistemological, ontological, and otherwise purely philosophical problem of reality-and-illusion, certainty-and-doubt, becomes infinitely more than a 'merely' philosophical problem. It becomes a high-powered tool for domination and a principal medium of political practice. (2004:49)

The violence of these regimes was thus clearly intended to attack not just bodies but also the selves and the minds, crushing opposition and making resistance inconceivable. Indeed, Franco (1999) underlines that political violence in Latin America since the 1950s has broken and destroyed every previously immune space that could be used for clandestine political activity, such as those associated with family and church. The political murders of women, children, nuns and priests reflect this penetration of safe zones. The chronic fear and uncertainty produced by these efforts have profoundly affected self-possession and social relationships. Indeed, as Diane Nelson notes;

> Guatemalans have a reputation in Central America for being *enconchados*, *encerrados*, closed off or turned inward like a snail in its shell. When asked about the effects of the war, many say it only increased these tendencies. 'People, families, they shut down. They don't talk about things. There's a generation gap because young people don't know what happened in their families, if people were involved', said a young ladina woman who had recently joined the URNG political party. (Nelson 2009:21)

The political violence of the internal conflict thus worked upon and strengthened fundamental aspects of ladino Guatemala sociality, such as the emphasis on self-containment and closing oneself off from the world (see e.g. Ystanes 2011, 2016). This has led to an increased isolation of the self, even in the midst of what ladino Guatemalans consider to be the most intimate of relations; the family.

The collective traumas produced by Latin American dirty wars thus forms the backdrop to contemporary political fears. While two former army members were recently sentenced for murder, rape and sexual enslavement of indigenous women during the civil war (BBC 2016), Guatemalans are still, to a large extent, being denied 'the right to the truth' (*el derecho a la verdad*). The right to the truth involves moving knowledge of isolated events from the private domain to the public sphere by official acknowledgement of them. Denying people this right has been an inherent part of the terrorizing of Latin American publics, as Ariel Dorfman emphasized with regards to Chile; 'by eliminating news, the Government hopes to eliminate reality' (cited in Manz 1995:154). Those who are victimized and terrorized by that reality cannot find peace of mind as long as it is not recognized, and they are forced to question their own experiences. Manz therefore identifies the right to the truth as fundamental for the process of healing and the formation of trust (1995:163; see also Zur 1994:14–15).

Because such acknowledgement is not forthcoming in Guatemala, the effects of terror continue to work among the population who are forced to question both their own experiences and those communicated by others. The profound uncertainty involved in experiencing and recounting violent occurrences therefore continues to yield complex and confusing narratives about what is going on and how to stay safe. The outcome is generalized political fear permeating the Guatemalan society, making the prospects for social 'healing' and cohesion bleak.

Contemporary Violence[9]

Although they now find themselves in a post-war situation, Guatemalans continue to maneuver a landscape of political fear created by violent crime and impunity (see also McNeish and López Rivera 2009; Nielsen 2014; O'Neill and Thomas 2011). Society is conceptualized as flung into violent chaos, and Guatemalan newspapers regularly documents that mundane day-to-day activities, such as taking the bus, are at times extremely dangerous.

For example, during my most recent fieldwork in 2007–2008, the public transportation system's passengers and workers found themselves constantly exposed to the possibility of violence. According to the transport business in Guatemala City, an estimated 187 buses were assaulted each day in the capital during this period. By the end of August 2008, 33 bus drivers and 3 driver's assistants (*ayudantes*) had been murdered that year, and 9 drivers had been injured (Méndez 2008). Some of these assaults were robberies, while others were instances of gangs or criminal organizations extorting bus companies and drivers. Everyone on the bus—drivers, assistants and passengers alike—is vulnerable in such situations and can easily come to harm. Sometimes the violence is exacerbated by passengers who carry their own guns for protection; shoot-outs have taken place inside buses.

Each day, Guatemalan newspapers covered the murders registered in the previous 24 hours, usually under the headline '*la journada de violencia*' (today's violence'). The way in which aggravated violence is thus characterized as a taken for granted day-to-day occurrence contributes to normalizing its presence in the minds of readers. Articles sometimes included photographs of victims' corpses and wailing next of kin, alongside speculation as to the motives of the crime. Revenge was often singled out as a probable motive, as was robbery. Whenever there were detainees, photographs of them were usually provided, alongside disclosure of their full names. In these photographs, detainees frequently appeared handcuffed, and if male, naked from the waist up, thus displaying tattoos indicating *mara* (gang) affinity. *Mara* detainees' aliases were also given. Although the pictures of detainees may have served to illustrate police success in fighting crime, most people were well aware that few murder cases actually lead to conviction. At the time, it was estimated that 90% of crimes went unpunished in Guatemala (UNICEF and CICIG 2009).

The press frequently quoted these statistics, alongside allegations that the corruption of members of the PNC (*Policía Nacional Civil*) and judges hinders the effective functioning of the justice system. The police and judges, however, may be under tremendous pressure by more powerful actors to obstruct the effective application of law and justice, as is thoroughly documented in Goldman's account of the efforts to bring Bishop Gerardi's murderers to trial (2007). Bishop Juan José Gerardi Conedera was murdered in his home in 1998, two days after publishing the report *Guatemala: Nunca más* (Guatemala: Never again) (ODHAG 1998). The report investigates civilian deaths and massacres during the internal conflict and overwhelmingly places responsibility for these abuses with the armed forces and paramilitary groups. It is widely assumed that Gerardi was murdered as retaliation for this report. After a long and difficult struggle to bring those responsible to justice, four men were eventually convicted for his murder in 2001. Three of them were military officers, two of whom were members of then President Alvaro Arzú's EMP (Estado Mayor Presidencial) Presidential Guard—active member Captain Byron Lima Oliva and former member Sergeant Major Jose Obdulio Villanueva Arevalo. After numerous appeals, the verdicts against them were finally upheld by the Constitutional Court in 2007 (Goldman 2007).

In 2006/2007, the general election campaign turned out to be the bloodiest so far in Guatemala's short democratic history. The Economist (2007) estimates that between 26 and 36 candidates and political activists were murdered between March 2006 and the beginning of August

2007. At that point, a month of campaigning remained. In response to these murders, there were speculations as to the possible ties between political parties and candidates, and organized crime (The Economist 2007, Cereser 2007). As the number of murdered candidates increased, the impression grew that only corruptible candidates were allowed to live. Graffiti in Flores, Petén, expressed this, denouncing Otto Peréz Molina, the presidential candidate for PP (Partido Patriota), as an assassin of bus drivers (*asesino de pilotos*)—a reference to the extortion practices of organized crime.

The new forms of violence have contributed to the widespread, generalized sense of political fear. Marta Elena Casaús Arzú, a Guatemalan sociologist and historian living in Spain, captures this well in an interview with the daily *Nuestro Diario*. When asked about the difference between living in Guatemala and Spain, she answers,

> In Spain, you leave the house and you don't ask yourself whether you will return. In Guatemala, you leave the house and you say, God willing, I will come back alive. This feeling of fear for your life disappears in Europe.[10] (Maldonado 2008)[11]

Here, Casaús Arzú summarizes succinctly the absence of trust in the world outside the home that permeates Guatemalan society (Ystanes 2011, 2016). If to experience social trust is to take one's safe movement outside the home for granted, then Guatemalans certainly do not have this luxury. The sentiment described by Casaús Arzú is widely shared, and people find confirmation of it in the media and in their daily conversations. It is difficult to separate oneself from the constant stream of information about violent acts and the prevalent 'talk of crime' (see Caldeira 2000 for a discussion of this phenomenon in the Brazilian context). The ensuing fear makes people worry about their journey to work, especially in Guatemala City, and many try to coordinate their activities so that they do not have to go anywhere alone unless absolutely necessary. This is particularly the case for women, and as such, there is a conflation of the moral and physical risks associated with them being *en la calle* (see also Franco 1999).[12]

However, although people try, it is difficult to control one's exposure to such events, as they have no choice but to make their bus rides to work and their trips to the market. Many try to rationalize the situation and adopt the view that violence is only targeted at those involved in criminal activities. For example, when in Petén a student was shot and killed while attending a class at the university; Rubén, who had many friends who were students, insisted that in general, it was not dangerous to attend classes. 'This sort of things only happens to those who are involved in something', he said.

Yet, things are not quite so simple. Murders often take place in front of witnesses in public places, such as the above-mentioned university lecture room, inside shops, at markets, on buses and on residential streets as people leave or enter their homes. Sometimes the victims are randomly selected as targets for muggings, whereas at other times they are victims of so-called *balas perdidas*, stray bullets aimed at someone else. Others still are specifically targeted for reasons of vengeance or holdups, because of their political activism or their refusal to comply with extortion.

Many Guatemalans understand the situation as the outcome of conflicts of interest that separate the upper classes and the political elite from the rest of the population. It is read against a background of hierarchized difference as a core principle for the organization of society. It is also understood as somehow controlled or at least accepted by the powerful Guatemalan elite, who use it to their advantage. In the midst of the chaos, politicians and activists are still being targeted, and organized crime seems unstoppable. Researchers concur with this perspective on the violence (e.g. McNeish and López Rivera 2009; Hurtado Paz y Paz 2007). In particular, many considered the former president Alfonso Portillo of the FRG party (2000–2004) as 'the one who had allowed organized crime to enter Guatemala'.[13]

In such ways, suspicion marks the relationship between the Guatemalan public and the political and economic elite. Those who face the possibility of violence every day as they step out of the house, use public transport or go to the market, without the luxury of armored cars and security guards, do not tend to believe that the powerful have their interests in mind. Even though elites also feel vulnerable to the violence, as the extensive use of armed guards indicates, they are nevertheless understood to be responsible for the dangers encountered *en la calle*. This conception draws on historical and contemporary hierarchization and thus places the present in continuity with the past. The lack of social cohesion and shared interests between the rulers and the ruled thus continues to give meaning to current events.

Hence, when I commented to Marco, a *profesional*[14] in his thirties, that the security situation in Guatemala appears to be much worse now than when I first started visiting in 1999, he dismissed the idea that the change had been that dramatic (although most people would agree that there has been a change for the worse). Instead, Marco pointed out that my experience was probably dictated by the fact that 'in the beginning you did not understand anything'. The presence of danger and violence is consequently perceived as continuity with the past, even though it now takes a different form, and is experienced as more prevalent by most of the people I have worked with. The common factor is that whereas before the violence was overwhelmingly committed on behalf of the government (ODHAG 1998; CDH 1999), it is now committed by other actors, who are nevertheless considered as operating with the government's blessing and the elite's interests in mind.

The Fear of Violence *en la calle* and the Penetration of Safe Zones

In Latin America, *la calle* (the street), the public domain, is often presented as a symbolic 'war of all against al' (DaMatta 1991:65); a space permeated by both playful and more serious challenges to the integrity of persons and groups (see also Ystanes 2011, 2016). Here, men can use their creative skills to flirt with women and establish friendship as well as relations of domination amongst themselves (see e.g. Limón 1989; Lauria 1964; Gutmann 1996). This public domain of outsiders and strangers is considered the location of mistrust, confrontation, conflict and moral risk. In contrast, family and kin are considered a realm of trust, respectability and intimacy. This conceptual boundary is often referred to as a distinction between *calle* (street) and *casa* (house), and it rests upon the assumption that close, mutually supportive relationships are more easily developed among kin. Conversely, it is considered that close relationships cultivated in the public domain may turn out to be deceptive (Ystanes 2011, 2016).

However, the metaphorical image of the street as a 'war of all against all' takes on a terrifyingly concrete meaning in light of the spiraling violence. Most people I know in Guatemala worry about leaving the house, especially on their own. An exception is the island of Flores, in Petén, or at least this was the case at the time of my main period of fieldwork there in 2007. During this time, *floreños* did not worry too much about security. Violent crime was mainly understood as taking place in the mainland twin towns of Santa Elena and San Benito, which are also considered to be poorer and to have more social problems than Flores (see also Schwartz 1990). The wealthier Flores, on the other hand, was conceptualized as an oasis of calm and security. It was also largely agreed that the problem of *maras* (gangs) and their violent activities was located in and isolated to Santa Elena and San Benito. Conceptually, then, danger and violence are not only associated with the morally ambiguous domain of *la calle* but also with poverty and marginality.

In Flores, people even let women in their company find their way home on their own after a night out drinking: '*aquí en la isla no pasa nada*' (here on the island nothing happens), they would say. In contrast, a business owner whose employees lived in Santa Elena and San Benito emphasized the terror they were exposed to: '*donde viven mis empleados hay muertos todos los días*' (where my employees live there are dead bodies every day). Towards the end of my stay, however, this feeling of separation between the safety of Flores and the danger of the mainland started to become blurred. There were more incidents and talk of armed robberies in shops and restaurants on the island, and the idea that the *maras* might be penetrating this former safe zone spread.

When I returned a few months later, in the spring of 2008, the situation had changed quite dramatically. People who had previously seen no problem with this now warned me against walking on my own after dark. There was a lot of talk about incidents where my interlocutors or people they knew had been robbed at gunpoint. In the few days that I was there, a young woman was threatened with a pistol to give up her mobile phone while making a call on the street, but escaped the situation by entering a nearby restaurant. She told me she was so shocked by what had happened that she did not think, just walked away. She was lucky to get away with this, as newspapers frequently report stories of people who are killed for refusing to give up their belongings in similar situations. It was clear from these accounts that violence and danger had now penetrated the safe zone of Flores in a way that was experienced as intimidating. This led to changes in behavior and precautions, thus blurring the separation between safe and dangerous zones. Similar ambiguities are also found in relation to the distinction between safe zones and dangerous zones elsewhere.

For example, Thomas et al. (2011) point to a tendency among Guatemalans to conceptualize urban areas as more dangerous than the countryside. However, Marisol, who lives in Carmelita, one of Petén's forest communities, considered '*falta de seguriad*' (lack of security) a problem in her village. Carmelita's community cooperative had for several years been involved in a struggle to maintain the existing forest conservation regime (Ystanes 2011, 2014). This model promotes both nature conservation and community development by granting of forest concessions to local communities within the protected area. So far, it has had promising results.[15]

The idea of overturning the existing conservation regime was first introduced in 2002, in a proposal put forward by the archaeological project excavating the ancient Mayan city El Mirador and their donors. This proposal sought to replace extraction activities with tourism as a means of forest preservation and vehicle for economic development. The story circulating in Petén is that the aforementioned President Alfonso Portillo (2000–2004) was flown to the excavation site by helicopter and was impressed by what he saw. Upon his return to the capital city, he promptly issued a presidential decree (Acuerdo Gobernativo 129–2002) overturning the existing legislation in favor of the tourism proposal. Concession communities feared for their livelihoods, and with the help of their umbrella organization ACOFOP (the Association of Forest Communities of Petén)[16] they challenged the validity of the decree. A long, conflict-ridden process followed. The Constitutional Court rejected the decree as unconstitutional in 2004, and President Oscar Berger finally revoked it in 2005. In the aftermath of these occurrences, a multisectorial discussion forum referred to as '*La Mesa*'[17] was established. The purpose was to institute consensus based decision-making, involving all of the so-called stakeholders. However, its workings were hampered by mutual mistrust and insurmountable power differences (see Ystanes (2011, 2014) for more details about this process).

At the time of Marisol's comment, La Mesa members debated the possibility of placing '*puestos de seguridad*' (police/security posts) in several places to monitor illegal activities within the protected forest areas. The plan involved the construction of a small police station in Carmelita. The most active members of the Carmelita cooperative were eager for this to materialize. Several claimed to be receiving death threats because of their work, in particular those who had denounced the unlawful sale of land within the concession area. During my fieldwork, at least two persons holding important positions within the cooperative decided to leave Carmelita due to such threats. These persons moved to San Benito or Santa Elena and continued to work for the cooperative while based there. In explaining to me why she considered it important to have a police presence in Carmelita, Marisol said,

> Here we are as far away from the authorities as one can get. If somebody wants to kill a person here, they can just go ahead and do it, and afterwards they can escape through the forest to Mexico, and it is as if nothing happened.

People in the area know the forest well, she says, so it is not hard for them to make it to the border. Hence, one can easily escape the consequences of a crime. Just like the apparently random violence encountered *en la calle*, the conflict within the community leading to these threats and the feeling of insecurity are interpreted against a backdrop of conflicting class interests. The cooperative is working within a framework of state ownership of the forest and community managed, communal access to its resources. The people opposing them reject this communal model and wish to have access to private ownership of the forest, and to dispose of the property as they wish. Cooperative members widely consider this group to be allied with the archaeological project and its elite donors, and as perceiving the community-based management model as a hindrance to their own potential economic success in tourism. Opposition to the cooperative and threats against cooperative members is therefore understood as yet another outcome of the conflict of interests between the elites and the rest of the population. The experience of fear that this situation gives rise to is repeatedly read into the social context of inequality and the use of violence by the powerful to protect their interests.

However, there is an ambiguity in Marisol's explanation, because she also claims that the presence of authorities would make her feel safer. She understands the people who are threatening her as protected by the Guatemalan elites, and hence authorities, yet call for the authorities to protect her. By indirect means, then, her plea for the right to live in her community without fear is a plea for ending the use of fear as a political instrument to maintain inequality.

The situation is complex, as are the narratives that circulate amongst people as they make sense of old and new forms of violence. Consuelo, another member of the Carmelita cooperative, told me that because of her role there, someone had broken into her house at night to intimidate her. The anniversary of the death of her husband, who had been killed by a stray bullet just outside her house, was also coming up. As she told me about this during lunch after a La Mesa meeting, she started crying from fear and grief. We were still sitting by the refectory table, surrounded by some of the people she, directly or indirectly, considered responsible for the threats she was receiving. For Consuelo, the dangers of the outside world had penetrated into the most intimate of safe spaces: her house. The intimidation was of course highly symbolic; the penetration of her house forewarned of a possible attack on her person, her body and her right to a mind of her own. The persons she held to be responsible for this violation were part of her community and the Mirador process, two entities that were now intrinsically tied together and in which Consuelo's existence is deeply embedded. Deprived of her husband by another violent occurrence just outside her home, she was left to fend for herself. Her safe zone had been shattered, and political fear now permeated her days and nights.

Concluding Remarks

Consuelo, Marisol and every Guatemalan engaged in political activism or simply making use of public space regularly experience 'fears that emanate from society or have consequences for society' (Robin 2004:2). The cases of Consuelo and Marisol illustrate that in Guatemala, political activism may still come with the price of intensified political fear. Depending on people's situation and activities, some manage to settle back into a more comfortable state of mind with relative ease, while others may find themselves living in a constant, low-intensity panic (Green 1999:60–61). Impunity is at the core of their struggle to make sense of the violence that mars their physical and mental landscapes, and the entanglements of the present with the past. It is perhaps in the interest of those who do not wish to grant Guatemalans the right to the truth that fear and complexity prevail. Rather than an emotion that catapults us into an enhanced state of action, consciousness and moral judgment, such fear is 'a symptom of pervasive conflict and political unhappiness' (Robin 2004:3) and 'a basic mode of social and political control' (2004:19). This does not mean that fear robs people of agency, but rather, as Zur points out, 'fear, suspicion and paranoia [do] not only result from impunity but are the psychological mechanisms which help to maintain it' (1994:13). The fear produced by violence is exacerbated by the perception of impunity and contributes to the maintenance of impunity—those who protest, risk losing the right to a self in a very concrete way. This situation is both an aspect of current circumstances and a continuity with the past marked by repressive military regimes and civil war. The trauma endured by the Guatemalan population is thus most productively understood as a collective and cumulative process of slow and persistent violence (see Chap. 1). While the individual effects of such violence are no doubt profound, so are the effects on the social body. Any notion of 'healing' must therefore address not just individual experiences but also the collective, societal aspects of terror. The recent conviction of two former militaries for sexual violence during the war (see BBC 2016) may fuel cautioned hopes, yet, so far, persistent impunity and denial of the right to the truth allow for the effects of terror to linger and reproduce.

Notes

1. In Spanish: *Guatemala, el país del eterno status quo.*
2. In Spanish: *Guatemala, el país de la eterna primavera.*
3. In Spanish: *El Acuerdo de Paz Firme y Duradera.*
4. In Spanish: Comité Coordinador de Asociaciones Agrícolas, Comerciales, Industriales y Financieras.
5. Original in Spanish: Actualmente, aunque con leyes, instituciones y políticas formales vigentes, los sectores económica y políticamente con más poder siguen imponiendo sus intereses particulares por encima de aquellos de la nación y de los sectores mayoritarios. La prosperidad de sus negocios ganaderos, agrícolas, madereros y algunos ilícitos como el narcotráfico, se fundamentan en la destrucción y degradación ambiental del departamento, en la inmutable pobreza de la mayoría de la población y, también, en el predominio de la ingobernabilidad, la corrupción y la anomia generalizada.
6. Original in Spanish: La Comisión Internacional de Juristas (CIJ) dijo que en Guatemala existe un 'pacto de impunidad' que incluye 'ataques sistemáticos en contra de operadores de justicia' dirigido por 'poderes fácticos.'
7. Civil Self Defence Patrols (*Patrullas de Autodefensa Civil*).
8. The numbers Zur and Nelson provide are not in agreement, as Zur states that PAC participation was mandatory for all males between 15 and 55 years of age (1994:13). I have nevertheless chosen to use Nelson's numbers here, as her publication is newer and it is likely that more accurate numbers have been established by the two truth commissions (CDH 1999, ODHAG 1998) produced after Zur published her article in 1994.
9. In the analysis of present-day violence, I draw upon two ethnographic fieldworks, one in Quetzaltenango in the western highlands in 2000, and the other in Petén in northern Guatemala in 2007–2008. The former focused on the conceptualization of risk and uncertainty in social relationships. The latter centered on the attempts to develop for tourism the ancient Mayan city of El Mirador in northern Petén, and at the same time; preserve the surrounding tropical forests. The ethnography thus spans both the intimate and public spheres.

10. Original Spanish: 'En España sales y no te preguntas si volverás a casa. En Guatemala sales y dices: 'Ojalá que pueda volver vivo'. Esa sensación de temor por tu vida desaparece en Europa'.
11. Accessed online at http://www.fygeditores.com/fglinajeyracismo01.htm.
12. See below for more on the conceptual separation between *casa* (house) and *calle* (street).
13. Since leaving office in 2004, Portillo has been on the run from and later standing trial for embezzlement charges in Guatemala. He was absolved of these charges in 2010, but the prosecution announced their intention to appeal the verdict. Since he was acquitted, Portillo was imprisoned in a US military base, waiting to stand trial in the USA where he was accused of money laundering (CNN México 2011, 2013). Portillo pleaded guilty to the charges during the 2014 trial. He was released from prison in February 2015, after serving his sentence, and has now returned to Guatemala (BBC 2015).
14. *Professional* refers to someone working in an occupation requiring university education and is associated with middle-class status.
15. See, for example, Cronkleton et al. (2008), Hay-Edie and Halverson (2006), Hurtado Paz y Paz (2007), Stoian and Rodas (2006), Taylor (2009), Taylor and Cheng (2009), Taylor et al. (2008).
16. Asociación de Comunidades Forestales de Petén.
17. The Multisectorial Roundtable for the Natural and Cultural Zone of Mirador/Río Azul (*La Mesa Multisectorial de la Zona Natural y Cultural Mirador/Río Azul*).

References

AFP. 2014. La impunidad es un 'cáncer' que corroe a guatemala, denuncia human rights watch. *El Periódico*, February 5. http://elperiodico.com.gt/es/20140205/pais/242150/.

Allison, M. 2013. Efraín ríos montt Becomes the First Head of State Tried and Convicted of Genocide in a Domestic Court. *Al Jazeera*, May 15. http://www.aljazeera.com/indepth/opinion/2013/05/201351591259267287.html.

BBC. 2015. Guatemala Ex-president Alfonso Portillo Freed from us Jail. *bbc.com*. http://www.bbc.com/news/world-latin-america-31633785.

———. 2016. Guatemala: Rape Sentences in Landmark Military Trial. *bbc.com*, February 27. http://www.bbc.com/news/world-35674893?SThisFB.

Broch-Due, V. 2005. Violence and Belonging: Analytical Reflections. In *Violence and Belonging. The Quest for Identity in Post-colonial Africa*, ed. Vigdis Broch-Due, 1–40. London: Routledge.

Caldeira, T.P.R. 2000. *City of Walls. Crime, Segregation, and Citizenship in São Paulo*. Berkeley: University of California Press.

CDH, C. p. e. E. H. 1999. *Guatemala memoria del silencio*. Guatemala City: CDH.

Cereser, L. 2007. Publicaciones extranjeras señalan violencia electoral. *La Prensa Libre*.

CNN México. 2011. La Justicia de Guatemala Absuelve al Expresidente Alfonso Portillo, May 10. http://mexico.cnn.com/mundo/2011/05/10/la-justicia-de-guatemala-absuelve-al-ex-presidente-alfonso-portillo

———. 2013. Alfonso Portillo, el Primer Expresidente de Guatemala Juzgado en EU, May 28. http://mexico.cnn.com/mundo/2011/11/17/alfonso-portillo-el-primer-expresidente-de-guatemala-juzgado-en-eu

Cronkleton, P., P.L. Taylor, D. Barry, S. Stone-Jovicich, and M. Schmink. 2008. *Environmental Governance and the Emergence of Forest-Based Social Movements, Cifor Occasional Paper no. 49*. Bogor, Indonesia: Center for International Forestry Research.

DaMatta, R. 1991. *Carnivals, Rogues, and Heroes. An Interpretation of the Brazilian Dilemma*. Notre Dame, IN: University of Notre Dame Press.

EFE—Guatemala. 2014. Comisión internacional de juristas asegura que en guatemala existe 'pacto de impunidad'. *El Espectador*, April 12. http://www.elespectador.com/noticias/elmundo/comision-internacional-de-juristas-asegura-guatemala-ex-articulo-486519.

Feitlowitz, M. 1998. *A Lexicon of Terror. Argentina and the Legacies of Torture*. Oxford: Oxford University Press.

Franco, J. 1999. Killing Priests, Nuns, Women, Children. In *Critical Passions. Selected Essays by Jean Franco*, eds. Mary Louise Pratt and Kathleen Newman, 9–17. Durham, NC: Duke University Press.

Goldman, F. 2007. *The Art of Political Murder. Who Killed the Bishop?* New York: Grove Press.

Grant, W. 2013. Guatemala annuls ríos montt's genocide conviction. *BBC*, May 21. http://www.bbc.co.uk/news/world-latin-america-22605022.

Green, L. 1999. *Fear as a Way of Life*. New York: Columbia University Press.

Gutmann, M.C. 1996. *The Meanings of Macho. Being a Man in Mexico City*. Berkeley: University of California Press.

Hale, C.R. 2006. *Más que un indio (More Than an Indian)*. In *Racial Ambivalence and Neoliberal Multiculturalism in Guatemala*. Santa Fe, NM: School of American Research Press.

Hay-Edie, T., and E. Halverson. 2006. *Acciones comunitarias para la conservación de la biodiversidad. Creación de vínculos entre la conservación del a biodiversidad y el desarrollo de mejores medios de sustento*. New York: Grupo de Ambiente y Energía del PNUD.

Hurtado Paz y Paz, M. 2007. *Sólo para medio vivir. La importancia actual de las actividades extractivas de recursos forestales no maderables en los hogares de car-*

melita y uaxactún, petén, Guatemala. Guatemala: FLACSO Guatemala/ Editorial de Ciencias Sociales.

Klein, N. 2007. *The Shock Doctrine: The Rise of Disaster Capitalism.* London: Penguin.

KUBARK. 1963. *Counterintelligence Interrogation.* CIA secret document, approved for release January 1997.

Lauria, A. 1964. 'Respeto', 'relajo' and Inter-personal Relations in Puerto Rico. *Anthropological Quarterly* 37(2): 53–67.

Limón, J.E. 1989. 'Carne, carnales', and the Carnivalesque: Bakhtinian 'batos', Disorder and Narrative Discourses. *American Ethnologist* 16(3): 471–486.

MacLean, E. and S. Beaudoin. 2015. Eighteen Months After Initial Conviction, Historic Guatemalan Genocide Trial Reopens but is Ultimately Suspended. *International Justice Monitor*, January 6. http://www.ijmonitor.org/2015/01/eighteen-months-after-initial-conviction-historic-guatemalan-genocide-trial-reopens-but-is-ultimately-suspended/.

Maldonado, G. 2008. Socióloga guatemalteca residente en españa. *Nuestro Diario/Edición Dominical, April* 6: 8–9.

Manz, B. 1995. Fostering Trust in a Climate of Fear. In *Mistrusting Refugeesi*, eds. E. Valentine Daniel and John Chr. Knudsen, 151–167. Berkeley: University of California Press.

McNeish, J.-A., and O. López Rivera. 2009. The ugly poetics of violence in post-accord Guatemala. *Forum for Development Studies* 36(1): 49–77.

Méndez, C. 2008. Inseguridad: Terror a bordo de ruta 40r. *La Prensa Libre.*

Nelson, D.M. 1999. *A Finger in the Wound. Body Politics in Quincentennial Guatemala.* Berkeley: University of California Press.

———. 2009. *Reckoning. The Ends of War in Guatemala.* Durham, NC: Duke University Press.

Nielsen, A. K. 2014. Managing the Threat of Violence in Guatemala. Violence as Part of Women's Everyday Lives. M.Phil thesis, Department of Social Anthropology, University of Bergen.

Norad. 2011. *Norads resultatrapport del 1: Bistand og konflikt.* Oslo: Norad.

O'Neill, K.L., and K. Thomas, eds. 2011. *Securing the City. Neoliberalism, Space and Insecurity in Postwar Guatemala.* Durham, NC: Duke University Press.

ODHAG, O.d.D.H.d.A.d.G. 1998. *Guatemala: Nunca más (Version Resumida).* Donostia: Tercera Prensa-Hirugarren Prentsa S.L.

Robin, C. 2004. *Fear. The History of a Political Idea.* New York: Oxford University Press.

Rodgers, D. 2002. Living in the Shadow of Death: Gangs, Violence and Social Order in Urban Nicaragua, 1996–2002. *Journal of Latin American Studies* 38(2): 267–292.

Schwartz, N.B. 1990. *Forest Society. A Social History of Petén, Guatemala.* Philadelphia: University of Pennsylvania Press.

Smith, C.A. 1990. Origins of the National Question in Guatemala: A Hypothesis. In *Guatemalan Indians and the State: 1540–1988*, ed. Carol A. Smith, 72–95. Austin: University of Texas.

———. 1995. Race-Class-Gender Ideology in Guatemala: Modern and Anti-modern Forms. *Comparative Studies in Society and History* 37(4): 723–749.

Stoian, D., and A. Rodas. 2006. Community Forest Enterprise in Guatemala: A Case Study of *cooperativa carmelita r.L.*: 1–21. CATIE-CeCoEco.s.

Taussig, M. 2004. Culture of Terror—Space of Death. Roger Casement's Putumayo Report and the Explanation of Torture. In *Violence in War and Peace. An Anthology*, eds. Nancy Scheper-Hughes and Philippe Bourgois, 39–53. Malden, MA: Blackwell.

Taylor, P.L. 2009. Conservation, Community, and Culture? New Organizational Challenges of Community Forest Concessions in the Maya Biosphere Reserve of Guatemala. *Journal of Rural Studies*. doi:10.1016/j.jrurstud.2009.09.006.

Taylor, P. L., and A. Cheng. 2009. Reflexive Resource Governance as Embedded Process: A Comparison of Two North American and Central American Community-Based Forestry Organizations. Conference on the Human Dimensions of Global Environmental Change, Amsterdam.

Taylor, P.L., P. Cronkleton, D. Barry, S. Stone-Jovicich, and M. Schmink. 2008. *'If you saw it with my eyes': Collaborative Research and Assistance with Central American Forest Steward Communities*. Bogor, Indonesia: Center for International Forestry Research.

The Economist. 2007. Guatemala's Pre-election Violence: The Bloodiest Election Campaign in the Country's History. *The Enonomist Newspaper*.

Thomas, K., K.L. O'Neill, and T. Offit. 2011. An Introduction. In *Securing the City: Neoliberalism, Space and Insecurity in Postwar Guatemalai*, eds. Kedron Thomas and O'Neill Kevin Lewis, 1–21. Durham, NC: Duke University Press.

UNICEF, and CICIG. 2009. Una generación marcada por la impunidad.

Whitehead, N.L. 2004. Introduction: Cultures, Conflicts, and the Poetics of Violent Practice. In *Violence*, ed. Neil L. Whitehead, 3–24. Santa Fe and Oxford: School of American Research Press and James Currey.

Ystanes, M. 2011. *Precarious Trust. Problems of Managing Self and Sociality in Guatemala*. Ph.D. thesis, University of Bergen.

———. 2014. Saving Guatemala's 'mayan forest': The Environmental Crisis and Contested Development. In *Crisis in the Nordic Nations and Beyond: At the Intersection of Environment, Finance and Multiculturalism*, eds. Kristín Loftsdóttir and Lars Jensen, 121–142. Farnham: Ashgate.

———. 2016. Unfixed Trust: Intimacy, Blood Symbolism, and Porous Boundaries in Guatemala. In *Trusting and Its Tribulations: Interdisciplinary Engagements with Intimacy, Sociality and Trusti*, eds. Vigdis Broch-Due and Margit Ystanes, 37–59. London: Berghahn Books.

Zur, J. 1994. The Psychological Impact of Impunity. *Anthropology Today* 10(3): 12–17.

CHAPTER 10

Laughter Without Borders: Embodied Memory, and Pan-Humanism in a Post-Traumatic Age

Nicolas Argenti

'Truly Beyond Culture': Communities of Suffering, Empires of Trauma

It was fashionable in the nineteenth and early twentieth centuries for anthropologists to title or subtitle their papers 'A little known people' of this or that region. (Evans-Pritchard is reported to have quipped that with so many people studying little known and even lesser known peoples, he should like to study a non-existent people). The rhetorical device of referring to exotic and impossibly remote social groups spoke to the self-image of the anthropologist as adventurer/explorer in search of radical cultural difference. In an inspiring recent article Joel Robbins (2013) adumbrates a turn that recently took place in the discipline—a fundamental shift away from the study of faraway peoples as examples of otherness first identified by Michel-Rolph Trouillot in 1991 (Trouillot 2003 [1991]). Robbins (2013) goes on to suggest that the new focus of anthropology—long in coming to fill the gap left by the turn away from 'the savage slot', as Trouillot (2003 [1991]) glibly referred to it—is now the suffering sub-

N. Argenti (✉)
Brunel University London, Uxbridge, UK

V. Broch-Due, B.E. Bertelsen (eds.), *Violent Reverberations*,
DOI 10.1007/978-3-319-39049-9_10

ject. From having been objects in the study of difference, other peoples have now become subjects similar to 'us' in a new empathetic embrace that seeks not to highlight human diversity or to emphasize difference but to establish communion in the universality of suffering. In espousing this new intimacy with other peoples, Robbins takes inspiration from Cathy Caruth's (1995) seminal work on trauma. As a literary critic, Caruth has been instrumental in taking the notion of trauma and post-traumatic stress from its clinical setting and introducing it into the realm of the humanities and the social sciences, simultaneously transforming its original use as a diagnosis of individual patients to a lament for the suffering of entire social groups across time and space.

The early psychological research on trauma from which Caruth draws her inspiration suggested that there was something about the experience of violence that placed it outside of memory, beyond the normal processes of remembering. According to this view, the psychic phenomenon of trauma itself engenders amnesia and silence. This view has been transmitted from early clinical theorists of trauma, through later generations of physicians such as Bessel van der Kolk (see van der Kolk and Grenberg 1987; van der Kolk and van der Hart 1991; Van der Kolk and Fisler 1995; Van der Kolk et al. 1996), to contemporary social scientists and literary critics, who have all dwelled on the silences and the aporia brought forth by violent pasts. These include many theorists in addition to Caruth (e.g. Agamben 1999; Bettelheim 1943; Caruth 1991a, b, c; Derrida 1976, 1986; Friedlander 1992; LaCapra 2001; Felman and Laub 1992; Laub 1991; Lyotard 1990; Unnold 2002; Vickroy 2002). According to the dominant theory of traumatic silence, one of the paradoxes of trauma is that those who live through events of excessive violence cannot react to them emotionally at the time of their occurrence. Janet and Freud also noted that the traumatic experiences of their patients, although absent from memory, clearly were present at some other level of consciousness, for, unaware as their patients were of the events that had precipitated their crises, they were compelled regularly to re-enact them with complete precision. Far from forgetting, these patients seemed to be suffering from the inability to forget or the failure to realize they were perpetually remembering. Where narrative memories are integrative, traumatic memories are intrusive and literal; they have no social component, but rather seem to spring upon their victims quite outside of their volition or control (Argenti and Schramm 2010; van der Kolk and van der Hart 1991; Langer 1991).

Highlighting the solipsistic nature of the condition, Derrida (1976) refers to traumatic memory as a 'crypt', a place hidden within or beneath another place, a place complete unto itself, but closed off from that outside itself of which it is nevertheless an inherent part. The crypt is formed in violence, and yet also in silence. Abraham (1975), Torok (1975), and Abraham and Torok (1976) similarly argue that the silence of incorporation reifies trauma as a presence that is then handed down from generation to generation. Children may thus incorporate the ghosts of their parents as bodily practices.[1] In the case of mass traumatic events, we are told by literary critics and anthropologists alike, these bodily memories may become established in the community as collective social practices (Abraham 1975:175–176, 1994:76; Alexander 2012; Alexander et al. 2004; Neal 1998; Caruth 1991; Das et al. 1997, 2000, 2001; Erikson 1991; Eyerman 2001; LaCapra 2001; Shaw 2002:5–6; Comaroff and Comaroff's 1992:38; Kleinman and Kleinman 1994:716–717). According to this model, phantoms or ghosts may take the form of bodily practices handed down as transgenerational traumatic memories, or transgenerational haunting.

Robbins convincingly demonstrates that these applications of trauma theory to ethnographic contexts are often paradoxically devoid of cultural specificity. Even when put to work by anthropologists working with 'faraway' or 'exotic' peoples, they overlook cultural difference, emphasizing instead the universal aspects of suffering that link the reader to the suffering subject of the study in a presumed universal language of pain. Reflecting on Valentine Daniel's (1996) work on the civil war in Sri Lanka, Robbins (2013:455) tells us that 'you would immediately accept Daniel's point that this kind of suffering and violence confronts you in your humanity and raises issues that you cannot help but feel are beyond culture'. 'Traumatic suffering', he adds, 'may truly be beyond culture' (ibid.). Robbins also points out that João Biehl's (2005) biographical monograph *Vita*, focusing on a single mentally ill woman in Brazil, similarly tells us little about Brazilian culture per se, the assumption being that the suffering subject is the same anywhere and everywhere in the world. Agreeing with Kleinman's blurb on the back of the book, that the book's protagonist Catarina has 'her humanity reaffirmed by the author', Robbins tells us that 'Biehl's telling of Catarina's story addresses its readers in their humanity—their ability to recognize suffering in its universal form' (2013:455).

But while Robbins is absolutely right in noting how Caruth and others have been instrumental in propagating the spread of trauma in scholarly writing across the disciplines, and charting the universalizing march of this discourse into anthropology itself, others have been more cautious of incorporating the theory into the social sciences and the humanities. In a critical review of trauma theory, Ruth Leys (2000) argues that there is in fact no consensus regarding the etiology or the symptoms of PTSD, that this syndrome is of 'dubious validity' as a psychological model (2000:7), and that its appropriation by poststructuralist literary critics and other humanists and social scientists is more problematic still. Leys finds the clinical model of traumatic memory reductionist in its depiction of the mind as a mechanistic entity in which unmediated memories can be lodged like computer files quite outside of symbolization (2000:229–265, 272–297). Similar critiques have been pioneered by Ian Hacking (1986, 1995), Derek Summerfield (1996, 1998), Alan Young (1995), and Peter Loizos (2008).

Didier Fassin and Richard Rechtman (2009) provide one of the most recent and comprehensive accounts of the escape of the trauma discourse from the laboratory or the analyst's couch into the population at large as it has gained the popular validity of what Ian Hacking refers to in another context as 'semantic contagion' (1995:238). Robbins devotes some time in his article to Fassin and Rechtman's identification of the potential for trauma to encapsulate our common humanity, but he downplays their critical interpretation of this phenomenon. In particular, Robbins ignores Fassin and Rechtman's warning of the analytical price one pays for this universalist empathy: Fassin and Rechtman emphasize above all the voraciousness of the trauma paradigm, which devours all difference as it spreads its tentacular grip across societies and—in its seductive vagueness—indiscriminately engulfs such disparate phenomena as slavery, the holocaust, the 11th September attacks, forced sterilization campaigns, the experience of a natural disaster or industrial accident, and discrimination. It is precisely in a critique of Cathy Caruth that Fassin and Rechtman (2009:18–19) argue that the methodology of trauma entails the abandonment of the search for other people's experience and its substitution for our own. This outward projection of a Western concern in the name of empathy, which Fassin and Rechtman expose as the 'empire of trauma', threatens to trivialize the category in the very process of proselytizing its blessings, identifying perpetrators and victims of violence as equally traumatized:

> The universalization of trauma results in its trivialization. In these models, every society and every individual suffers the traumatic experience of their past. Not only do scales of violence disappear, but their history is erased. (Fassin and Rechtman 2009:19)

Robbins is aware of one of the costs of the new pan-humanism in anthropology: the abrogation of the potential for critical evaluation of other cultures as different from ours, and the abandonment of the original utopian ideal that drove the ethnographic search for alternative cultural worlds in the West since the Renaissance. My own reservation regarding the deployment of the trauma paradigm in our discipline has to do not with the loss of a critical sense of difference but with the implicit assumption in trauma theory that the only means people have of dealing with oppression and violence throughout the world is to be subjected to its terror, destroyed as functioning social agents by its crushing power, and rendered mute patients in need of the diagnosis and therapeutic attention of Western specialists. The trauma paradigm is by definition not a social theory but an atomizing one: it singles out the patient not only as an individual but as an individual irremediably isolated from his or her social world, doomed to live in perpetuity in the frozen time of their original trauma, as they repeat as unmediated experience the violence that they have failed to mediate as memory. The current understanding of trauma in the West—just over a hundred years old as a clinical concept and half that age as a popular one—is of questionable cross-cultural validity. Linked as it is to processes of industrialization, capitalist individuation, and total war, it is not an analytical model but a cultural and historical phenomenon. More importantly, it does not describe a social process but a process of putative social disintegration and atomization, in which overwhelming violence has destroyed all semblance of the social ties linking individuals to one another into a cultural whole. In a word, trauma confronts the utopian anthropological ideal of Shakespearean brave new worlds with the dystopian surrender to a Huxleyan Brave New World.

In what follows, I look back at my own engagement with trauma theory in my work in Cameroon and delineate my current approach to memories of violence in the Aegean island of Chios where I now work. I suggest that we can keep hold of the pan-humanist ideal in recent anthropology that Robbins is defending without relinquishing the critical focus on cultural difference that he is also at pains to defend. It is our research participants who have shown us how to do this without any need for the cultural agent orange of trauma theory, which desiccates everything it touches in its unreflexive production of universal victimhood and its monochrome histories of the vanquished (Koselleck 2002). In thrall to suffering and terror, we have ignored the social power of ritual laughter.

Thunder in the Mountains: Masking, Terror, and Desire

My own work has had the air of an uneasy *pas de deux* with the trauma paradigm. Conducting research on political hierarchy in the highland kingdoms of the Cameroon Grassfields in the 1990s, my attention was drawn to the awesome displays of wealth and power invested in the royal courts and their associated secret societies. Arriving as I had in the kingdom of Oku, where I would spend the subsequent two years, in the midst of the first royal investiture since 1956, I spent the first months confronted by all of the palace masks, which were brought out during the protracted mourning period in processions, sacrificial rites, and performances not seen for a generation (Argenti 2007). Cloaked in gowns of human hair, their faces concealed behind rough jute sacking, their formless and hunched bodies draped with medicinal amulets, forest plants, and the fleeces or stuffed carcasses of wild animals, sporting monstrous masks so large they often had to be carried like headloads, armed with massive cudgels, spears, and cutlasses, enraged and demonically belligerent, they often had to be restrained by stout lianas that groups of warriors from the palace regulatory society struggled to keep hold of as the masks rampaged unchecked through the throngs of people attending the obsequies at the palace. So frightening were these embodiments of unbridled rage and malevolent power that the assembled throngs would turn their backs so as not to set eyes on the masks as they trod ominously past, or would flee in panicked waves, running over each other to save themselves as the faceless beings lunged at them, brandishing their rough-hewn weapons.

These untamed sylvan beasts (it was forbidden to refer to them as masks) were said to have emerged from the realm of the dead in the inaccessible depths of the virgin forest that crested the isolated mountaintops and sacred crater lake of the kingdom's highest peaks, and to be at the beck and call of the palace authorities, who would let them loose on their citizens for sport on occasions of state. One of them, with the masker's lowered face obscured in a jute sack, a porcupine quill stuck through his nose, his hunched and hooded head surmounted by the mask of a grimacing ape, its body bristling with the long brown feathers of the plundering raptor, and armed with a sinister cudgel and several spears, was remembered with particular dread as having been the palace executioner until the advent of the colonial era. The hawkish lilting whistle that it emitted as it negotiated the forest paths with its peculiarly hesitant simian gate and the accompanying discordant clashing of the broken double-bell that its gleefully ululating acolytes pounded behind it were enough to send men, women, and children fleeing pell-mell into the bush at its approach. Horrific, ominous, violent, and frankly dangerous as these masks were, they nevertheless represented a source of grim fascination to the people of the outlying villages of the kingdom, who thronged to the palace in their thousands during the months of the interregnum; in part at least to witness and to subject themselves to the depredations of these rampaging embodiments of palatine power, grief, and rage.

At home in their village compounds, the untitled commoners at the base of the kingdom's hierarchy emulated the palace's predilection for attracting the beasts of the forest—luring them, it was said, into the compound courtyard with the seductively aqueous and plangent sound of the xylophone music that the reticent creatures couldn't resist. Once enticed out of their mountain redoubts, these wild spirit beings were entrapped in the compound mask house from which, like those of the palace, they were only ever permitted to emerge to mourn a death in the family. Unlike the palatine masks, however, the village masks were not a source of unmitigated fear and loathing. They were not violent and antisocial, but seen by all as beautiful, seductive, and enticing. When they came out mournfully at night, wailing disconsolately at the death of a member of their secret society, women would secret themselves in their houses to avoid the barrenness or insanity that would result from seeing them in their unmasked nocturnal state; but even then young women were peculiarly moved by the masks' bestial howls of pain, sorrow, and loss, and inexplicably attracted to the susurrations of their speaking in tongues and the lascivious low growls and eerie modulated, buzzing cries they emitted at the barricaded door as—demented with grief and rutting in their sudden liberty—they sought to seduce the young women into letting them in. The next morning a lone mask—its arms crossed over its chest in mourning—would make its way listlessly to the graveside of the deceased before the earth had been filled in over the body and the men of the compound had stamped it down in rhythmic unison to the accompaniment of their ribald songs. Now wearing the carved wooden 'head' it had lacked in the night (at which point the hooded faces of the maskers make them appear like headless stumps), the mask was no longer the impassioned source of danger and fear it had been in the darkness but an embodiment of the sorrow and pain experienced by all the assembled family and friends of the deceased; and it acted for all of them when it clasped a handful of the red earth and let it fall desultorily into the open sepulcher. But when, on the anniversary of the death, the entire group came out of the compound mask house to celebrate the memory of the deceased, it was a different matter: gone were the 'obsequies of tears' of the burial, and in their place the 'obsequies of dancing' had begun.

Beautiful were the masks as they danced with their beaded earrings, their cowry-shell headdresses, their parti-colored gowns, and their flying whisks as their rattle-clad ankles slammed down to the rhythm of the xylophone and the drums. Unforgettable were those days of unrestrained celebration, of communion, and of commensality as extended families came together from across the country to banish the specter of death that had been hanging for so many months over the afflicted house. As the compounds' masks—unmentionable but known to all as the young men of the compound—danced to the enchanting and mesmeric music of their beloved and captivating xylophone, the elders would push coins into their palms while the women danced on the periphery, clapping, shaking their 'spear hands', and ululating with unrestrained pride and giddy elation. The boldest among them might take hold of the sharp iron blade of a masks' spear, leading it round the xylophone ensemble as the mask danced obediently behind her holding the spear haft. Other women would take it upon themselves to lure the leader of the masks, known as 'the captain' in pidgin, into the ring when it was proving too skittish or diffident to lead its troupe into the dance space. Writhing slowly and seductively round to the rhythmic pulse in coy circles, a young woman would unbind her brightly-printed headscarf and wave it gracefully in front of the pulsating line of hulking masks, dancing as if for fractions of eternity in and out towards the stubborn captain, luring him in step by step despite himself till he suddenly came bursting forth like a charging buffalo—'breaking the stones beneath his feet!'—the gathered men would enthuse as they recalled the dance in the days that followed. As enthralling as the masks of the palace were in their ghastliness and macabre horror, so were the village masks every bit as enchanting in their beauty and seduction, and the more subjugated and belittled one had been by the palace masks, all the more intense was the pleasure taken in the magnificence of one's own compound masks.

Never were the people of Oku more oppressed and terrified, and never more elated and triumphant than in the presence of their masks. And yet, despite the stark contrast between the belligerent and threatening masks of the palace on the one hand and the attractive and celebratory masks of the village lineages on the other, one choreographic element remained fundamental to all these masks alike when they performed in a group to the music of the xylophone. Although they all emerged alone to 'display' (*ʃiɛŋə*), as their uncontained and sinister rampages were euphemistically referred to, some of the palace masks also united on occasion to dance as a group around the palace xylophone. This performance was not the unmitigated source of collective rejoicing and aesthetic delight that lured commoners exuberantly into the dancing ring in the euphoric performances of village masks, but rather an offputtingly ominous shuffle that only members of the palace secret societies dared to approach. Closely packed in single file, the palace masks trudged mirthlessly round the palace courtyard to the pounding xylophone rhythm of the secret society members in their midst, who for their part all bit medicinal plants between tightly clenched teeth to ward off the poisonous effects of the masks' offensive magic. The palace masks, albeit terrifying on their own, were now themselves hounded by another mask running alongside them as they trod laboriously on, harried by their tormenting guardian with its drawn cutlass if they slowed or fell out of step. Their merciless nemesis was none other than Mabu, the executioner mask. Mabu, the armed guard who harried his masks mercilessly on, was known as the *kəʃiɛŋɛnɛ*, 'the one who displays'—of the palace masking group. He performed alongside the obedient coffle of the palace masks the feats of war-like agonism and violence for which those palatine masks are all famed when performing on their own. His role was not unique to the palace group masquerade, however, but also an essential part of every village masking group. Less sinister in the village groups, the *kəʃiɛŋɛnɛ* would appear in a spirit of contrasting playfulness and of jubilant pride, running with a spear or cutlass alongside the dancing masks, and rounding up the wayward and the slow so that they should not fall out of the single-file procession or lose the rhythm of the dance. In the safety of one's village and compound, banished and forgotten was the fear and horror of the palatine procession, replaced now with the gaiety and seduction of the commoners' celebrations that it had paradoxically inspired.

In contemplating the marriages of opposites—beauty and violence, pleasure and terror, seduction and denigration, oppression and transcendence, mourning and celebration, melancholy and mirth—that the masks of Oku seemed paradoxically to embody, I turned my attention to a modern performance by a dance group named Air Youth that was not masked, but which performed in track suits and red berets, executing self-consciously modernist dance steps, re-enacted gestures of state ceremony and pomp, and appropriated acrobatic martial arts moves, all to the unusual and exotic accompaniment of blow-pipes and drums (Argenti 1998). What I realized about this group's mimetic appropriation of alternative realities would eventually lead to my understanding of the traditional masquerades of Oku: in their dances, they were re-enacting episodes of extreme violence that had befallen the village at the hands of the paramilitary police a few years earlier, when gendarmes had stabbed a woman to death and rampaged through the village firing automatic weapons at the people as they fled. The red berets and army boots of the dancers were those worn by the gendarmes; their standing to attention, swagger sticks, salutes, and marching re-enacting the military bearing of these hated figures of government oppression. And yet, the key to the whole performance was what would happen after it was over: during informal get-togethers, when the dancing had ended, the mood would sometimes shift from a marshal and competitively agonistic one to one of calm and quiet serenity. At such moments, the band would play a slower rhythm, and the women who had been watching from the side-lines would break with the conservative protocol of Grassfields decorum and join in with the men, hugging them and bursting into fits of laughter as they lolloped and skipped mesmerically along together like carefree gamboling youths. Curiously denuded of their years as they embodied this episode of their past, the women who had been so cruelly assaulted by the gendarmes now danced in adoring embrace with the red-hatted and black-booted embodiments of the very soldiers who had attacked them. Audaciously wrapped arm in arm with their siblings, husbands, sons, and lovers, they swayed and laughed illicitly with them, confounding local norms of propriety as they transformed memories of massacre into unashamed celebrations of desire, of pleasure, and of tenderness.

Writing a book a decade after my research in Oku (Argenti 2007), my fascination with the ineffable eeriness of the masked dances I had studied was deepened by a growing unease at the unplumbed silence with which my questions regarding the violence of the past had always been met by my friends and acquaintances. It was only by chance, after I had known one of the victims of the debacle of the gendarmes (a woman in whose compound I lived and in whose kitchen I had spent nearly every evening for 18 months), that she told me one night that she had been shot on that day, laconically pulling up her waistcloth to show me the circular scar on her leg where the bullet had torn through her flesh. My friends were equally elusive about the more distant past, of the depredations of the slave trade that had affected the area so catastrophically over so many centuries. So secretive were people about this untold past that it was an offence finable by the palatine authorities to refer to anyone's slave ancestry, and I would never learn the word for slave (*kəkɔs*, from the root *kɔɔ* 'to catch') during my entire two-year first stay in the kingdom (Argenti 2007: Chap. 3). Was this a region in which history—the history of the transatlantic slave trade into which the region possibly fed more human beings than any other in Africa, and of forced colonial labor that produced more deaths than any industrialized war—had been forgotten?

It was with both of these unresolved impressions—the uncanniness of the dances and the silence of the past—that in the course of writing the monograph I suddenly came across a throwaway aside in a colonial diary that hit me with the force of a physical blow. The author of the diary was Marie Pauline Thorbecke, wife of a German ethnographer exploring the region in the early twentieth century. She was recording her frustrations with the tedium of the caravan of forced laborers carrying their supplies (Argenti 2007:102). In order to ensure that their starving porters did not escape into the bush, the Thorbecks—like the German traders in the region and the slave traders before them whom they now employed as their labor recruiters—kept armed guards at the front and back of the column, while another ran up and down the line of porters, whipping those who wandered out of the line. The image was a perfect description of the choreography of the mask groups of the Cameroon Grassfields; the leaders of which are called 'captains' to this day, and the meandering masks of which are mercilessly hunted down during the performance by a figure with a cudgel who threatens and bullies them back into the line—the role played by the hooded and simian executioner mask at the palace.

Reading the diary a decade after having witnessed the dances, I suddenly realized that, just like the paramilitary violence at the dark heart of the joyous dances of Air Youth, the memories of the slave coffle and the porters' caravans were not spoken of because they had always been embodied; they were not remembered because, with every performance of the palatine masks, they were repeated: the sinister parade that they enacted could be none other than the belated succedaneum of the slave coffles of the precolonial period and the catastrophically deadly marches of forced laborers of the early colonial era.

Is not the recurring somatic enactment of an original experience the definition that Freud gave to trauma when he first afforded the term its psychic dimension? Is not the inability to articulate experiences so far outside of normal human experience that they are not cognized, not experienced, as they first happen at the core of the PTSD diagnosis? A society in which the people were doomed to repeat in lugubrious and mournful performances what they could not remember because it had 'always already fallen outside of memory' (Blanchot 1995, Langer 1991:38) seemed to be a society of trauma par excellence—or did it? The dancers inside the masks were not catatonically repeating a physical or psychic blow that they had personally suffered; they were performing a dance that they had voluntarily learned, which they chose to perform in appropriate contexts, in which they took pride and pleasure, and by which they were not haunted beyond the arena of the dance space. In other words, the dance repeated the originary event, but now as pleasure and as triumph, introducing laughter where once there had been only pain.

Traumatic Memory and Carnival Laughter

Having now transposed my research focus from Cameroon to Greece, I have been working on collective memory on the Aegean island of Chios. Very different in many respects of its history and social structure from the kingdoms of the Grassfields, the island shares with this region a past of political violence and of slavery. In particular, the island is sadly remembered in the annals of Modern Greek history for an unprecedented massacre that took place there in the spring of 1822, at the start of the Greek war of Independence. Following the landing of a band of agents provocateurs from the neighboring island of Samos who proceeded to force the small Ottoman garrison of Chios into their fortress—mainly ... by yelling at them' (Calvocoressi 1994:16)—and there to lay siege to them, the Ottoman Navy sailed to Chios with a massive fleet. The punitive expedition that ensued lasted for six months and resulted in the massacre or sale into slavery of nine tenths of the island's inhabitants, leaving 10,000 survivors in a population of 120,000 and sparking an exodus from the island that would become the *cause celebre* of its day, galvanizing philhellenic sentiment throughout Western Europe and the USA (Argenti 1932;

Calvocoressi 1994). Chios had not become part of the new Greek state following independence but remained an Ottoman possession following the massacre right up to its invasion by Greek troops during the Balkan wars in 1912. Then, just ten years after independence, the island was flooded with refugees fleeing the 1922 catastrophe of Smyrna across the narrow straits in Asia Minor, with further groups arriving in boats as part of the exchange of populations between Greece and Turkey in 1923–24 (Clark 2006:46, Clogg 1992:91–93; Demetriou 2013; Hirschon 1989:9, 2003; Housepian 1966; Llewellyn-Smith 1973:88–91, 303–319). In the Second World War the island suffered again as the occupation by the Germans and the ensuing allied blockade of the Mediterranean resulted in a catastrophic famine, with thousands dying from starvation (Argenti 1966; Hionidou 2006).

In 2010, as the Greek sovereign debt crisis took hold, the violence and suffering of past ages seemed to come to life again, transfixing the people of Chios with the horror of their resurrection: the massacre of the people of the island in the nineteenth century, the 1922 Catastrophe of Smyrna and the forced exchange of populations between Greece and Turkey, the famine during the occupation of the island by the Germans—all time and all suffering seemed to walk again in the fearful premonitions of the victims of the current crisis (Argenti forthcoming). While all of these events are spoken of explicitly today in the context of the on-going crisis, memories of other episodes of violence from a more distant past no longer form part of discursive memory but are still remembered on the island as non-discursive, embodied practices. In the period of the Byzantine Empire and afterwards, during the Genovese occupation of Chios, the island—famed for its wealth as it had been since antiquity—had always been subject to raids by Barbary corsairs (Green 2010). As a result, the villages were always built away from the shoreline, separated from their adjoining harbors by a line of hills to hide them from view from the sea. Settlements were fortified, with the houses of the outer perimeter adjoining each other in an unbroken windowless wall that served as a defensive palisade at times of attack. Villagers reserved the ground floor of their houses for livestock and storage so that, as the invaders were breaking in, they could escape through their roofs, running along the tops of the adjoining houses all the way to the fortified tower at the center of the village that served as the place of refuge in which they would barricade themselves until help could arrive from neighboring villages. Try as they might to take precautions, the villagers were nonetheless cruelly harried by the corsairs and often lost victims to them who would be taken to the ports of North Africa and sold as slaves or ransomed back to their families. An annual re-enactment of these attacks takes place annually in the village of Thymiana where, during the carnival festivities of *apokries (αποκριεσ)* preceding Easter, some of the villagers dress up as pirates and storm the village, with others coming to the defense of the settlement as they engage in a mock battle with the intruders.

Despite the many depredations and losses incurred during the centuries of attacks, the villagers of Thymiana remember this period of their history with a unique (and perhaps apocryphal) victory. There are many versions of the story. According to one, when a ship of corsairs was seen approaching the village one night of apokries in the Genovese period, the villagers all went to hide, leaving out the stores of wine that they had readied for their own festivities. (According to other versions of the story, they invited them to join them in their revelries). Then, when the corsairs had been drinking and carousing all night and were in no state for a fight, the villagers set upon them, capturing them and leading them to the village square with cries of 'βρε!, μωρί! μωρί! (meaning something like 'Oh! You poor fools!') In the village square they hanged them and left their bodies on display for three days (according to other versions they decapitated them and impaled their heads on spikes). Because of the public, demonstrative nature of the executions, the event came to be known as μόστρα; from the Italian for an exhibition, show, or spectacle. The following year, it is said, the villagers re-enacted the battle, and they have continued doing so ever since, with the five guilds[2] of the village taking over control of the festivities.

Starting on the Friday evening, villagers of Thymiana begin their carnival revelries. When I arrived in the village in 2012 it was about eight-thirty in the evening and the festivities were already well in train. We could hear the drums and recorders of the marching band from a distance as we walked up the darkened streets towards the central square where the corsairs had been hanged, and then we began to come across the revelers in their fright wigs, rubber masks, and home-made comic costumes. The maskers were mostly young men, though many women and older men were also among them. Passers-by offered us nuts and raisins and we fell in step with the band as they made their way slowly down the street playing a high-pitched island song. Almost every one of the young men in attendance was cross-dressing that night. Some of them had opted for the grotesque; their hairy legs and potbellies grossly at odds with the shiny leotards, fishnet stockings and undersized glittery swimsuits they wore. The more ephebic bachelors, graced with svelte physiques, had shaved their legs, put on high-heels and miniskirts, and donned plausible wigs of long, wavy blond hair. Their handsome faces were beautifully made up, they wore false eyelashes, and they carried themselves with great confidence, poise, and a certain graceful allure. As they chatted nonchalantly to one another, handbag or cigarette in hand, or swayed imperturbably to the music that emanated from the open doorways, they were disturbingly convincing; fascinating men and women alike with their studied ambiguity. As we moved on, a woman adorned in the disorientatingly life-like costume of a hauntingly beautiful fallow deer emerged furtively from the darkness and passed soundlessly by, the delicate spider webs and moss caught in her antlers fluttering behind her in the warm sea breeze.

Under the arches of the medieval ramparts, posters had been put up with photographs of past μόστρα in Thymiana, some of them from the 1960s and 1970s. Alongside these were satirical cartoons, including depictions of Angela Merkel scolding the prime minister or, in another collage, teaching a minister to read the word μνημόνιο (memorandum—i.e. the bailout agreements or 'memoranda of understanding' as they are officially known). As the band walked on through the streets, the revelers crying 'βρε! μωρί, μωρί!' in their wake, some picked up sticks with which they engaged in mock sabre fights, moving as if in slow motion to the sound of the music and clapping their sabers together to the rhythm of the drums. In their extravagant women's outfits, children throwing confetti over them as they performed their half-fight, half-dance, they made unlikely pirates, but they amused the crowd of onlookers all the more. At last we came to a school playground in front of the main church where plastic tables and chairs had been set out. Traditional island dance music played on the PA system, and the revelers began their slow, demure local dances; their effortless courteousness, grace, and restraint in pleasant disequilibrium with the irreverence of their costumes. Transgender Turkish women of the seraglio coyly held hands with cannibals, comic-book bones protruding from their improbably large afros. A group of women had donned matching pink plastic bottoms and wore signs on their backs that read 'They even got my nickers!' in reference to the punitive austerity measures the government had recently implemented. In the ring of dancers, a sumo wrestler in a fat suit cavorted with a man in false breasts, fishnet stockings, and a shiny red nylon one-piece swimsuit with a devil's tail protruding from the rear. Among the bystanders on the edge of the ring, the fallow deer briefly reappeared, shyly eyeing the dancers before melting silently back into the enshrouding obscurity.

Thirty-six hours later, on the Sunday of μόστρα 40 days before Easter, each of the churches in Thymiana held a service at the same time in the morning, attended by the villagers in their traditional costumes and the pirates with gold earrings and black skullcaps. After the service at Aghios Dimitrios, during which the priest had asked the congregation to pray for God to bless the nation's politicians with the gift of wisdom they so sorely lacked, ouzo and food were served on the doorstep of the church. Some of the villagers told me that the μόστρα, and apokries in general, have their origins in Bacchanalian feasts of the classical era. One local told me that the Thymianousi still carried on the Dyonisia in the modern era, and that they had been involved in the rites when the ill-fated pirates had attacked them. In each of the churches, some of the youths were dressed as pirates, others in the traditional costume of the village. After the feasting, the pirates and the villagers in traditional costume lined up in procession, making their way through the church cemetery to a drum and flute ensemble, again as in the Dionisia of ancient Greece, where they propitiated the dead by pouring libations of ouzo onto the graves in remembrance of lost souls—an ancient tradition known as σπονδή that involved the pouring of good wine on a grave. Many of the dead in the church, I was told, were from the stonemasons' guild and had taken part in the μόστρα in their youth.

Two flag bearers, one carrying the flag of Greece, the other the flag of the church, then led the procession down the hill toward the village. As they went, the man carrying the Greek flag came across a friend of his coming up the hill, and called out to him ironically 'You see what things have come to [in the current crisis]: I'm now reduced to carrying this flag about to make ends meet!' On the way, we reached a crossroads where we waited for the congregation of the builders' guild to join us from the church of St John. A young boy handed out small glasses of ouzo, another passed round a basket of the traditional chickpea and peanut snack. Many of the men had picked sprigs of olive on their way that they had tucked behind their ears. A few bearded transvestites came ambling up from the village to keep our spirits up and share our drinks. Then a cry of 'βρε! μωρί, μωρί!' announced the arrival of the congregation from St John. Most of them were dressed as pirates, and waved their sabers over their heads as they saw us. The two flag bearers were joined by a third with a giant black jolly roger. The young men from the two congregations separated into pirates and villagers, the pirates taking the lead down the hill, and the villagers following ten meters behind them. Every so often, as the drums and flutes played on, they stopped to engage in choreographed sabre fights to the rhythm of the drums. Following the same cycle of slow steps each time, they first dragged the tips of their steel sabers noisily along the ground as they approached each other, then jumping up to the beat of the drum, one dancer would strike the other's sabre three times as the other held his with both hands above his head. The two then switched roles and performed the moves again. Finally, one would skip backward in rhythmic steps, dragging his sabre along the flagstones with a metallic ringing, while the other lunged toward him, thrusting the point of his sabre toward his opponent in a rocking motion. Their duel over, they each returned to their group, and another pair took their place.

The dance took place at intervals all the way to the center of the village, the balconies of the medieval houses providing the vantage points from which the villagers enjoyed this playful re-enactment of a mortal conflict. The local tradition of the μόστρα then gave way to the modern, national tradition of the carnival as the pirates and their opponents dispersed to be replaced by a procession of floats. Almost all of these explicitly addressed the crisis. The first of the floats represented the Dionysian king of the carnival; a traditional Greek soldier from the regiment of the elite guard of the tomb of the unknown soldier (εύζωνες) but coiffed with a Mohican of Euro notes. A young woman in a blond bob and spectacles—Angela Merkel—stood behind him with a giant pair of scissors that she snapped ominously shut, preparing to give him the 'hair cut' that the economists had been warning the Greek economy was to receive at the hands of the troika. Another float depicted a hotdog stand, the villainous cook of which was referred to as the 'doctor of famine' (γιατρός τις πείνας)—the famine of the Second World War that everyone now feared would be returning (Argenti forthcoming; Knight 2012a). Another float depicting the tale of Alice in Wonderland, a larger-than-life model of the Queen of Hearts gushing blood from her mouth and heart, satirized the politicians' misrepresentation of the true state of the economy prior to the crash. Alice, in blond wig and blue dress with a white pinafore, threw handfuls of confetti merrily to the crowd. A sign on the back of her cart read 'Greece: the land of deceit'. (Ελλάδα: Η χώρα της απάτης, a play on words, where απάτης [short-change, deceit] replaced θαυμάτων [wonders]). Children in hats of gold and wearing gowns made of the Greek flag on one side and a rainbow on the other walked behind the float carrying cautionary placards, one of which read simply 'stop watching the news' (σταματήστε να βλέπετε ειδήσεις).

A giant mock-up of a grinning and lascivious Big Bad Wolf came next, representing the bogeyman of the EU/Greek government about to devour the Little Red Riding Hood of the innocent Chiots. In her red miniskirt and matching hood, she threw matching rose petals to the crowd, oblivious of the wolf's claws that embraced her from behind. The next float addressed a local dimension of the crisis: depicting a traditional Chiot house of the Genovese style from the famed citrus orchards of the Kampos and a mandarin tree, it referred to the fury in the village that the local bottling plant, once an important employer, had stopped buying Chiot fruit to make its juice, replacing it with imported frozen concentrate from Brazil. The theme of national corruption, international interference, and local impoverishment was carried on in subsequent floats with people being 'pressed like olives' by a man in a suit in one float, while another depicted the Greek expression 'something's burning' (κάτι καίγει, i.e. 'something's fishy') with children—the principle victims of the bailout program in many people's minds—in a cooking pot, the word 'Elections' painted on the burning kitchen wall behind them.

The last two floats descended into bacchanalian humor, one of them mimicking a recent television advert for iridescent condoms, the other carrying transvestites throwing water-filled condoms at the crowd. As the last of the floats passed by, the celebrants closed in behind them, following them to the village square where they sat down to eat, drink, and dance again as they had on the Friday evening.

Pan-Humanism and the Festive World

So it is that the abductions and power structures in the highlands of Cameroon that fed the transatlantic slave trade and the depredations of Barbary corsairs in the Aegean are remembered today in non-discursive practices that keep these events alive in the bodies of the people descended from the original victims of those violent upheavals. The masked dances of the Cameroon Grassfields and the revelries of the Chiot μόστρα have this in common despite the differences of their social and historical contexts: that they revive on a perpetual basis events that are seldom if ever spoken of explicitly, and that they enact them wordlessly; subjugating to physical experience and action what remains unspoken in daily life. We can propose that such behavior is suggestive of traumatic re-enactment; constituting the return of the repressed, Derrida's encryption, Abraham's ghostliness (1975), or Freud's *Nachträlichkeit*. In another example that I do not have the space to describe here in full, Chios has also been noted by folklorists since the nineteenth century for the popular tradition of αγασ (Politis, in

Herzfeld 1986:147, note 9). This carnival performance, which continues to take place to this day in a few of the southern villages of the island during apokries, re-enacts the trials and court hearings held by the local Ottoman potentate, the Αγας, during the period of Ottoman suzerainty. Feared for his power though he undoubtedly was, the Αγας of the carnival re-enactment appears as a jocund pantomime buffoon who is married off to a local man dressed as a Turkish *hanim* before proceeding merrily to hold court in the village square with her at his side. In the course of the hearing over which he presides, all the villagers bring forth those against whom they have had a grievance that year. Liberally deploying obscenities and insinuations in the course of his inquisition (in one ceremony I attended he punctuated his judgments with a bright red dildo he slammed on the table in lieu of a gavel), the Αγας eventually determines a punishment for the accused, which is summarily carried out on the spot by his appointed henchmen.

At the time that the folklorist Politis noted the performance of this event on Chios in 1909, the massacres of 1822 had taken place less than a century earlier and the island was still under Ottoman suzerainty; its population well below what it had been just prior to the catastrophe. Again, it would seem in this case that the horrors of previous generations—unspeakable under continued Ottoman control—return to this day with their full force as action because, having been encrypted, they cannot be spoken. The details of the performances of the masked dances of Oku and the μόστρα of Chios do not support the original clinical definition of traumatic re-enactment, however. Traumatic memories are meaningless and involuntary repetition—recurrences of the event taking place as it were in a perpetual present—always for the first time—as experience and not as memory. Like Funes, the hapless hero of Borges' tale *The Man With Perfect Memory*, the trauma patient remembers every detail of every day (without knowing that he does), but it takes him another entire day to recount one. Far from being memories, traumatic re-enactments represent the integral return of the originary experience.[3] These masked dances and carnival performances, on the contrary, are learned, they are pleasurable, and far from being intrusive, they are voluntarily performed in socially appropriate contexts. Neither the masked dancers of the Grassfields nor the pirates and villagers of the μόστρα could be said to be suffering from a trauma—individual or collective—without stretching the original definition of the term beyond any relation to its original meaning.

One might argue that I have erected a straw man argument: that there is no collective trauma in my examples not because of any limit to the theory, but because I have chosen examples of memories originating too far in the past for them to constitute any probable source of contemporary suffering: slavery and pirate raids are simply too distant and too quaint to be real sources of collective anxiety any longer (though it must be said that in the courts of the Grassfields cases of slavery continued to be heard into the 1930s, and that Chios did not attain independence until 1912). But as it happens each of these case studies involves an originary experience of much closer chronological proximity to the present re-enactment: the dancers of the Grassfields not only repeat the abductions of past slave traders, but also—in the performance of the Air Youth group—the attacks by paramilitary forces that occurred in the dancers' own lifetimes. And just as a syncretic, modernist dance addresses contemporary experiences of political violence in Oku, likewise in Chios, the second half of the carnival festivities are given over to the modernist floats, which in turn address the contemporary sovereign debt crisis.

There is no doubt that the restructuring program being imposed on Greece is having such deleterious consequences on people's well-being that it constitutes a form of structural violence, with unemployment rising steeply, pensions and salaries slashed, benefits cut, medical services reduced, and suicide rates spiking to their highest ever recorded level (Alexandrakis 2016; Brekke et al. 2014; Couroucli 2013; Dalakoglou 2013, Vournelis 2016). The collapse of the government and its replacement by EU-appointed technocrats, and at the local level in Chios the opening of soup kitchens for the first time since the aftermath of the Second World War, now evoke the eschatological specter of famine that islanders presumed had been forever banished 60 years ago (η πείνα—the same word used for occupation in Chios since the German occupation/famine of the Second World War). As mentioned above, the sudden proximity of hunger has triggered the return of memories of past disasters that befell the island—the massacres of 1822, the earthquake of 1881, the Asia Minor catastrophe of 1924, the exchange of populations between Greece and Turkey, and the occupation of the Second World War all now seem like resurgent events with a new urgency, the cloak of time that made them distant and past suddenly torn away by the current crisis (Argenti forthcoming; c.f. Knight 2012a, b, 2013).

It would be tempting to fit these reminiscences into the trauma discourse, to see in the effects of the crisis but a trigger for the involuntary resurgence of traumatic sequelae in the social body of the island. In doing so, we would recognize the suffering wrought by the effects of restructuring programs on the nations of the fringes of Europe. But we would recognize suffering at the cost of erasing agency: if the people of Greece recall the violence of the past today, it is not involuntarily as victims of a mass psychic disorder but as a willed contribution to a discourse in the making that promises to make sense of the ineffable violence of the present. Real as the collective anxiety is in Chios today regarding the effects of the on-going austerity measures and the political instability of the country, its collective representations, like those by Air Youth of the calamities that befell their own community, are not mere involuntary repetitions of the disaster. They are mimetic appropriations of it that transform the original event in the very act of its representation: the representation of the trauma is not the return of the trauma—rather, it marks the social response that transforms the unmediated event into collective memory. In their exultant obscenity, their disdain for authority, their rejection of the establishment, and their jubilant ridiculing of political power, the floats introduce something new to a collective experience of social crisis: where the experience is one of pain, loss, anguish, anger, and of abject subjection, its representation reproduces it as a source of carnival laughter, of pleasure, and of seminal fecundity. In Chios, the communion of the people lies not in their suffering and abjection, but in their ritual laughter and collective mobilization. What Bakhtin (1968:7) perceived in classical European bacchanalia and medieval carnival perdures in the social body to this day:

> Carnival is not a spectacle seen by the people; they live in it, and everyone participates because its very idea embraces all the people. While carnival lasts, there is no other life outside it. During carnival time life is subject only to its laws … the laws of its own freedom. It has a universal spirit; it is a special condition of the entire world, of the world's revival and renewal, in which all take part. Such is the essence of carnival.

Bakhtin's profound insight into the transcendent nature of carnival laughter is generalizable across cultures far less reductionistically than is the trauma paradigm. The ambiguous, unbounded nature of carnival, which is not a play on a stage, not a representation, but seeks always to overflow into the confines of 'serious' life and reality, is just as true—in its own way—in the Grassfields as it is in Greece. In the kingdoms of the Grassfields, the ribald grotesqueries and monstrous travesties of the masks—by turns terrifying, hilarious, and seductive—spill over to the young men at burials as they sing out hilarious, death-defying obscenities while stamping the corpse into the earth as they dance upon it—the earth that swallows up and gives birth—and it infects the young women who turn their faces to the wall in their darkened houses, but stifle giggles of excitement as the masks huddle outside in the night, crying for them to let them in. Carnival laughter is ambivalent: it is happy and triumphant, but mocking and deriding. 'It asserts and denies, it buries and revives' (Bakhtin 1968:11–12). Such is the laughter of carnival: its collective mirth holds the memory that all power emanates from the people, and for this reason it renders all that is bodily grandiose. In carnival, laughter is suffused with images of growth, fertility, and abundance, 'it is the fruitful earth and the womb. It is always conceiving' (Bakhtin 1968:21). Medieval carnival represented terror as comic monsters who were defeated by laughter. In this way, terror was turned into something comic and almost risible, a source of collective euphoria. This alchemical transformation was not a mockery of the political—it was political. To the chronology of the state, unilineal and static in the self-important pomposity of its patriotic memorializations, it introduced a radical new chronotope that deconstructed official versions of time and space. 'Ritual based on laughter', Bakhtin tells us, 'existed in all the countries of medieval Europe …'

> [It] offered a completely different, nonofficial, extraecclesiastical and extrapolitical aspect of the world, of man, and of human relations; [it] built a second world and a second life outside officialdom, a world in which all medieval people participated … in which they lived. (Bakhtin 1968:5–6)

Bakhtin writes chronologically of the development of carnival laughter through the ages, identifying a putative golden age from which we are now sadly fallen, the present epoch marking the apparent imprisonment of laughter into circumscribed spheres of life and strictly demarcated calendric periods. But Bakhtin was using temporality as a literary trope in his oeuvre: Rousseau before him in his *Social Contract* had identified a golden age of humanity before the onset of private property had divided society, but he had done so not as a proto-evolutionist, but to elaborate a thought experiment through which we could imagine a social life outside the confines of class distinctions. In the same manner, Bakhtin sets the classical age of carnival laughter in an imagined past that is not truly temporal, but which lives in an *illo tempore* that represents an alternative, potential, or utopian dimension of the possible at all times. The timeless dimension of Bakhtin's insight, which obtains its profundity precisely from the fact that it is not historical, is brought out in Bergson's philosophical work on laughter, which highlights the shared, social dimension of the comic in all times and places:

> One would not experience the comic if one were isolated. Laughter needs an echo. Listen to it closely: it is not an articulate, neat, finished sound; it would prolong itself, echoing from place to place, beginning with a sudden burst to roll on in diminishing waves, like thunder in the mountains. (Bergson 1940:4–5 my trans.)

In Rabelaisian France and in classical Rome, in slave-era Cameroon and in crisis-stricken Greece: amongst the arid boulders of timeless stability ritual laughter—thunder in the mountains—watered the saplings of change, renewal, and regeneration.

The ambiguity of carnival—its propensity always to go beyond itself and to break out of the bounds set for it (for the animalistic but crypto-human masks to break out of the circle and run amok, for the drunken pirates not to stick to the parade route, for the flag carrier to mock his predicament, for the transvestites to hover between genders, for the floats to traduce the troika)—is relevant for the trauma discourse today because it reveals that representations of past episodes of violence are not merely replayed as the unmediated return of the event, but that the hilarity and the ecstasy of carnival infuse trauma with an additional element that was absent from its first occurrence. In denuding the monster of its terror and representing it as farce, carnival makes the grotesque stately and the stately grotesque.

The trauma discourse bears witness to human suffering, but it does so at the cost of reducing our interlocutors to isolated psychiatric patients stripped of cultural context and in need of therapy. Trauma theory has been of use to anthropology in helping the discipline to highlight the suffering of the world, but a new paradigm is called for that will recognize not only the torment but also the everyday heroism, the social solidarity, and the political engagement of the oppressed, the marginalized, the unemployed, and the disaffected. Where trauma replaced the object of difference with a subject of empathy, a new theory of shared humanity could now supplant the paternalism of communion with a celebration of ritual laughter. Our role as anthropologists will then move from affirming the humanity of silent sufferers to celebrating the struggles of the marginalized.

Acknowledgments I extend my heartfelt thanks for the opportunity to write this paper and for help in thinking through it to Bjørn Enge Bertelsen, Vigdis Broch-Due, Roy Dilley, Katie Gianakaki, Tim Ingold, Daniel Knight, Stavroula Pipirou, and Anna Portisch. I gratefully acknowledge the support of the ESRC in funding the research in Greece referred to in this chapter.

Notes

1. One of the best depictions of this trans-generational process comes not from ethnography but from fiction, in Toni Morrison's novel *Beloved*, which traces the haunting by the young girl Seth, killed by her slave mother, through subsequent generations of her African American family.
2. The stonemasons, the stone carvers, the builders, the ironsmiths, and the nailers. Each had their own church in Thymiana. The patron saint of stonemasons is St John, and their church bears the same name. The builders' church is Aghios Dimitrios, the ironsmiths' is St Theodore, the nailers' was St George, in the neighbouring village of Karfas (this was the only church without its own graveyard).
3. As Charlotte Delbo has said of the concentration camps that she survived in the second World War, 'Auschwitz is there, fixed and unchangeable, but wrapped in the impervious skin of memory that segregates itself from the present "me"' (Delbo, in Langer 1991:5)—encryption by any other name.

References

Abraham, Nicolas. 1994 [1975]. Notes on the Phantom: A Complement to Freud's Metapsychology. In *The Shell and the Kernel*. Trans. T. Rand and eds. Nicolas Abraham and Maria Torok, 171–176. Chicago, IL: University of Chicago Press. (Also published in Meltzer (ed.), *The Trial(s) of Psychoanalysis*, pp. 75–80.)

Abraham, N., and M. Torok. 1976. *Cryptonymie: Le Verbier de l'Homme aux Loups*. Paris: Aubier Flammarion.

Agamben, G. 1999. *Remnants of Auschwitz: The Witness and the Archive*. New York: Zone Books.

Alexander, Jeffrey C. 2012. *Trauma: A Social Theory*. Malden, MA: Polity.

Alexander, Jeffrey C., Ron Eyerman, Bernard Giesen, Neil J. Smelser, and Piotr Sztompka. 2004. *Cultural Trauma and Collective Identitity*. Berkeley: University of California Press.

Alexandrakis, Othon. 2016. Transformative Connections: Trauma, Cooperative Horizons, and Emerging Political Topographies in Athens, Greece. *History and Anthropology* 27(1): 32–44.

Argenti, P. 1932. *The Massacres of Chios Described in Contemporary Diplomatic Reports*. London: John Lane, the Bodley Head.

———. 1966. *The Occupation of Chios by the Germans and Their Administration of the Island, 1941–44*. Cambridge: Cambridge University Press.

Argenti, N. 1998. Air Youth: Performance, Violence and the State in Cameroon. *Journal of the Royal Anthropological Institute* 4(4): 753–782.

———. 2007. *The Intestines of the State: Youth, Violence and Belated Histories in the Cameroon Grassfields*. Chicago, IL: University of Chicago Press.

———. Forthcoming. *The Greek Crisis of Memory*. Bloomington: Indiana University Press.

Argenti, N., and K. Schramm, eds.2010. *Remembering Violence: Anthropological Perspectives on Intergenerational Transmission*. New York: Berghahn.

Bakhtin, M. 1968. *Rabelais and His World*. Trans. Helene Iswolski. Cambridge, MA, M.I.T. Press.

Bergson, Henri. 2012 [1940]. *Le rire: essai sur la signification du comique*. Paris: Presses Universitaires de France.

Bettelheim, B. 1943. Individual and Mass Behaviour in Extreme Situations. *The Journal of Abnormal and Social Psychology* 38: 417–452.

Biehl, J. 2005. *Vita: Life in a Zone of Social Abandonment*. Berkeley: University of California Press.

Blanchot, M. 1995. *The Writing of the Disaster*. Trans. Ann Smock. Lincoln: University of Nebraska Press.

Brekke, J.K., D. Dalakoglou, C. Filippidis, and A. Vradis, eds.2014. *Crisis-Scapes: Athens and Beyond*. Athens, GA: Synthesi.

Calvocoressi, P. 1994. *Threading My Way*. London: Gerald Duckworth.

Caruth, C. 1991a. Unclaimed Experience: Trauma and the Possibility of History. *Yale French Studies* 79(4): 181–192.

———. 1991b. Introduction: Psychoanalysis, Culture and Trauma. *American Imago* 48(1): 1–12.

———. 1991c. Introduction: Psychoanalysis, Culture and Trauma II. *American Imago* 48(4): 417–424.

———. 1995. Introduction. In *Trauma: Explorations in Memory*, ed. C. Caruth, 3–12. Baltimore, MD: Johns Hopkins University Press.

Clark, Bruce. 2006. *Twice a Stranger: How Mass Explusion Forged Modern Greece and Turkey*. London: Granta.

Clogg, R. 1992. *A Concise History of Greece*. Cambridge: Cambridge University Press.

Comaroff, Jean, and John Comaroff. 1992. *Ethnography and the Historical Imagination*. Boulder, CO: Westview Press.

Couroucli, M. 2013. L'européanisme mis en question: récits ethno-orientalistes de la crise grecque. *Société d'Ethnologie*. Conférence Eugène Fleischmann VII.

Dalakoglou, D. 2013. The Crisis Before 'the Crisis'. *Social Justice* 39(1): 24–42.

Daniel, E. Valentine. 1996. *Charred Lullabies: Chapters in an Anthropography of Violence*. Princeton, NJ: Princeton University Press.

Das, Veena, Margaret M. Lock, and Arthur Kleinman. 1997. *Social Suffering*. Berkeley: University of California Press.

Das, Veena, Arthur Kleinman, Mamphela Ramphele, and Pamela Reynolds. 2000. *Violence and Subjectivity*. Berkeley: University of California Press.

Das, Veena, Arthur Kleinman, Margaret M. Lock, Mamphela Ramphele, and Pamela Reynolds. 2001. *Remaking a World: Violence, Social Suffering and Recovery*. Berkeley: University of California Press.

Demetriou, Olga. 2013. *Capricious Borders: Minority, Population, and Counter-Conduct Between Greece and Turkey*. Oxford: Berghahn.

Derrida, J. 1976. Fors: Les Mots Anglés de Nicolas Abraham et Maria Torok. Preface by Nicolas Abraham and Maria Torok, 7–73. In *Cryptonymie: Le Verbier de l'Homme aux Loups*. Paris: Aubier Flammarion.

———. 1986. *Schibboleth: Pour Paul Celan*. Paris: Galilée.

Erikson, K. 1991. Notes an Trauma and Community. *American Imago* 48(4): 455–472.

Eyerman, R. 2001. *Cultural Trauma: Slavery and the Formation of African American Identity*. Cambridge: CUP.

Fassin D., and R. Rechtman. 2009 [2007]. *The Empire of Trauma: An Inquiry into the Condition of Victimhood*. Trans. Rachel Gomme. Princeton, NJ: Princeton University Press.

Felman, Shoshana, and Dori Laub. 1992. *Testimony: Crises of Witnessing in Literature, Psychoanalysis, and History*. London: Routledge.

Friedlander, S. 1992. Trauma, Transference, and 'Working Through' in Writing the History of the *Shoah*. *History and Memory* 4(1): 39–59.

Green, Sarah. 2010. Performing Border in the Aegean. *Journal of Cultural Economy* 3(2): 261–278.

Hacking, I. 1995. *Rewriting the Soul: Multiple Personality and the Sciences of Memory*. Princeton, NJ: Princeton University Press.

Herzfeld, M. 1986. *Ours Once More: Folklore, Ideology, and the Making of Modern Greece*. New York: Pella.

Hionidou, V. 2006. *Famine and Death in Occupied Greece, 1941–1944*. Cambridge: Cambridge University Press.

Hirschon, R. 1989. *Heirs of the Greek catastrophe: The social life of Asia Minor refugees in Piraeus*. Oxford: Berghahn.

———. 2003. *Crossing the Aegean: An Appraisal of the 1923 Compulsory Population Exchange Between Greece and Turkey*. Oxford: Berghahn.

Housepian, M.D. 1966. *Smyrna 1922: The Destruction of a City*. London: Faber.

Kleinman, A., and J. Kleinman. 1994. How Bodies Remember: Social Memory and Bodily Experience of Criticism, Resistance, and Delegitimation Following China's Cultural Revolution. *New Literary History* 25: 708–723.

Knight, D. 2012a. Cultural Proximity: Crisis, Time and Social Memory in Central Greece. *History and Anthropology* 23(3).

———. 2012b. Turn of the Screw: Narratives of History and Economy in the Greek Crisis. *Journal of Mediterranean Studies* 21(1): 53–76.

———. 2013. The Greek Economic Crisis as Trope. *Focaal—Journal of Global and Historical Anthropology* 65: 147–159.

Koselleck, R. 2002. *The Practice of Conceptual History: Timing History, Spacing Concepts.* Stanford, CA: Stanford University Press.

LaCapra, D. 2001. *Writing History, Writing Trauma.* Baltimore, MD: Johns Hopkins University Press.

Langer, L. 1991. *Holocaust Testimonies: The Ruins of Memory.* New Haven, CT: Yale University Press.

Laub, D. 1991. Truth and Testimony: The Process and the Struggle. *American Imago* 48(1): 75–91.

Leys, R. 2000. *Trauma: A Genealogy.* Chicago, IL: University of Chicago Press.

Llewellyn-Smith, M. (Sir). 1973. *Ionian Vision: Greece in Asia Minor 1919–1922.* London: Hurst.

Loizos, P. 2008. *Iron in the Soul: Displacement, Livelihood and Health in Cyprus.* Oxford: Berghahn.

Lyotard, J.-F. 1990. *Heidegger and 'the Jews'.* Trans. Andreas Michel and Mark S. Roberts. Minneapolis: University of Minnesota Press.

Neal, A. 1998. *National Trauma and Collective Memory: Major Events in the American Century.* Armonk, NY: M.E. Sharpe.

Robbins, J. 2013. Beyond the Suffering Subject: Toward an Anthropology of the Good. *Journal of the Royal Anthropological Institute* 19(3): 447–462.

Shaw, R. 2002. *Memories of the Slave Trade: Ritual and the Historical Imagination in Sierra Leone.* Chicago, IL: University of Chicago Press.

Summerfield, D. 1996. The Impact of War and Atrocity on Civilian Populations: Basic Principles for NGO Interventions and a Critique of Psychological Trauma Projects, Network Paper 14, Relief and Rehabilitation Network.

———. 1998. The Social Experience of War and Some Issues for the Humanitarian Field. In *Rethinking the Trauma of War*, eds. P. Bracken and C. Petty, 9–37. London: Free Association Books.

Torok, M. 1994 [1975]. Story of Fear: The Symptoms of Phobia—The Return of the Repressed or the Return of the Phantom? In *The Shell and the Kernel.* Trans. T. R. Nicholas and eds. Nicolas Abraham and Maria Torok, 177–186. Chicago, IL: University of Chicago Press.

Trouillot, M.R. 2003 [1991]. Anthropology and the Savage Slot: The Poetics and Politics of Otherness. In *Global Transformations: Anthropology and the Modern World*, ed. M.R. Trouillot, 7–28. Chicago, IL: University of Chicago Press.

Unnold, Y.S. 2002. *Representing the Unrepresentable: Literature of Trauma Under Pinochet in Chile*. New York: Peter Lang.

Van der Kolk, B., and M. Grenberg. 1987. The Psychobiology of the Trauma Response: Hyperarousal, Constriction, and Addiction to Traumatic Reexposure. In *Psychological Trauma*, ed. B. van der Kolk, 63–88. Washington, DC: American Psychiatric Publishing.

Van der Kolk, B., and R. Fisler. 1995. Dissociation and the Fragmentary Nature of Traumatic Memories: Overview and Exploratory Study. *Journal of Traumatic Stress* 8(4): 505–525.

Van der Kolk, B., and O. van der Hart. 1991. The Intrusive Past: The Flexibility of Memory and the Engraving of Trauma. *American Imago* 48(1): 425–454.

Van der Kolk, B., A. McFarlane, and L. Weisath. 1996. *Traumatic Stress: The Effects of Overwhelming Experience on Mind, Body, and Society*. New York: Guilford Press.

Vickroy, L. 2002. *Trauma and Survival in Contemporary Fiction*. Charlottesville and London: University of Virginia Press.

Vournelis, Leonidas. 2016. Alexander's Great Treasure: Wonder and Mistrust in Neoliberal Greece. *History and Anthropology* 27(1): 121–133.

Young, A. 1995. *The Harmony of Illusions: Inventing Post-Traumatic Stress Disorder*. Princeton, NJ: Princeton University Press.

Index

V. Broch-Due, B.E. Bertelsen (eds.), *Violent Reverberations*,
DOI 10.1007/978-3-319-39049-9

H

I

P

Q

R